See also Index of *DSM-IV* Psychiatric Diagnoses on p xv.

Nursing Diagnoses in Psychiatric Nursing:
A Pocket Guide for Care Plan Construction

Fourth Edition

MARY C. TOWNSEND, RN, MN, CS
Assistant Professor
Kramer School of Nursing
Oklahoma City University
Oklahoma City, Oklahoma

Certified Clinical Nurse Specialist
Adult Psychiatric/Mental Health Nursing

 F.A. DAVIS COMPANY • Philadelphia

F. A. Davis Company
1915 Arch Street
Philadelphia, PA 19103

Printed in the United States of America

Last digit indicates print number: 10 9 8 7 6 5 4 3 2 1

Publisher, Nursing: Robert G. Martone
Production Editor: Nancee A. Morelli
Cover Designer: Steven R. Morrone

Library of Congress Cataloging in Publication Data

Townsend, Mary C., 1941–
    Nursing diagnoses in psychiatric nursing : a pocket guide for
care plan construction/Mary C. Townsend.—4th ed.
    p. cm.
Includes bibliographical references and indexes.
ISBN 0-8036-0290-1 (pbk)
1. Psychiatric nursing—Handbooks, manuals, etc. 2. Mental
illness—Diagnosis—Handbooks, manuals, etc. 3. Nursing
diagnosis—Handbooks, manuals, etc.   I. Title.
    [DNLM: 1. Mental Disorders—nursing—handbooks.
2. Nursing Diagnosis—handbooks. 3. Patient Care Planning—
handbooks.   WY 39
T749n 1997]
RC440.T69 1997
610.73'68—dc21
DNLM/DLC
for Library of Congress   96-45615
                                                          CIP

THIS BOOK IS DEDICATED:

To my husband, Jim, who has encouraged and supported me throughout this project and whose love continues to nurture and sustain me, even after 35 years.

To my daughters, Kerry and Tina, who have brought joy that only a parent could understand, frustrations that only a parent could tolerate, happiness that only a parent could appreciate, and tears that only a parent could endure. You are truly loved.

To my faithful and beloved companions, Cocoa, Buddy, and Affie, whose warm, furry bodies at my feet helped to make the long hours of writing more tolerable and enjoyable.

And finally, to my father and mother, Francis and Camalla Welsh, who reared my sister Francie and me without knowledge of psychology or developmental theories but with the kind of unconditional love I have come to believe is so vital to the achievement and maintenance of emotional wellness.

MCT

ACKNOWLEDGMENTS

My special thanks and appreciation:

To Bob Martone, who patiently provided essential editorial assistance and guidance throughout the project.

To the editorial and production staffs of the F. A. Davis Company, who are always willing to provide assistance when requested and whose consistent excellence in publishing makes me proud to be associated with them.

To the gracious individuals who read and critiqued the original manuscript, providing valuable input into the final product.

And finally, a special acknowledgment to the nurses who staff the psychiatric units of the clinical agencies where nursing students go to learn about psychiatric nursing. To those of you who willingly share your knowledge and expertise with, and act as role models for, these nursing students. If this book provides you with even a small amount of nursing assistance, please acknowledge it as my way of saying, "thanks."

MCT

CONSULTANTS

Maude H. Alston, RN, PhD
Assistant Professor of Nursing
University of North Carolina at Greensboro
Greensboro, North Carolina

Betty J. Carmack, RN, EdD
Assistant Professor
University of San Francisco
School of Nursing
San Francisco, California

Doris K. DeVincenzo, PhD
Professor
Lienhard School of Nursing
Pace University
Pleasantville, New York

Mary Jo Gorney-Fadiman, RN, PhD
Assistant Professor
San Jose State University
School of Nursing
San Jose, California

Mary E. Martucci, RN, PhD
Associate Professor and Chairman
Saint Mary's College
Notre Dame, Indiana

Sheridan V. Mc Cabe, BA, BSN, MSN, PhD
Assistant Professor of Nursing
University of Virginia
School of Nursing
Charlottesville, Virginia

Elizabeth Anne Rankin, PhD
Psychotherapist and Consultant
The University of Maryland
School of Nursing
Baltimore, Maryland

Judith M. Saunders, DNS, FAAN
Postdoctoral Research Fellow
University of Washington
School of Nursing
Seattle, Washington

Gail Stuart, RN, CS, PhD
Associate Professor
Medical University of South Carolina
College of Nursing
Charleston, South Carolina

TABLE OF CONTENTS

INDEX OF *DSM-IV* PSYCHIATRIC DIAGNOSES

Chapter 1

NURSING DIAGNOSES IN PSYCHIATRIC NURSING

HOW TO USE THIS BOOK

In an attempt to standardize clinical nursing practice, the North American Nursing Diagnosis Association (NANDA) has published a list of nursing diagnoses that have been approved through the 12th National Conference on Classification of Nursing Diagnosis in 1996. Standardization of nursing actions and common terminology are important in the provision of consistent care over time, among nurses, across shifts, and even between different health-care agencies.

There are those individuals who believe that NANDA's list is incomplete. My intent is not to judge the completeness of this list, but to suggest the need for clinical testing of what is available. NANDA encourages nurses to submit new nursing diagnoses for consideration by the group, after they have conducted testing and research of that diagnosis in the clinical setting.

There are three essential components in a nursing diagnosis, which have been referred to as the *PES format* (Gordon, 1987). The "P" identifies the health problem, the "E" represents the etiology (or cause) of the problem, and the "S" describes a cluster of signs and symptoms, or what has come to be known as "defining characteristics." These three parts are combined into one statement by the use of "connecting words." The diagnosis would then be written in this manner: Problem "related to" etiology "evidenced by" signs and symptoms (defining characteristics).

The problem can be identified as the human response to actual or potential health problems as assessed by the nurse. The etiology may be represented by past experiences of the individual, genetic influences, current environmental factors, or pathophysiologic changes. The defining characteristics describe what the client says and what the nurse observes that indicate the existence of a particular problem.

Nursing diagnoses, then, become the basis for the care plan. This book may be used as a guide in the construction of care plans for various psychiatric clients. The concepts are presented in such a manner that they may be applied to various types of health-care settings: inpatient hospitalization, outpatient clinic, home health, partial hospitalization, and private practice, to name a few. Major divisions in the book have been identified by psychiatric diagnostic categories, according to the order in which they appear in the *Diagnostic and Statistical Manual of Mental Disorders, 4th Edition* (*DSM-IV*, 1994). The use of this format is not to imply that nursing diagnoses are based on, or flow from, medical diagnoses, but is meant only to enhance the usability of the book. In addition, I am not suggesting that those nursing diagnoses presented with each psychiatric category are all-inclusive.

It is valid, however, to state that certain nursing diagnoses are indeed common to individuals with specific psychiatric disorders. The diagnoses presented in this book are meant to be used as guidelines for construction of care plans that must be individualized for each client, based on the nursing assessment. The interventions can also be used in areas where interdisciplinary treatment plans take the place of the nursing care plan.

Each chapter begins with an overview of information related to the medical diagnostic category, which may be useful to the nurse as background assessment data. This section includes:

1. **The Disorder.** A definition and common types or categories that have been identified.
2. **Predisposing Factors.** Information regarding theories of etiology, which the nurse may use in formulating the "related to" portion of the nursing diagnosis, as it applies to the client.
3. **Symptomatology.** Subjective and objective data identifying behaviors common to the disorder. These behav-

iors, as they apply to the individual client, may be pertinent to the "evidenced by" portion of the nursing diagnosis.

Information presented with each nursing diagnosis includes the following:

1. **Definition.** The approved NANDA definition is used with those nursing diagnoses for which a NANDA definition exists. I have suggested definitions for clarification of the other nursing diagnoses, and these are identified by brackets [ ].
2. **Possible Etiologies ("related to").** This section suggests possible causes for the problem identified. Those not approved by NANDA are identified by brackets [ ]. **Related/Risk Factors** are given for diagnoses for which the client is at risk.
3. **Defining Characteristics ("evidenced by").** This section includes signs and symptoms that may be evident to indicate that the problem exists. Again, as with definitions and etiologies, those not approved by NANDA are identified by brackets [ ].
4. **Goals/Objectives.** These statements are made in client behavioral objective terminology. They are measurable, short- and long-term goals, to be used in evaluating the effectiveness of the nursing interventions in alleviating the identified problem. There may be more than one short-term goal, and they may be considered "stepping stones" to fulfillment of the long-term goal. For purposes of this book, "long-term," in most instances, is designated as "by discharge," whether the client is in an inpatient or outpatient setting.
5. **Interventions with Selected Rationales.** Only those interventions that are appropriate to a particular nursing diagnosis within the context of the psychiatric setting are presented. Rationales for selected interventions are included to provide clarification beyond fundamental nursing knowledge, and to assist in the selection of appropriate interventions for individual clients.
6. **Outcome Criteria.** These are behavioral changes that can be used as criteria to determine the degree to which the nursing diagnosis has been resolved.

To use this book in the preparation of psychiatric nursing care plans, find the section in the text applicable to the client's psychiatric diagnosis. Review background data pertinent to the diagnosis, if needed. Complete a biopsychosocial history and assessment on the client. Select and prioritize nursing diagnoses appropriate to the client. Using the list of NANDA-approved nursing diagnoses, be sure to include those that are client specific, and not just those that have been identified as "common" to this particular medical diagnosis. Select nursing interventions and outcome criteria appropriate to the client for each nursing diagnosis identified. Write all of this information on the care plan, with a date for evaluating the status of each problem. On the evaluation date, document success of the nursing interventions in achieving the goals of care, using the desired client outcomes as criteria. Modify the plan as required.

This book helps to familiarize the nurse with the current NANDA-approved nursing diagnoses and provides suggestions for their use within the psychiatric setting. It is designed to be used as a quick reference in the preparation of care plans, with the expectation that additional information will be required under each nursing diagnosis as the nurse individualizes care for psychiatric clients.

NURSING DIAGNOSES ACCEPTED BY NANDA (Through 12th Conference)

Activity Intolerance
Activity Intolerance, risk for
Adaptive Capacity, intracranial, decreased
Adjustment, impaired
Airway Clearance, ineffective
Anxiety (specify level)
Aspiration, risk for

Body Image Disturbance
Body Temperature, altered, risk for
Bowel Incontinence
Breastfeeding, effective
Breastfeeding, ineffective
Breastfeeding, interrupted
Breathing Pattern, ineffective

Cardiac Output, decreased
Caregiver Role Strain
Caregiver Role Strain, risk for
Communication, impaired, verbal

Community Coping, enhanced, potential for
Community Coping, ineffective
Confusion, acute
Confusion, chronic
Constipation
Constipation, colonic
Constipation, perceived
Coping, defensive
Coping, individual, ineffective

Decisional Conflict (specify)
Denial, ineffective
Diarrhea
Disuse Syndrome, risk for
Diversional Activity Deficit
Dysreflexia

Energy Field Disturbance
Environmental Interpretation Syndrome, impaired

Family Coping, ineffective: compromised
Family Coping, ineffective: disabling
Family Coping: potential for growth
Family Process, altered: alcoholism
Family Processes, altered
Fatigue
Fear
Fluid Volume Deficit
Fluid Volume Deficit, risk for
Fluid Volume Excess

Gas Exchange, impaired
Grieving, anticipatory
Grieving, dysfunctional
Growth and Development, altered

Health Maintenance, altered
Health-Seeking Behaviors (specify)
Home Maintenance Management, impaired
Hopelessness
Hyperthermia
Hypothermia

Incontinence, functional
Incontinence, reflex
Incontinence, stress

Incontinence, total
Incontinence, urge
Infant Behavior, disorganized
Infant Behavior, disorganized, risk for
Infant Behavior, organized, potential for enhanced
Infant Feeding Pattern, ineffective
Infection, risk for
Injury, risk for

Knowledge Deficit (specify)

Loneliness, risk for

Memory, impaired

Noncompliance (specify)
Nutrition, altered, less than body requirements
Nutrition, altered, more than body requirements
Nutrition, altered, risk for more than body requirements

Oral Mucous Membrane, altered

Pain
Pain, chronic
Parental Role Conflict
Parent/Infant/Child Attachment, altered, risk for
Parenting, altered
Parenting, altered, risk for
Perioperative Positioning Injury, risk for
Peripheral Neurovascular Dysfunction, risk for
Personal Identity Disturbance
Physical Mobility, impaired
Poisoning, risk for
Post-Trauma Response
Powerlessness
Protection, altered

Rape-Trauma Syndrome
Rape-Trauma Syndrome: compound reaction
Rape-Trauma Syndrome: silent reaction
Relocation Stress Syndrome
Role Performance, altered

Self-Care Deficit (specify): feeding, bathing/hygiene, dressing/grooming, toileting
Self-Esteem, chronic low

Self-Esteem Disturbance
Self-Esteem, situational low
Self-Mutilation, risk for
Sensory-Perceptual Alterations (specify): visual, auditory, kinesthetic, gustatory, tactile, olfactory
Sexual Dysfunction
Sexuality Patterns, altered
Skin Integrity, impaired
Skin Integrity, impaired, risk for
Sleep Pattern Disturbance
Social Interaction, impaired
Social Isolation
Spiritual Distress (distress of the human spirit)
Spiritual Well-Being, enhanced, potential for
Spontaneous Ventilation, inability to sustain
Suffocation, risk for
Swallowing, impaired

Therapeutic Regimen: community, ineffective management
Therapeutic Regimen: families, ineffective management
Therapeutic Regimen: individual, effective management
Therapeutic Regimen: individual, ineffective management
Thermoregulation, ineffective
Thought Processes, altered
Tissue Integrity, impaired
Tissue Perfusion, altered (specify): renal, cerebral, cardiopulmonary, gastrointestinal, peripheral
Trauma, risk for

Unilateral Neglect
Urinary Elimination, altered
Urinary Retention

Ventilatory Weaning Response, dysfunctional (DVWR)
Violence, risk for, directed at self/others

Chapter 2

NURSING PROCESS: ONE STEP TO PROFESSIONALISM

Nursing has struggled for many years to achieve recognition as a profession. Out of this struggle has emerged an awareness for the need to do the following:

1. Define the boundaries of nursing (What is nursing?).
2. Identify a scientific method for the delivery of nursing care.

In its statement on social policy, the American Nurses' Association (ANA) has presented the following definition: "Nursing is the diagnosis and treatment of human responses to actual or potential health problems" (ANA, 1980).

The nursing process has been identified as nursing's scientific methodology for the delivery of nursing care. The curricula of most nursing schools now include nursing process as a component of their conceptual frameworks. The National Council of State Boards of Nursing (NCSBN) uses the nursing process as the basis for the Registered Nurse State Board Test Pool Examination (NCSBN, 1985). Questions that relate to nursing behaviors in a variety of client situations are presented according to the steps of the nursing process:

1. **Assessment.** Establishing a database about a client
2. **Diagnosis.** Identifying the client's health-care needs and selecting goals of care
3. **Outcome Identification.** Establishing criteria for measuring achievement of desired outcomes

4. **Planning.** Designing a strategy to achieve the goals established for client care
5. **Implementation.** Initiating and completing actions necessary to accomplish the defined goals
6. **Evaluation.** Determining the extent to which the goals of care have been achieved

By following these six steps, the nurse has a systematic framework for decision making and problem solving in the delivery of nursing care. The nursing process is dynamic, not static. It is an ongoing process that continues for as long as the nurse and client have interactions directed toward change in the client's physical or behavioral responses. Figure 2–1 presents a schematic of the ongoing nursing process.

Nursing diagnosis is an integral part of the nursing process. In this step, the nurse identifies the "human responses to actual or potential health problems." In some states, diagnosing is identified within the Nurse Practice Acts as a legal responsibility of the professional nurse. Shoemaker has stated, "Nursing diagnosis provides the basis for prescriptions for definitive therapy for which the nurse is accountable" (Kim et al, 1984).

As an inherent part of the nursing process, nursing di-

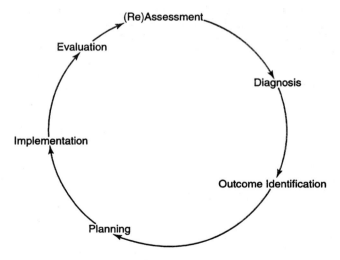

FIGURE 2–1   The ongoing nursing process.

agnosis is also reflected in the ANA Standards of Practice. These standards provide one broad basis for evaluating practice and reflect a recognition of the rights of the person receiving nursing care (ANA, 1991).

Nursing diagnosis can no longer be recognized as part of nursing's future. Nursing diagnosis is now. This provides a challenge for nursing educators and administrators to assist not only the nursing students of today but also those registered nurses currently staffing health-care agencies who were never introduced to nursing diagnosis in their basic educational programs and who are now being told they must conform. The purpose of this book is to provide that assistance to students and staff nurses as they endeavor to provide high-quality nursing care to their psychiatric clients.

This chapter includes one example of a nursing history and assessment tool that may be used to gather information about the client during the assessment phase of the nursing process. Also presented is a sample case study using this assessment tool to formulate the client database, followed by a care plan developed from the assessment information.

NURSING HISTORY AND ASSESSMENT TOOL*

GENERAL INFORMATION

Client Name: _____

Room Number: _____

Doctor: _____

Age: _____

Sex: _____

Race: _____

Dominant Language: _____

Marital Status: _____

Chief Complaint: _____

_____

_____

Allergies: _____

Diet: _____

Height/Weight: _____

Vital Signs: TPR/BP _____

Name and Phone No. of
    Significant Other: _____

_____

City of Residence: _____

Diagnosis (Admitting &
    Current): _____

_____

Conditions of Admission

Date: _____   Time: _____

Accompanied by: _____

Route of Admission (wheelchair, ambulatory, cart): _____

Admitted from: _____

PREDISPOSING FACTORS

Genetic Influences

Family Configuration (use genograms):

Family of Origin: Present Family:

Family Dynamics (describe significant relationships be-
    tween family members): _____

    _____

    _____

    _____

    _____

_____

*Modified with permission from Nursing Faculty, Butler County Com-
munity College, El Dorado, Kansas, who formulated this tool in Au-
gust 1984, based on the concept of stress adaptation.

Medical/Psychiatric History: _____
  Client: _____

_____

Family Members: _____

_____

Other GENETIC influences affecting present adaptation.
(This might include effects specific to gender, race, appearance [such as genetic physical defects], or any other factor related to genetics that is affecting the client's adaptation that has not been mentioned elsewhere in this assessment.)

_____
_____
_____
_____
_____

Past Experiences

Cultural and Social History
Environmental Factors (family living arrangements, type of neighborhood, special working conditions): _____

_____

Health Beliefs and Practices (personal responsibility for health; special self-care practices): _____

_____

Religious Beliefs and Practices: _____

_____

Educational Background: _____

_____

Significant Losses/Changes (include dates): _____

_____

Peer/Friendship Relationships: _____

_____

Occupational History: _____

_____
_____

Previous Pattern of Coping with Stress: _____

_____

Other Lifestyle Factors Contributing to Present Adaptation:

_____

_____

Existing Conditions

Stage of Development (Erikson)
Theoretically: _____
Behaviorally: _____
Rationale: _____

_____

Support Systems: _____

_____

Economic Security: _____

_____

Avenues of Productivity/Contribution:
Current Job Status: _____

_____

Role Contributions and Responsibility for Others: _____

_____

PRECIPITATING EVENT
Describe the situation or events that precipitated this illness/hospitalization: _____

_____

_____

CLIENT'S PERCEPTION OF THE STRESSOR
Client's and/or family member's understanding or description of stressor/illness and expectations of hospitalization/treatment: _____

_____

_____

_____

ADAPTATION RESPONSES

Psychosocial

Anxiety Level (circle level, and check the behaviors that apply):

Mild   Moderate   Severe   Panic
Calm _____ Friendly _____ Passive _____ Alert _____
Perceives environment correctly _____ Cooperative _____
Impaired attention _____ "Jittery" _____
Unable to concentrate _____ Hypervigilant _____
Tremors _____ Rapid speech _____ Withdrawn _____
Confused _____ Disoriented _____ Fearful _____
Hyperventilating _____ Misinterpreting the environment
(hallucinations/delusions) _____ Depersonalization _____
Obsessions _____ Compulsions _____ Somatic
complaints _____ Excessive hyperactivity _____
Other _____
_____

Mood/Affect (circle as many as apply):
Happiness   Sadness   Dejection   Despair
Elation   Euphoria   Suspiciousness
Apathy (little emotional tone)   Anger/Hostility

Ego Defense Mechanisms (describe how used by client):
Projection: _____
Suppression: _____
Undoing: _____
Displacement: _____
Intellectualization: _____
Rationalization: _____
Denial: _____
Repression: _____
Isolation: _____
Regression: _____
Reaction Formation: _____
Splitting: _____
Religiosity: _____
Sublimation: _____
Compensation: _____

Level of Self-Esteem (circle one):
Low   Moderate   High
Things client likes about self: _____
_____
Things client would like to change about self: _____
_____
Objective assessment of self-esteem:
  Eye contact: _____
  General appearance: _____
_____

Personal hygiene: _____
Participation in group activities and interactions with
others: _____
_____
_____

Stage and Manifestations of Grief (circle one):
   Denial   Anger   Bargaining   Depression   Acceptance
Describe client's behaviors that are associated with this
stage of grieving in response to loss or change: _____
_____
_____
_____

Thought Processes (circle as many as apply):
Clear   Logical   Easy to follow   Relevant
Confused   Blocking   Delusional   Rapid flow of
thoughts   Slowness in thought association
Suspicious
Memory: Recent (circle one):   Loss   Intact
              Remote (circle one):   Loss   Intact
Other: _____
_____

Communication Patterns (circle as many as apply):
Clear   Coherent   Slurred speech   Incoherent
Neologisms   Loose associations   Flight of ideas
Aphasic   Perseveration   Rumination
Tangential speech   Loquaciousness
Slow, impoverished speech
Speech impediment (describe): _____
Other: _____
_____

Interaction Patterns (describe client's pattern of interpersonal interactions with staff and peers on the unit, e.g.,
manipulative, withdrawn, isolated, verbally or physically
hostile, argumentative, passive, assertive, aggressive,
passive-aggressive, other): _____
_____
_____
_____
_____

Reality Orientation (check those which apply):

Oriented to: Time _____ Person _____

Place _____ Situation _____

Ideas of Destruction to Self/Others? Yes No

If yes, consider plan; available means: _____

_____

_____

_____

Physiologic

Psychosomatic Manifestations (describe any somatic complaints that may be stress-related): _____

_____

_____

_____

Drug History and Assessment:

Use of Prescribed Drugs:

Name	Dosage	Prescribed for	Results

Use of Over-the-Counter Drugs:

Name	Dosage	Used for	Results

Use of Street Drugs and/or Alcohol:

Name	Amount Used	How Often Used	When Last Used	Effects Produced

Pertinent Physical Assessments:

Respirations: Normal: _____ Labored: _____
Rate: _____ Rhythm: _____
Skin: Warm: _____ Dry: _____ Moist: _____ Cool: _____
Clammy: _____ Pink: _____ Cyanotic: _____
Poor turgor: _____ Edematous: _____
Evidence of: Rash: _____ Bruising: _____
Needletracks: _____ Hirsutism: _____ Loss of hair: _____
Other: _____

Musculoskeletal status: Weakness: _____ Tremors: _____
Degree of range of motion (describe limitations): _____
_____
Pain (describe): _____
Skeletal deformities (describe): _____
Coordination (describe limitations): _____

Neurologic status:
History of (check all that apply): Seizures: _____
(describe method of control): _____
Headaches (describe location and frequency): _____
_____
Fainting spells: _____ Dizziness: _____
Tingling/numbness (describe location): _____

Cardiovascular: BP: _____ Pulse: _____
History of (check all that apply):
Hypertension: _____ Palpitations: _____
Heart murmur: _____ Chest pain: _____
Shortness of breath: _____ Pain in legs: _____
Phlebitis: _____ Ankle/leg edema: _____
Numbness/tingling in extremities: _____
Varicose veins: _____

Gastrointestinal:
Usual diet pattern: _____
Food allergies: _____
Dentures? _____ Upper: _____ Lower: _____
Any problems with chewing or swallowing? _____
Any recent change in weight? _____
Any problems with:
  Indigestion/heartburn? _____
    Relieved by: _____

Nausea/vomiting? _____
    Relieved by: _____
Loss of appetite? _____
History of ulcers? _____
Usual bowel pattern: _____
    Constipation: _____ Diarrhea: _____
    Type of self-care assistance provided for either of the
above problems: _____

Genitourinary/Reproductive:
Usual voiding pattern: _____
Urinary hesitancy: _____ frequency: _____
Nocturia: _____ Pain/burning: _____
Incontinence: _____
Genital lesions: _____
    Discharge: _____ Odor: _____
History of venereal disease: _____ If yes, explain: _____
_____
Any concerns about sexuality/sexual activity: _____
_____
_____
Method of birth control used: _____
    Females:
    Date of last menstrual cycle: _____
    Length of cycle: _____
    Problems associated with menstruation: _____
_____
    Breasts: Pain/tenderness: _____
        Swelling: _____ Discharge: _____
        Lumps: _____ Dimpling: _____
    Practice self-breast examination: _____
        Frequency: _____
    Males:
    Penile discharge: _____
    Prostate problems: _____

Eyes:	Yes	No	Explain
Glasses	_____	_____	_____
Contacts	_____	_____	_____
Swelling	_____	_____	_____
Discharge	_____	_____	_____
Itching	_____	_____	_____
Blurring	_____	_____	_____
Double vision	_____	_____	_____

Ears:	Yes	No	Explain
Pain	___	___	_____
Drainage	___	___	_____
Difficulty hearing	___	___	_____
Hearing aid	___	___	_____
Tinnitus	___	___	_____

Medication Side Effects:
Symptoms that may be attributed to current medication usage: _____
_____
_____

Altered Laboratory Values and Possible Significance:
_____
_____

Activity/Rest Patterns:
Exercise (amount, type, frequency): _____
_____

Leisure time activities: _____
_____

Patterns of sleep: Number of hours per night: _____
　　　　　　　　　Use of sleep aids: _____
　　　　　　　　　Pattern of awakening during the
　　　　　　　　　night: _____
　　　　　　　　　_____

　　　　　　　　　Feel rested on awakening: _____

Personal Hygiene/Activities of Daily Living:
Patterns of self-care: Independent _____
Requires assistance with: Mobility _____
　　　　　　　　　　　　Hygiene _____
　　　　　　　　　　　　Toileting _____
　　　　　　　　　　　　Feeding _____
　　　　　　　　　　　　Dressing _____
　　　　　　　　　　　　Other _____
Statement describing personal hygiene and general appearance: _____
_____
_____

Other pertinent physical assessments: _____
_____
_____

SUMMARY OF INITIAL PSYCHOSOCIAL/
PHYSICAL ASSESSMENT

Knowledge Deficits Identified

Nursing Diagnoses Indicated

SAMPLE: Nursing History/Assessment and Care Plan

GENERAL INFORMATION

Sam is a 45-year-old white male admitted to the psychiatric unit of a general medical center by his family physician, Dr. Jones, who reported that Sam had become increasingly despondent over the last month. His wife reported that he had made statements such as, "Life is not worth living," and "I think I could just take all those pills Dr. Jones prescribed at one time, then it would all be over." He was admitted at 6:40 PM, via wheelchair from admissions, and accompanied by his wife. He reports no known allergies. Vital signs upon admission were temperature, 97.9°F; P, 80; respirations, 16; and BP, 132/77. He is 5 feet 11 inches tall and weighs 160 lb. He was referred to the psychiatrist on call, Dr. Smith. Orders include suicide precautions, level I; regular diet; chemistry profile and routine urinalysis in AM; Desyrel, 200 mg tid; Dalmane, 30 mg hs prn for sleep.

PREDISPOSING FACTORS

GENETIC INFLUENCES

Family Configuration

Family of Origin:

(Father) 65 1985 MI

(Mother) 70

45 (Client) 43 (Sister) 41 (Brother) 39 (Brother)

Present Family:

45 (Client) 43 (Wife)

18 (Daughter) 16 (Son)

Dynamics: Sam says he loves his wife and children and does not want to hurt them, but feels they no longer need him. He states, "They would probably be better off without me." His wife appears to be very concerned about his condition, though in his despondency, he seems oblivious to her feelings. His mother lives in a neighboring state, and he sees her infrequently. He admits that he is somewhat bitter toward her for allowing him and his siblings to "suffer from the physical and emotional brutality of their father." His siblings and their families live in distant states, and he sees them rarely, during holiday gatherings. He feels closest to the older of the two brothers.

Medical/Psychiatric History

Sam's father died 5 years ago at age 65 of a myocardial infarction. Sam and both his brothers have a history of high cholesterol and triglycerides from approximately age 30. During his regular physical examination 1 month ago, Sam's family doctor recognized symptoms of depression and prescribed Elavil. Sam's mother has a history of depressive episodes. She was hospitalized once about 7 years ago for depression, and she has taken various antidepressant medications over the years. Her family physician has also prescribed Valium for her on numerous occasions for her "nerves." No other family members have a history of psychiatric problems.

PAST EXPERIENCES

Sam was the first child in a family of four. He is 2 years older than his sister and 4 years older than the third child, a brother. He was 6 years old when his youngest sibling, also a boy, was born. Sam's father was a career Army man, who moved his family many times during their childhood years. Sam attended 15 schools from the time he entered kindergarten until he graduated from high school.

Sam reports that his father was very autocratic and had many rules that he expected his children to obey without question. Infraction resulted in harsh discipline. Because Sam was the oldest child, his father believed he should assume responsibility for the behavior of his siblings. Sam describes the severe physical punishment he received from his father when he or his siblings allegedly violated one of the rules. It was particularly intense when Sam's father had been drinking, which he did most evenings and weekends.

Sam's mother was very passive. Sam believes she was afraid of his father, particularly when he was drinking, so she quietly conformed to his lifestyle and offered no resistance, even though she did not agree with his disciplining of the children. Sam reports that he observed his father physically abusing his mother on a number of occasions, most often when he had been drinking.

Sam states that he had very few friends when he was growing up. With all the family moves, he gave up trying to make new friends because it became too painful to give them up when it was time to leave. He took a paper route when he was 13 years old and then worked in fast food restaurants from age 15 on. He was a hard worker and never seemed to have difficulty finding work in any of the places where the family relocated. He states that he appreciated the independence and being away from home as much as his job would allow. "I guess I can honestly say I hated my father, and working was my way of getting away from all the stress that was going on in that house. I guess my dad hated me, too, because he never was satisfied with anything I did. I never did well enough for him in school, on the job, or even at home. When I think of my dad now, the memories I have are of being criticized and beaten with a belt."

On graduation from high school, Sam joined the Navy, where he learned a skill that he used after discharge to obtain a job in a large aircraft plant. He also attended the local university at night, where he earned his accounting degree. When he completed his degree, he was reassigned to the administration department of the aircraft company, and he has been in the same position for 12 years without a promotion.

Sam says he believes in God but does not attend a church. He drinks socially but does not smoke. He has regular physical, dental, and eye examinations.

Significant losses include loss of self-esteem due to being passed over for promotion, and loss of a satisfactory father-son relationship.

His previous pattern of coping with stress has been to develop a migraine headache, to escape into sleep, excessive use of suppression, or to become mildly depressed and withdrawn until the stressor was relieved.

EXISTING CONDITIONS

Stage of Development

Sam is in the generativity versus self-absorption stage. Most of the time he is fulfilling the tasks of generativity (successful at work and in community; rearing children). However, when depressed, he becomes very self-absorbed and his behaviors are focused inward.

Sam has a strong support system in his wife and children. He is currently holding a position of responsibility in the aircraft company, his wife teaches elementary school, and they have sufficient insurance to cover medical expenses. He has fulfilled his responsibilities on the job and in the home until recently, when his despondency began to interfere with social and occupational functioning.

PRECIPITATING EVENT

Over the last 12 years, Sam has watched while a number of his peers were promoted to management positions. Sam has been considered for several of these positions but has never been selected. Last month a management position became available for which Sam felt he was qualified. He applied for this position, believing he had a good chance of being promoted. However, when the announcement was made, the position had been given to a younger man who had been with the company only 5 years. Sam seemed to accept the decision, but over the last few weeks he has become more and more withdrawn. He speaks to very few people at the office and is becoming more and more behind in his work. At home, he eats very little, talks to family members only when they ask a direct question, withdraws to his bedroom very early in the evening, and does not come out until time to leave for work the next morning. Today, he refused to get out of bed or to go to work. His wife convinced him to talk to their family doctor, who admitted him to the hospital.

CLIENT'S PERCEPTION OF THE STRESSOR

Sam states that all his life he has "not been good enough at anything. I could never please my father. Now I can't seem to please my boss. What's the use of trying? I came to the hospital because my wife and my doctor are afraid I might try to kill myself. I must admit the thought has crossed my mind more than once. I seem to have very little motivation for living. I just don't care any more.''

ADAPTATION RESPONSES

PSYCHOSOCIAL

1. Anxiety level is moderate. Client is alert and cooperative, though attention seems to be impaired at times and client has difficulty concentrating. No misinterpretation of the environment noted.
2. Mood is one of dejection and despair. Affect is sad, flat, with little emotional tone.
3. Ego defense mechanisms employed:
   a. ***Displacement:*** Client is displacing anger at parents and boss onto self.
   b. ***Regression:*** Client is withdrawing into self and becoming socially isolated.
4. Level of self-esteem is very low. Client speaks of himself as never having been able to please the important people in his life. Feels as though family would be better off without him. Eye contact is poor. Client looks at hands in lap while talking. Hygiene appears to be appropriate, but general appearance is disheveled. Clothes are wrinkled, hair is uncombed. Interaction with others is virtually nil.
5. Regarding stage of grief, client appears to be fixed in the anger stage of the grieving process, and the anger is turned inward on the self. Manifestations include feelings of low self-esteem and despair at what he perceives as a lack of accomplishment in his life.
6. Thought processes are clear and logical, though there is some slowness in thought association.
7. Communication patterns are clear and coherent, but with some ruminations regarding his inability to please his parents and boss.
8. Interaction patterns: withdrawn; isolated; passive; no attempt to interact with others.
9. Client is oriented to time, person, place, and situation.
10. Client admits to having thoughts of killing self at this time. He had previously considered taking an overdose of Elavil, which had been prescribed by his family physician. He does not have the Elavil with him in the hospital.

PHYSIOLOGIC

1. Sam states that he sometimes experiences migraine headaches (HA). He has not noticed if they occur more often during periods of stress.

2. **Drug History and Assessment**
   a. *Use of Prescribed Drugs*
      - Elavil, 50 mg bid, for depression. No improvement.
      - Fiorinal #3, 1 capsule q 8 hr as needed for headache pain. Relief obtained.
      - Robaxin, 750 mg prn for back pain. Relief obtained.

   b. *Use of Over-the-Counter Drugs*
      - Aspirin, 2 tablets prn for headache. Relief obtained.
      - Actifed, 1 tablet prn for sinus drainage. Relief obtained.
      - Mylanta, 2 tablets prn for heartburn. Relief obtained.

   c. *Use of Street Drugs and/or Alcohol*
      - Denies use of street drugs. Social drinking and two beers or glasses of wine in the evenings. Last consumed two nights ago. "Relaxes me and helps me sleep."

3. **Pertinent Physical Assessments**
   a. ***Respirations:*** Normal; rate 16; rhythm regular.
   b. ***Skin:*** Warm and dry; pink in color; diminished turgor; no noticeable edema; 3-inch scar on right thigh from childhood injury.
   c. ***Range of Motion:*** Full.
   d. ***Neurologic Status:*** Migraine headache about once a month; pain is usually unilateral, behind eye, in temple, and at base of skull. Fiorinal #3 provides some relief, but usually has to sleep until pain subsides.
   e. ***Cardiovascular:*** BP, 132/77; P, 80. Denies pain or any numbness or tingling.
   f. ***Gastrointestinal:*** Usually eats a light breakfast and lunch with heaviest meal in the evening. Lately, has been able to eat very little. Has no desire to eat. Has lost about 10 lb in the last 3 weeks. Denies any food allergies. Experiences heartburn 3 to 4 times per week, which is relieved by two Mylanta tablets. No history of peptic ulcers. Denies problems with constipation. Reports daily bowel movement; however, with loss of appetite, has a bowel movement every 2 to 3 days.

g. *Genitourinary/Reproductive:* Denies any problems with voiding. Denies concerns about sexuality; however, reports decrease in libido with feelings of depression. Vasectomy performed when client was 32 years old.

h. *Eyes:* Wears bifocal glasses for both close and distant vision. Complained of occasional blurred vision.

i. *Ears:* Denies problems with ears or hearing. Reports occasional mild tinnitus with aspirin use.

j. *Medication Side Effects:* Client complains of dry mouth and blurred vision (both common side effects of Elavil).

k. *Altered Laboratory Values and Possible Significance:*

Serum albumin, 3.5 g% (normal, 4 to 4.5), possibly caused by malnourished condition

BUN, 16 mg/100 mL (normal, 10 to 15), may be caused by mild dehydration

Cholesterol, 275 mg/dL (150 to 250), familial hypercholesterolemia

Sodium, 143 mEq/L (normal, 136 to 142), possible dehydration and insufficient water intake

l. *Activity/Rest Patterns:* Exercises very little; enjoys walking, but does not seem to have the energy lately. Used to play bridge in leisure time, but has not socialized much in last couple of months. Sleeps at least 8 hours per night. Lately, since depressed, some nights falls asleep right after dinner (or even before) and sleeps till morning. Still has very little energy.

m. *Personal Hygiene/ADL:* Functions independently in ADL. Client is clean, with no noticeable body odor. Clothes are clean, but wrinkled (as though they had been slept in). Hair is not combed. Has about 2 days' growth of beard.

SUMMARY OF INITIAL PSYCHOSOCIAL/PHYSICAL ASSESSMENT

A 45-year-old gentleman admitted to the psychiatric unit by family physician after expressing suicidal ideations. He is very despondent and admits to having thoughts of suicide. He is lethargic and unkempt. He maintains minimal eye contact. There is no evidence of psychotic behaviors. Thinking process is slow, but intact. Client is withdrawn, with minimal verbalizations, but is cooperative with admission process.

KNOWLEDGE DEFICITS IDENTIFIED

Client needs to learn:

- Available resources when feeling suicidal.
- Ways to increase self-esteem.
- Side effects of Desyrel.
- Methods of relaxation.
- Assertiveness techniques.
- More appropriate ways of coping with stress.

NURSING DIAGNOSES INDICATED

1. Risk for self-directed violence related to depressed mood and expressions of having nothing to live for.
2. Dysfunctional grieving related to unresolved losses (promotion and satisfactory father-son relationship) evidenced by anger turned inward on self and desire to end life.
3. Chronic low self-esteem related to lack of positive feedback and learned helplessness evidenced by a sense of worthlessness, lack of eye contact, social isolation, and negative/pessimistic outlook.
4. Social isolation related to depressed mood and feelings of worthlessness evidenced by withdrawal and desire to be alone; uncommunicative.
5. Powerlessness related to lack of positive feedback evidenced by apathy, passivity, and statements, "I was never able to please my father; now I can't please my boss. What's the use of trying? I just don't care anymore."
6. Alteration in nutrition, less than body requirements related to decreased food intake because of depressed mood and loss of appetite evidenced by loss of weight (10 lb in 3 weeks), diminished skin turgor, decreased serum albumin, increased serum sodium.

Nursing Diagnoses and Interventions for Sam

RISK FOR SELF-DIRECTED VIOLENCE

Related/Risk Factors ("related to")
Depressed mood
Expressions of having nothing to live for

Goals/Objectives
Short-Term Goal
Client will seek out staff when ideas of suicide occur.

Long-Term Goal
Client will not harm self during hospitalization.

Interventions with *Selected Rationales*
1. Ask client directly: "Have you thought about killing yourself? If so, what do you plan to do? Do you have the means to carry out this plan?" *The risk of suicide is greatly increased if the client has developed a plan, and particularly if means exist for the client to execute the plan.*
2. Create a safe environment for the client. Remove all potentially harmful objects from client's access (sharp objects, straps, belts, ties, glass items). *Client safety is a nursing priority.*
3. Formulate a short-term verbal contract with the client that he will not harm himself during next 24 hours. When that contract expires, make another, and so forth. *Discussion of suicidal feelings with a trusted individual provides a degree of relief to the client. A contract gets the subject out in the open and places some of the responsibility for his safety with the client. An attitude of acceptance of the client as a worthwhile individual is conveyed.*
4. Secure a promise from the client that he will seek out a staff member if thoughts of suicide emerge. *Suicidal clients are often very ambivalent about their feelings. Discussion of feelings with a trusted individual may provide assistance before the client experiences a crisis situation.*
5. Encourage verbalizations of honest feelings. Through exploration and discussion, help client to identify symbols of hope in his life (participating in activities he finds satisfying outside of his job).
6. Allow client to express angry feelings within appropriate limits. Encourage use of exercise room and punching bag each day. Help client to identify true source of anger, and

work on adaptive coping skills for use outside the hospital (e.g., jogging, exercise club available to employees of his company). *Depression and suicidal behaviors may be viewed as anger turned inward on the self. If this anger can be verbalized in a nonthreatening environment, the client may be able to resolve these feelings, regardless of the discomfort involved. Physical activities relieve pent-up tension.*

7. Identify community resources that the client may use as a support system and from whom he may request help if feeling suicidal (e.g., suicidal or crisis hotline; psychiatrist or social worker at community mental health center; hospital "HELP" line). *Having a concrete plan for seeking assistance during a crisis may discourage or prevent self-destructive behaviors.*

8. Introduce client to support and education groups for adult children of alcoholics (ACOA). *The purpose of these ACOA groups is to help members overcome the guilt, depression, low self-esteem, and other characteristics common to adults who grew up in homes with an alcohol-dependent parent.*

9. Most important, spend time with the client. *This provides a feeling of safety and security, while also conveying the message, "I want to spend time with you because I think you are a worthwhile person."*

Outcome Criteria
1. Client verbalizes no thoughts of suicide and expresses some hope for the future.
2. Client is able to verbalize names of resources outside the hospital from whom he may request help if feeling suicidal.

DYSFUNCTIONAL GRIEVING

Possible Etiologies ("related to")
Unresolved losses (job promotion and satisfactory father-son relationship)

Defining Characteristics ("evidenced by")
Anger turned inward on self and desire to end life

Goals/Objectives
Short-Term Goal
Client will verbalize anger toward boss and parents within 1 week.

Long-Term Goal
Client will verbalize own position in grief process and begin movement in the progression toward resolution by discharge.

Interventions with *Selected Rationales*
1. Client is fixed in anger stage of grieving process. Discuss behaviors associated with this stage with him. *Accurate baseline assessment data are necessary to effectively plan care for the grieving client.*
2. Develop trusting relationship with client. Show empathy and caring. Be honest and keep all promises. *Trust is the basis for a therapeutic relationship.*
3. Convey an accepting attitude—one in which client is not afraid to express feelings openly. *An accepting attitude conveys to the client that you believe he is a worthwhile person. Trust is enhanced.*
4. Allow client to verbalize feelings of anger. Initial expression of anger may be displaced on nurse or therapist. Do not become defensive if this should occur. Assist client to explore angry feelings so that they may be directed toward the intended persons. *Verbalization of feelings in a nonthreatening environment may help client come to terms with unresolved issues.*
5. Assist client to discharge pent-up anger through participation in large motor activities (brisk walks, jogging, physical exercises, volleyball, punching bag, exercise bike, or other equipment). *Physical exercise provides a safe and effective method for discharging pent-up tension.*
6. Explain normal stages of grief, and the behaviors associated with each stage. Help client to understand that feelings such as guilt and anger toward boss and parents are appropriate and acceptable during this stage of the grieving process. Help him also to understand that he must work through these feelings and move past this stage in order to eventually feel better. *Knowledge of acceptability of the feelings associated with normal grieving may help to relieve some of the guilt that these responses generate. Knowing why he is experiencing these feelings may also help to resolve them.*
7. Encourage client to review relationship with his parents. With support and sensitivity, point out reality of the situation in areas in which misrepresentations are expressed. Explain common roles and behaviors of members in an alcoholic family. *Client must give up desire for idealized family and accept the reality of his childhood situation*

and the effect it has had on his adult life, before the grief process can be completed.

8. Assist client in problem solving as he attempts to determine methods for more adaptive coping. Suggest alternatives to anger turned inward on the self when negative thinking sets in (e.g., thought-stopping techniques). Provide positive feedback for strategies identified and decisions made. *Positive feedback increases self-esteem and encourages repetition of desirable behaviors.*

9. Encourage client to reach out for spiritual support during this time in whatever form is desirable to him. Assess spiritual needs of client, and assist as necessary in the fulfillment of those needs.

Outcome Criteria
1. Client is able to verbalize normal stages of grief process and behaviors associated with each stage.
2. Client is able to identify own position within the grief process and express honest feelings related to loss of job promotion and satisfactory parent-child relationship.
3. Client is no longer manifesting exaggerated emotions and behaviors related to dysfunctional grieving and is able to carry out activities of daily living independently.

CHRONIC LOW SELF-ESTEEM

Possible Etiologies ("related to")
Lack of positive feedback and learned helplessness

Defining Characteristics ("evidenced by")
A sense of worthlessness, lack of eye contact, social isolation and negative, pessimistic outlook

Goals/Objectives
Short-Term Goal
Client will discuss feelings about self, and when these feelings were developed, with staff nurse by 1 week.

Long-Term Goal
Client will exhibit increased feelings of self-worth by discharge, as evidenced by verbal expression of positive aspects about self, past accomplishments, and future prospects.

Interventions with *Selected Rationales*
1. Be accepting of client and his negativism. *An attitude of acceptance enhances feelings of self-worth.*

2. Spend time with client *to convey acceptance and contribute toward feelings of self-worth.*

3. Help client to recognize and focus on strengths, accomplishments, and experiences that create good feelings about himself. Minimize attention given to past (real or perceived) failures. *Self-esteem is enhanced by recognition and discussion of positive aspects of self. Lack of attention to negative ruminations may help to eliminate them.*

4. Encourage participation in group activities from which client may receive positive feedback and support from peers. *Recognition and acceptance increase self-esteem.*

5. Help client identify realistic aspects he would like to change about himself and assist with problem solving toward this effort. *Low self-worth may interfere with client's perception of own problem-solving ability. Assistance may be required.*

6. Ensure that client is not becoming increasingly dependent and that he is accepting responsibility for his own behaviors. *Client must be able to function independently if he is to be successful within the less-structured community environment.*

7. Ensure that therapy groups offer client simple methods of achievement within a short period of time. Offer recognition and positive feedback for actual accomplishments. *Successes and recognition increase self-esteem.*

8. Teach assertiveness techniques: The ability to recognize the differences among passive, assertive, and aggressive behaviors; the importance of respecting the human rights of others while protecting one's own basic human rights. *Self-esteem is enhanced by the ability to interact with others in an assertive manner.*

9. Teach effective communication techniques, such as the use of ''I'' messages and placing emphasis on ways to avoid making judgmental statements.

10. Assist client to perform aspects of self-care where required. Offer positive feedback for tasks performed independently. *Successful accomplishments and positive feedback enhance self-esteem and encourage repetition of desirable behaviors.*

Outcome Criteria
1. Client is able to verbalize positive aspects about self.
2. Client is able to communicate assertively with others.
3. Client expresses some optimism and hope for the future.

SOCIAL ISOLATION

Possible Etiologies ("related to")
Depressed mood and feelings of worthlessness

Defining Characteristics ("evidenced by")
Withdrawal and desire to be alone; uncommunicative

Goals/Objectives
Short-Term Goal
Client will develop trusting relationship with one staff nurse by end of first week of hospitalization.

Long-Term Goal
Client will voluntarily spend time with other clients and staff members in group activities on the unit by discharge.

Interventions with *Selected Rationales*
1. Spend time with client. This may mean just sitting in silence for a while. *Presence of the nurse will help improve client's perception of self as a worthwhile person.*
2. Develop a therapeutic nurse-client relationship through frequent, brief contacts and an accepting attitude. Show unconditional positive regard. *The nurse's presence, acceptance, and conveyance of positive regard will enhance the client's feelings of self-worth.*
3. After client feels comfortable in one-to-one relationship, encourage attendance in group activities. May need to attend with him the first few times to offer support. Accept client's decision to remove himself from group situation if anxiety becomes too great. *The presence of a trusted individual provides emotional security for the client.*
4. Verbally acknowledge client's absence from any group activities. *Knowledge that his absence was noticed may reinforce the client's feelings of self-worth.*
5. Teach client assertiveness techniques. Interactions with others may be discouraged by client's use of passive or aggressive behaviors. *Knowledge and use of assertive techniques may increase self-confidence and improve client's relationships with others.*
6. Provide lots of structure in client's daily activities. Devise a time schedule of therapeutic activities and provide client with a written copy. Try to schedule most of his activities for afternoon and early evening. *Depressed clients must have lots of structure in their lives because of impair-*

ment in decision-making and problem-solving ability. The written schedule provides a concreteness from which the client can derive some security. Severely depressed clients feel their worst early in the morning and better as the day progresses.

7. Teach skills that client may use to approach others in a socially acceptable manner. Practice these skills with client through role playing.

8. Provide positive reinforcement for client's voluntary interactions with others. *Positive reinforcement enhances self-esteem and encourages repetition of desirable behaviors.*

Outcome Criteria

1. Client demonstrates willingness or desire to socialize with others.
2. Client voluntarily attends group activities.
3. Client approaches others in appropriate manner for one-to-one interaction.

POWERLESSNESS

Possible Etiologies ("related to")
Lack of positive feedback

Defining Characteristics ("evidenced by")
"I could never please my father. Now I can't seem to please my boss. What's the use of trying? . . . I just don't care anymore."

Goals/Objectives
Short-Term Goal
Client will take charge of own ADL within 1 week.

Long-Term Goal
Client will be able to effectively problem-solve ways to take control of own life situation by discharge, thereby decreasing feelings of powerlessness.

Interventions with *Selected Rationales*
1. Allow client to take as much responsibility as possible for own self-care practices. *Providing client with choices will increase his feelings of control.* Examples:
   a. Include client in setting the goals of care he wishes to achieve.

   b. Allow client to establish own schedule for self-care activities.
   c. Provide client with privacy as need is determined.
   d. Provide positive feedback for decisions made. Respect client's right to make those decisions independently, and refrain from attempting to influence him toward those which may seem more logical.
2. Assist client to set realistic goals for himself. *Goals that are unrealistic set the client up for failure, reinforcing feelings of powerlessness.*
3. Help client identify areas of life situation that he can control (employment situation). *Client's emotional condition interferes with his ability to problem solve. Assistance is required to accurately perceive the benefits and consequences of available alternatives.*
4. Help client identify areas of life situation that are not within his ability to control (loss of satisfactory father-son relationship). Encourage verbalization of feelings related to this inability *in an effort to deal with unresolved issues and accept what cannot be changed.*
5. Identify ways in which client can achieve. Encourage participation in these activities and provide positive reinforcement for participation, as well as achievement. *Positive reinforcement enhances self-esteem and encourages repetition of desirable behaviors.*

Outcome Criteria
1. Client verbalizes choices he has made in a plan to maintain control over his own life situation.
2. Client verbalizes honest feelings about life situations over which he has no control.
3. Client is able to verbalize system for problem solving as required for adequate role performance.

ALTERED NUTRITION, LESS THAN BODY REQUIREMENTS

Possible Etiologies ("related to")
Decreased food intake because of depressed mood and loss of appetite.

Defining Characteristics ("evidenced by")
Loss of weight (10 lb in 3 weeks), diminished skin turgor, decreased serum albumin, increased serum sodium

Goals/Objectives
Short-Term Goal
By third hospital day, client will eat regular meals and snacks
  as provided on each shift.

Long-Term Goal
By discharge, client will exhibit no signs or symptoms of malnutrition.

Interventions with *Selected Rationales*
1. In collaboration with dietitian, determine number of calories required to provide adequate nutrition and realistic
   weight gain.
2. Ensure that diet includes foods high in fiber content to
   prevent constipation. Encourage client to increase fluid
   consumption and physical exercise to promote normal
   bowel functioning. Fluid is also required to correct mildly
   dehydrated condition. *Depressed clients are particularly
   vulnerable to constipation brought on by psychomotor
   retardation. Abnormal laboratory values indicate possible mild dehydration.*
3. Perform strict documentation of intake, output, calorie
   count. *This information is necessary to make an accurate nutritional assessment and maintain client safety.*
4. Weigh client daily. *Weight loss or gain is important assessment information.*
5. Determine client's likes and dislikes and collaborate with
   dietitian to provide favorite foods. Encourage wife to bring
   in foods that he has enjoyed in the past. *Client is more
   likely to eat foods that he particularly enjoys.*
6. If client continues to experience loss of appetite, it may
   be desirable to provide small, frequent feedings, including
   a bedtime snack, rather than three larger meals. *Large
   amounts of food may be objectionable, or even intolerable, to an anorexic client.*
7. Stay with client during meals to assist as needed, and to
   offer support and encouragement. *Mealtime is a social
   time, and the presence of a trusted individual can provide needed security.*
8. Monitor laboratory values, and report significant changes
   to physician. Monitor serum albumin, sodium, and blood
   urea nitrogen for return to normal levels. *Laboratory values provide objective data regarding nutritional status.*
9. Teach the importance of adequate nutrition and fluid intake. *Client may have inadequate or inaccurate knowledge regarding the contribution of good nutrition to
   overall wellness.*

Outcome Criteria

1. Client has shown a slow, progressive weight gain during hospitalization.
2. Vital signs, blood pressure, and all laboratory serum studies are within normal limits.
3. Client is able to verbalize importance of adequate nutrition and fluid intake.

Chapter 3

CONCEPTS OF PSYCHOBIOLOGY

INTRODUCTION

The 101st legislature of the United States designated the 1990s as the "decade of the brain." With this legislation comes the challenge for studying the biologic basis of behavior. In keeping with this "neuroscientific revolution," greater emphasis is placed on the study of the organic basis for psychiatric illness. Certain mental illnesses are being looked on as "physical illnesses characterized by, or resulting from, malfunctions and/or malformations of the brain" (Peschel and Peschel, 1991).

This is not to imply that psychosocial and sociocultural influences are totally discounted. The systems of biology, psychology, and sociology are not mutually exclusive but are interacting systems. This is clearly indicated by the fact that individuals experience biologic changes in response to various environmental events. Indeed, each of these disciplines may at various times be most appropriate for explaining behavioral phenomena.

This chapter presents an overview of neurophysiologic, neurochemical, and endocrine influences on psychiatric illness. Various diagnostic procedures used to detect alterations in biologic function that may contribute to psychiatric illness are identified.

NEUROPHYSIOLOGIC INFLUENCES

THE BRAIN

Following is a summary of the major structures of the brain and their primary functions. Diagrams of these structures are presented in Figures 3–1, 3–2, and 3–3.

1. **The Forebrain.** The forebrain is composed of the cerebrum and the diencephalon.

   a. *Cerebrum.* The cerebrum is composed of two hemispheres separated by a deep groove that houses a band of 200 million neurons called the *corpus callosum.* The outer shell is called the *cortex.* It is extensively folded and consists of billions of neurons. The left hemisphere appears to be dominant in most people. It controls speech, comprehension, rational-

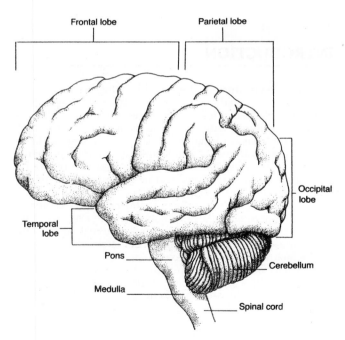

FIGURE 3–1 The human brain: Cerebral lobes, cerebellum, and brain stem. (From Scanlon and Sanders, 1995, with permission.)

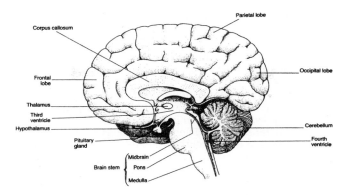

FIGURE 3–2 The human brain: Midsagittal surface. (From Scanlon and Sanders, 1995, with permission.)

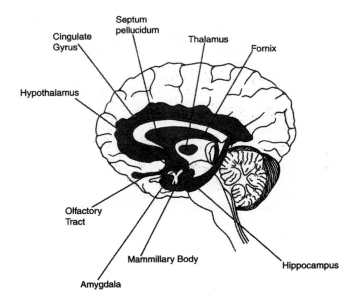

FIGURE 3–3 Structures of the limbic system. (Adapted from Scanlon and Sanders, 1995, with permission.)

ity, and logic. The right hemisphere is nondominant in most people. Sometimes called the "creative" brain, it is associated with affect, behavior, and spacial perceptual functions. Each hemisphere is divided into four lobes.

- *Frontal Lobes.* The frontal lobes control voluntary body movement, including movements that permit speaking, thinking and judgment formation, and expression of feelings.
- *Parietal Lobes.* The parietal lobes control perception and interpretation of most sensory information (including touch, pain, taste, and body position).
- *Temporal Lobes.* The temporal lobes are concerned with hearing, short-term memory, sense of smell, and expression of emotions through connection with the limbic system.
- *Occipital Lobes.* The occipital lobes are the primary area of visual reception and interpretation.

b. *Diencephalon.* The diencephalon connects the cerebrum with lower brain structures. Its major structures include the thalamus, hypothalamus, and limbic system.

- *Thalamus.* The thalamus integrates all sensory input (except smell) on its way to the cortex. The thalamus also has some involvement with emotions and mood.
- *Hypothalamus.* The hypothalamus regulates the anterior and posterior lobes of the pituitary gland. It exerts control over the actions of the autonomic nervous system, and regulates appetite and temperature.
- *Limbic System.* The limbic system consists of medially placed cortical and subcortical structures and the fiber tracts connecting them with one another and with the hypothalamus. These structures include the hippocampus, mammillary body, amygdala, olfactory tract, hypothalamus, cingulate gyrus, septum pellucidum, thalamus, and fornix. The limbic system, which is sometimes called the "emotional brain," is associated with feelings of fear and anxiety; anger and aggression; love, joy, and hope; and with sexuality and social behavior.

2. **The Midbrain.** The main structures of the midbrain are called the mesencephalon.

a. *Mesencephalon.* Structures of major importance in the mesencephalon include nuclei and fiber tracts.

They extend from the pons to the hypothalamus and are responsible for the integration of visual, auditory, and balance ("righting") reflexes.

3. **The Hindbrain.** The hindbrain consists of the pons, the medulla, and the cerebellum.

   a. *Pons.* The pons is responsible for regulation of respiration and skeletal muscle tone. Ascending and descending fiber tracts of the pons connect the brain stem with the cerebellum and cortex.

   b. *Medulla.* The medulla provides a pathway for all ascending and descending fiber tracts. It contains vital centers that regulate heart rate, blood pressure, and respiration, and reflex centers for swallowing, sneezing, coughing, and vomiting.

   c. *Cerebellum.* The cerebellum regulates muscle tone and coordination and maintains posture and equilibrium.

NERVE TISSUE

The tissue of the central nervous system (CNS) consists of nerve cells called neurons that generate and transmit electrochemical impulses. The structure of a neuron is composed of a cell body, an axon, and dendrites. The cell body contains the nucleus and is essential for the continued life of the neuron. The dendrites are processes that transmit impulses toward the cell body, and the axon transmits impulses away from the cell body. Cells called *afferent* (or *sensory*) *neurons* carry impulses from the periphery to the CNS, where they are interpreted into various sensations. The *efferent* (or *motor*) *neurons* carry impulses from the CNS to the muscles and glands of the periphery. A third type of cell, called *interneurons*, exists entirely within the CNS. Ninety-nine percent of all nerve cells belong to this group. They may carry only sensory or motor impulses, or they may serve as integrators in the pathways between afferent and efferent neurons. They account in large part for thinking, feelings, learning, language, and memory.

Some messages may be processed through only a few neurons, while others may require thousands of neuronal connections. The neurons that transmit the impulses do not actually touch each other. The junction between two neurons is called a *synapse*. The small space between the axon terminals of one neuron and the cell body or dendrites of another is called the *synaptic cleft*. Chemicals called *neu-*

rotransmitters are stored in the axon terminals of presynaptic neurons. Electrical impulses cause the release of these chemicals into the synaptic cleft. The neurotransmitter combines with receptor sites on the postsynaptic neuron, resulting in a determination of whether or not another electrical impulse is generated.

NEUROCHEMICAL INFLUENCES

NEUROTRANSMITTERS

Neurotransmitters are responsible for essential functions in the role of human emotion and behavior. They are also the target for the mechanism of action of many of the psychotropic medications.

After a neurotransmitter has performed its function in the synaptic cleft, it either returns to the vesicles in the axon terminals to be stored and used again, or it is inactivated and dissolved by enzymes. The process of being stored for reuse is called *reuptake*, a function that holds significance for understanding the mechanism of action of certain psychotropic medications.

Many neurotransmitters exist within the central and peripheral nervous systems, but only a limited number have implications for psychiatry. Major categories include the cholinergics, monoamines, amino acids, and neuropeptides. The location, function, and implications of these neurotransmitters are described in Table 3–1.

ENDOCRINE INFLUENCES

Human endocrine functioning has a strong foundation in the CNS, under the direction of the hypothalamus, which has direct control over the pituitary gland. The pituitary gland has two major lobes—the anterior lobe (also called the *adenohypophysis*) and the posterior lobe (also called the *neurohypophysis*). The pituitary gland is only about the size of a pea. However, despite its size and because of the powerful control it exerts over endocrine functioning in humans, it is sometimes called the "master gland." Many of the hormones subject to hypothalamus-pituitary regulation may have implications for behavioral functioning. Discussion of these hormones is summarized in Table 3–2.

A summary of various psychiatric disorders and the possible biologic influences discussed in this chapter (with the addition of possible genetic influences) is presented in Table 3–3.

DIAGNOSTIC PROCEDURES USED TO DETECT ALTERED BRAIN FUNCTIONING

A number of diagnostic procedures are used to detect alteration in biologic functioning that may contribute to psychiatric disorders. Following is an explanation of various examinations, the technique used, the purpose of the examination, and possible findings.

1. **Electroencephalography (EEG)**
   a. *Technique.* Electrodes are placed on the scalp in a standardized position. Amplitude and frequency of beta, alpha, theta, and delta brain waves are graphically recorded on paper by ink markers for multiple areas of the brain surface.
   b. *Purpose/Possible Findings.* Measures brain electrical activity; identifies dysrhythmias, asymmetries, or suppression of brain rhythms; used in the diagnosis of epilepsy, neoplasm, stroke, metabolic, or degenerative disease.

2. **Computerized EEG Mapping**
   a. *Technique.* EEG tracings are summarized by computer-assisted systems in which various regions of the brain are identified and functioning is interpreted by color coding or gray shading.
   b. *Purpose/Possible Findings.* Measures brain electrical activity; used largely in research to represent statistical relationships between individuals and groups or between two populations of subjects (e.g., clients with schizophrenia vs. control subjects).

3. **Computed Tomographic (CT) Scan**
   a. *Technique.* May be used with or without contrast medium. X-rays are taken of various transverse planes of the brain while a computerized analysis produces a precise reconstructed image of each segment.
   b. *Purpose/Possible Findings.* Measures accuracy of brain structure to detect possible lesions, abscesses, areas of infarction, or aneurysm. CT has also identi-

TABLE 3–1 Neurotransmitters in the Central Nervous System

Neurotransmitter	Location/Function	Possible Implications for Mental Illness
I. Cholinergics A. Acetylcholine	ANS: Sympathetic and parasympathetic presynaptic nerve terminals; parasympathetic postsynaptic nerve terminals. CNS: Cerebral cortex, hippocampus, limbic structures, and basal ganglia. Functions: Sleep, arousal, pain perception, movement, memory.	Increased levels: Depression. Decreased levels: Alzheimer's disease, Huntington's chorea, Parkinson's disease.
II. Monoamines A. Norepinephrine	ANS: Sympathetic postsynaptic nerve terminals. CNS: Thalamus, hypothalamus, limbic system, hippocampus, cerebellum, cerebral cortex. Functions: Mood, cognition, perception, locomotion, cardiovascular functioning, and sleep and arousal.	Decreased levels: Depression. Increased levels: Mania, anxiety states, schizophrenia.
B. Dopamine	Frontal cortex, limbic system, basal ganglia, thalamus, posterior pituitary, and spinal cord. Functions: Movement and coordination, emotions, voluntary judgment, release of prolactin.	Decreased levels: Parkinson's disease and depression. Increased levels: Mania and schizophrenia.
C. Serotonin	Hypothalamus, thalamus, limbic system, cerebral cortex, cerebellum, spinal cord. Functions: Sleep and arousal, libido, appetite, mood, aggression, pain perception, coordination, judgment.	Decreased levels: Depression. Increased levels: Anxiety states.
D. Histamine	Hypothalamus	Decreased levels: Depression.

III. Amino Acids

A. Gamma Aminobutyric Acid (GABA)

Hypothalamus, hippocampus, cortex, cerebellum, basal ganglia, spinal cord, retina.

Functions: Slowdown of body activity.

Decreased levels: Huntington's chorea, anxiety disorders, schizophrenia, and various forms of epilepsy.

Toxic levels: "glycine encephalopathy," decreased levels are correlated with spastic motor movements.

B. Glycine

Spinal cord and brainstem.

Functions: Recurrent inhibition of motor neurons.

C. Glutamate and aspartate

Pyramidal cells of the cortex, cerebellum, and the primary sensory afferent systems; hippocampus, thalamus, hypothalamus, spinal cord.

Functions: Relay of sensory information and in the regulation of various motor and spinal reflexes.

Increased levels: Huntington's chorea, temporal lobe epilepsy, spinal cerebellar degeneration.

IV. Neuropeptides

A. Endorphins and enkephalins

Hypothalamus, thalamus, limbic structures, midbrain, and brain stem. Enkephalins are also found in the gastrointestinal tract.

Functions: Modulation of pain and reduced peristalsis (enkephalins).

Modulation of dopamine activity by opioid peptides may indicate some link to the symptoms of schizophrenia.

B. Substance P

Hypothalamus, limbic structures, midbrain, brainstem, thalamus, basal ganglia, and spinal cord; also found in gastrointestinal tract and salivary glands.

Function: Regulation of pain.

Decreased levels: Huntington's chorea.

C. Somatostatin

Cerebral cortex, hippocampus, thalamus, basal ganglia, brain stem, and spinal cord.

Function: Inhibits release of norepinephrine; stimulates release of serotonin, dopamine, and acetylcholine.

Decreased levels: Alzheimer's disease.

Increased levels: Huntington's chorea.

From Townsend, 1996, p. 70, with permission.

TABLE 3–2 Hormones of the Neuroendocrine System

Hormone	Location and Stimulation of Release	Target Organ	Function	Possible Behavioral Correlation to Altered Secretion
Antidiuretic hormone (ADH)	Posterior pituitary; release stimulated by dehydration, pain, stress	Kidney (causes increased reabsorption)	Conservation of body water and maintain blood pressure	Polydipsia; altered pain response; modified sleep pattern
Oxytocin	Posterior pituitary; release stimulated by end of pregnancy; stress; during sexual arousal	Uterus; breasts	Contraction of the uterus for labor; release of breast milk	May play role in stress response by stimulation of ACTH
Growth hormone (GH)	Anterior pituitary; release stimulated by growth hormone releasing hormone from hypothalamus	Bones and tissues	Growth in children; protein synthesis in adults	Anorexia nervosa
Thyroid-stimulating hormone (TSH)	Anterior pituitary; release stimulated by thyrotropin releasing hormone from hypothalamus	Thyroid gland	Stimulation of secretion of thyroid hormones needed for metabolism of food and regulation of temperature	Increased levels: insomnia, anxiety, emotional lability Decreased levels: fatigue, depression

Adrenocorticotropic hormone (ACTH)	Anterior pituitary; release stimulated by corticotropin releasing hormone from hypothalamus	Adrenal cortex	Stimulation of secretion of cortisol, which plays a role in response to stress	Increased levels: mood disorders, psychosis Decreased levels: depression, apathy, fatigue
Prolactin	Anterior pituitary; release stimulated by prolactin releasing hormone from hypothalamus	Breasts	Stimulation of milk production	Increased levels: depression, anxiety, decreased libido, irritability
Gonadotropic hormones	Anterior pituitary; release stimulated by gonadotropin releasing hormone from hypothalamus	Ovaries and testes	Stimulation of secretion of estrogen, progesterone, and testosterone; role in ovulation and sperm production	Decreased levels: depression and anorexia nervosa Increased testosterone: increased sexual behavior and aggressiveness
Melanocyte-stimulating hormone (MSH)	Anterior pituitary; release stimulated by onset of darkness	Pineal gland	Stimulation of secretion of melatonin	Increased levels: depression

From Townsend, 1996, p. 73, with permission.

TABLE 3–3 Biological Implications of Psychiatric Disorders

Anatomic Brain Structures Involved	Neurotransmitter Hypothesis	Possible Endocrine Correlation	Possible Genetic Link
Schizophrenia Frontal cortex, temporal lobes, limbic system	Dopamine hyperactivity	Decreased prolactin levels	Twin, familial, and adoption studies suggest a genetic link
Depressive Disorders Frontal lobes, limbic system, temporal lobes	Decreased levels of norepinephrine, dopamine, and serotonin	Increased cortisol levels; thyroid hormone hyposecretion; increased melatonin	Twin, familial, and adoption studies suggest a genetic link
Bipolar Disorder Frontal lobes, limbic system, temporal lobes	Increased levels of norepinephrine, dopamine, and serotonin in acute mania	Some indication of elevated thyroid hormones in acute mania	Twin, familial, and adoption studies suggest a genetic link

Disorder (Area of Brain)	Biochemical Influences	Neuroendocrine Influences	Genetic Influences
Panic Disorder Limbic system, midbrain	Increased levels of norepinephrine; decreased GABA activity	Elevated levels of thyroid hormones	Twin and familial studies suggest a genetic link
Anorexia Nervosa Limbic system, particularly the hypothalamus	Decreased levels of norepinephrine, serotonin, and dopamine	Decreased levels of gonadotropins and growth hormone; increased cortisol levels	Twin and familial studies suggest a genetic link
Obsessive Compulsive Disorder Limbic system, basal ganglia (specifically caudate nucleus)	Decreased levels of serotonin	Increased cortisol levels	Twin studies suggest a possible genetic link
Alzheimer's Disease Temporal, parietal and occipital regions of cerebral cortex; hippocampus	Decreased levels of acetylcholine, norepinephrine, serotonin, and somatostatin	Decreased corticotropin-releasing hormone	Familial studies suggest a genetic predisposition; early onset disorder linked to marker on chromosome 21

From Townsend, 1996, p. 81, with permission.

fied various anatomic differences in clients with schizophrenia, organic mental disorders, and bipolar disorder.

4. **Magnetic Resonance Imaging (MRI)**
    a. ***Technique.*** Within a strong magnetic field, the nuclei of hydrogen atoms absorb and re-emit electromagnetic energy that is computerized and transformed into image information. No radiation or contrast medium is used.
    b. ***Purpose/Possible Findings.*** Measures anatomic and biochemical status of various segments of the brain; detects brain edema, ischemia, infection, neoplasm, trauma, and other changes such as demyelination. Morphological differences have been noted in brains of clients with schizophrenia as compared with control subjects.

5. **Positron Emission Tomography (PET)**
    a. ***Technique.*** The client receives an intravenous injection of a radioactive substance (type dependent on brain activity to be visualized). The head is surrounded by detectors that relay data to a computer that interprets the signals and produces the image.
    b. ***Purpose/Possible Findings.*** Measures specific brain functioning, such as glucose metabolism, oxygen utilization, blood flow, and, of particular interest in psychiatry, neurotransmitter/recepter interaction.

6. **Single Photon Emission Computed Tomography (SPECT)**
    a. ***Technique.*** The technique is similar to PET, but a longer-acting radioactive substance must be used to allow time for a gamma camera to rotate about the head and gather the data, which are then computer assembled into a brain image.
    b. ***Purpose/Possible Findings.*** Measures various aspects of brain functioning, as with PET; has also been used to image activity or cerebrospinal fluid circulation.

SUMMARY

The "medicalization of psychiatry" necessitates that nurses be cognizant of the interaction between physical and mental factors in the development and management of psychiatric illness. These current trends have made it essential for nurses to increase their knowledge about the structure and functioning of the brain. This includes the processes of neurotransmission and the function of various neurotransmitters. This is especially important in light of the increasing role of psychotropic medication in the treatment of psychiatric illness. Because the mechanism of action of many of these drugs occurs at synaptic transmission, nurses must understand this process so that they may predict outcomes and safely manage the administration of psychotropic medications.

The endocrine system plays an important role in human behavior through the hypothalamic-pituitary axis. Hormones influence a number of physiologic and psychologic life-cycle phenomena, such as moods, sleep-arousal, stress response, appetite, libido, and fertility.

It is also important for nurses to keep abreast of the expanding diagnostic technologies available for detecting alterations in physical functioning. These technologies are facilitating the growth of knowledge linking mental illness to disorders of the brain.

Chapter 4

DISORDERS USUALLY FIRST DIAGNOSED IN INFANCY, CHILDHOOD, OR ADOLESCENCE

BACKGROUND ASSESSMENT DATA

Several common psychiatric disorders may arise or become evident during infancy, childhood, or adolescence. Essential features of many disorders are identical, regardless of the age of the individual. Examples include the following:

Cognitive Disorders
Schizophrenia
Schizophreniform
   Disorder
Adjustment Disorder
Sexual Disorders
Personality Disorders

Substance-Related
   Disorders
Mood Disorders
Somatoform Disorders
Psychological Factors
   Affecting Medical
   Conditions

There are, however, several disorders that appear during the early developmental years and are identified according to the child's ability or inability to perform age-appropriate tasks or intellectual functions. Selected disorders are presented here. It is essential that the nurse working with these clients understand normal behavior patterns characteristic of the infant, childhood, and adolescent years.

MENTAL RETARDATION

DEFINED

Mental retardation is defined by deficits in general intellectual functioning and adaptive functioning, and identified by an intelligence quotient (IQ) of approximately 70 or below on an individually administered IQ examination (APA, 1994). Mental retardation is further categorized (by IQ level) as mild (IQ of 50 to 70), moderate (IQ of 35 to 49), severe (IQ of 20 to 34), and profound (below 20).

PREDISPOSING FACTORS

1. **Physiologic**
   a. About 5% of cases of mental retardation are caused by hereditary factors, such as Tay-Sachs disease, phenylketonuria, and hyperglycemia. Chromosomal disorders, such as Down's syndrome and Klinefelter's syndrome, have also been implicated.
   b. Events that occur during the prenatal period, such as maternal ingestion of alcohol or other drugs, maternal infections, toxemia, and uncontrolled diabetes, and perinatal period, such as birth trauma or premature separation of the placenta, can result in mental retardation.
   c. Mental retardation can occur as an outcome of childhood illnesses, such as encephalitis or meningitis, or be the result of poisoning or physical trauma in childhood.
2. **Psychosocial**
   a. Fifteen percent to 20 percent of cases of mental retardation are attributed to deprivation of nurturance and social, linguistic, and other stimulation, and to severe mental disorders, such as autistic disorder (APA, 1994).

SYMPTOMATOLOGY (Subjective and Objective Data)

1. At the mild level (IQ of 50 to 70), the individual can live independently, but with some assistance. He or she is capable of sixth-grade-level work and can learn a vo-

cational skill. Social skills are possible, but the individual functions best in a structured, sheltered setting. Coordination may be slightly affected.

2. At the moderate level (IQ of 35 to 49), the individual can perform some activities independently, but requires supervision. Academic skill can be achieved to about the second grade level. The individual may experience some limitation in speech communication and in interactions with others. Motor development may be limited to gross motor ability.

3. The severe level of mental retardation (IQ of 20 to 34) is characterized by the need for complete supervision. Systematic habit training may be accomplished, but the individual does not have the ability for academic or vocational training. Verbal skills are minimal and psychomotor development is poor.

4. The profoundly mentally retarded individual (IQ of less than 20) has no capacity for independent living. Constant aid and supervision are required. No ability exists for academic or vocational training. There is a lack of ability for speech development, socialization skills, or fine or gross motor movements. The individual requires constant supervision and care.

COMMON NURSING DIAGNOSES AND INTERVENTIONS

(Interventions are applicable to various health care settings, such as inpatient and partial hospitalization, community outpatient clinic, home health, and private practice.)

RISK FOR INJURY

Definition: *A state in which the individual is at risk of injury as a result of environmental conditions interacting with the individual's adaptive and defensive resources.*

Related/Risk Factors ("related to")
Altered physical mobility
Aggressive behavior

Goals/Objectives
Short-/Long-Term Goal
Client will not experience injury.

Interventions with *Selected Rationales*
1. *To ensure client safety:*
   a. Create a safe environment for the client. Remove small items from the area where the client will be ambulating and move sharp items out of his or her reach.
   b. Store items that client uses frequently within easy reach.
   c. Pad side rails and headboard of client with history of seizures.
   d. Prevent physical aggression and acting out behaviors by learning to recognize signs that client is becoming agitated.

Outcome Criteria
1. Client has experienced no physical harm.
2. Client responds to attempts to inhibit agitated behavior.

SELF-CARE DEFICIT

Definition: *A state in which the individual experiences an impaired ability to perform or complete [activities of daily living] independently.*

Possible Etiologies ("related to")
Altered physical mobility
Lack of maturity

Defining Characteristics ("evidenced by")
[Unwillingness or inability to keep self clean]
[Uncombed hair; offensive body and breath odor]
[Inability to obtain adequate nutrition without assistance]
[Inability to dress or groom self without assistance]
[Inability to toilet self without assistance]
[Incontinence]

Goals/Objectives
Short-Term Goal
Client will be able to participate in aspects of self-care.

Long-Term Goal
Client will have all self-care needs met.

Interventions with *Selected Rationales*

1. Identify aspects of self-care that may be within the client's capabilities. Work on one aspect of self-care at a time. Provide simple, concrete explanations. *Because clients' capabilities vary so widely, it is important to know each one individually, and to ensure that no client is set up to fail.*
2. Offer positive feedback for efforts at assisting with own self-care. *Positive reinforcement enhances self-esteem and encourages repetition of desirable behaviors.*
3. When one aspect of self-care has been mastered to the best of the client's ability, move on to another. Encourage independence but intervene when client is unable to perform. *Client comfort and safety are nursing priorities.*

Outcome Criteria

1. Client assists with self-care activities to the best of his or her ability.
2. Client's self-care needs are being met.

IMPAIRED VERBAL COMMUNICATION

Definition: *The state in which an individual experiences a decreased or absent ability to use or understand language in human interaction.*

Possible Etiologies ("related to")
Developmental alteration

Defining Characteristics ("evidenced by")
Speaks or verbalizes with difficulty
Difficulty forming words or sentences
Difficulty expressing thought verbally
Inappropriate verbalizations
Does not or cannot speak

Goals/Objectives
Short-Term Goal
Client will establish trust with caregiver and a means of communication of needs.

Long-Term Goals
1. Client's needs are being met through established means of communication.

2. If client cannot speak or communicate by other means, needs are met by caregiver's anticipation of client's needs.

Interventions with *Selected Rationales*
1. Maintain consistency of staff assignment over time. *This facilitates trust and the ability to understand client's actions and communication.*
2. Anticipate and fulfill client's needs until satisfactory communication patterns are established. Learn (from family, if possible) special words client uses that are different from the norm.
3. Identify nonverbal gestures or signals that client may use to convey needs if verbal communication is absent. Practice these communication skills over and over. *Some mentally retarded children, particularly at the severe level, can only learn by systematic habit training.*

Outcome Criteria
1. Client is able to communicate with consistent caregiver.
2. (For client who is unable to communicate): Client's needs, as anticipated by caregiver, are being met.

IMPAIRED SOCIAL INTERACTION

Definition: *The state in which an individual participates in an insufficient or excessive quantity or ineffective quality of social exchange.*

Possible Etiologies ("related to")
Speech deficiencies
Difficulty adhering to conventional social behavior (because of delayed maturational development)

Defining Characteristics ("evidenced by")
Observed use of unsuccessful social interaction behaviors
Dysfunctional interaction with peers, family, and/or others
Observed discomfort in social situations

Goals/Objectives
Short-Term Goal
Client will attempt to interact with others in the presence of trusted caregiver.

Long-Term Goal
Client will be able to interact with others using behaviors that are socially acceptable and appropriate to developmental level.

Interventions with *Selected Rationales*
1. Remain with client during initial interactions with others on the unit. *The presence of a trusted individual provides a feeling of security.*
2. Explain to other clients the meaning behind some of the client's nonverbal gestures and signals. *Others may be more accepting of the client's differentness if they have a better understanding of his or her behavior.*
3. Use simple language to explain to client which behaviors are acceptable and which are not. Establish a procedure for behavior modification that offers rewards for appropriate behaviors and renders an aversive reinforcement in response to the use of inappropriate behaviors. *Positive, negative, and aversive reinforcements can contribute to desired changes in behavior. The privileges and penalties are individually determined as staff learns the likes and dislikes of the client.*

Outcome Criterion
1. Client interacts with others in a socially appropriate manner.

AUTISTIC DISORDER

DEFINED
Autistic disorder is characterized by a withdrawal of the child into the self and into a fantasy world of his or her own creation. Activities and interests are restricted and may be considered somewhat bizarre. The disorder is rare, but occurs 4 to 5 times more often in males than in females. Onset of symptoms is prior to age 3. The course is chronic and often persists into adulthood.

PREDISPOSING FACTORS

1. **Physiologic**
   a. *Genetics.* An increased risk of autistic disorder exists among siblings of individuals with the disorder (APA, 1994). Some studies suggest an increased risk

as high as 50 times greater than the general population.

b. *Neurologic Factors.* Certain developmental problems, such as postnatal neurologic infections, congenital rubella, phenylketonuria, and fragile X syndrome, have also been implicated.

2. **Psychosocial**
   a. *Psychodynamic Theory.* Mahler and coworkers (1975) have suggested that the autistic child is fixed in the presymbiotic phase of development. The child does not achieve a symbiotic relationship with, nor differentiate self from, mother. Ego development is delayed; the child does not communicate or form relationships.
   b. *Theory of Family Dynamics.* Very early interaction patterns have been suggested as important in the predisposition to autistic disorder. In this theory, parents of autistic children were described as aloof and distant, with little emotional attachment to the child. Kanner (1973) coined the term *refrigerator parents* to describe their lack of warmth and affectionate behavior.

SYMPTOMATOLOGY (Subjective and Objective Data)

1. Failure to form interpersonal relationships, characterized by unresponsiveness to people; lack of eye contact and facial responsiveness; indifference or aversion to affection and physical contact. In early childhood, there is a failure to develop cooperative play and friendships.
2. Impairment in communication (verbal and nonverbal) characterized by absence of language or, if developed, often an immature grammatical structure, incorrect use of words, echolalia, or inability to use abstract terms. Accompanying nonverbal expressions may be inappropriate or absent.
3. Bizarre responses to the environment, characterized by resistance or extreme behavioral reactions to minor occurrences; abnormal, obsessive attachment to peculiar objects; ritualistic behaviors.
4. Extreme fascination for objects that move (e.g., fans, trains). Special interest in music, playing with water, buttons, or parts of the body.
5. Unreasonable insistence on following routines in pre-

cise detail (e.g., insisting that exactly the same route always be followed when shopping).
6. Marked distress over changes in trivial aspects of environment (e.g., when a vase is moved from its usual position).
7. Stereotyped body movements (e.g., hand flicking or twisting, spinning, head banging, complex whole-body movements).

COMMON NURSING DIAGNOSES AND INTERVENTIONS

(Interventions are applicable to various health-care settings, such as inpatient and partial hospitalization, community outpatient clinic, home health, and private practice.)

RISK FOR SELF-MUTILATION

Definition: A state in which an individual is at risk to perform an act upon the self to injure, not kill, which produces tissue damage and tension relief.

Related/Risk Factors ("related to")
[Unfulfilled tasks of trust vs. mistrust]
[Fixation in presymbiotic phase of development]
[Neurologic changes occurring in response to certain physical conditions, such as postnatal infections, congenital rubella, phenylketonuria, and fragile X syndrome]
[Inadequate parental nurturing]
[History of self-mutilative behaviors in response to increasing anxiety]
[Obvious indifference to environment or hysterical reactions to changes in the environment]

Goals/Objectives
Short-Term Goal
Client will demonstrate alternative behavior (e.g., initiating interaction between self and nurse) in response to anxiety within specified time. (Length of time required for this objective will depend on severity and chronicity of disorder.)

Long-Term Goal
Client will not inflict harm on self.

Interventions with *Selected Rationales*
1. Intervene to protect child when self-mutilative behaviors, such as head banging or other hysterical behaviors, become evident. *The nurse is responsible for ensuring client safety.*
2. A helmet may be used to protect against head banging, hand mitts to prevent hair pulling, and appropriate padding to protect extremities from injury during hysterical movements.
3. Try to determine if self-mutilative behaviors occur in response to increasing anxiety, and if so, to what the anxiety may be attributed. *Mutilative behaviors may be averted if the cause can be determined.*
4. Work on one-to-one basis with child *to establish trust.*
5. Offer self to child during times of increasing anxiety, *in order to decrease need for self-mutilative behaviors and provide feelings of security.*

Outcome Criteria
1. Anxiety is maintained at a level at which client feels no need for self-mutilation.
2. When feeling anxious, client initiates interaction between self and nurse.

IMPAIRED SOCIAL INTERACTION

Definition: The state in which an individual participates in an insufficient or excessive quantity or ineffective quality of social exchange.

Possible Etiologies ("related to")
Self-concept disturbance
Absence of available significant others
[Unfulfilled tasks of trust vs. mistrust]
[Neurologic changes occurring in response to certain physical conditions, such as neurologic infections, congenital rubella, phenylketonuria, and fragile X syndrome]
[Inadequate parental nurturing]

Defining Characteristics ("evidenced by")
[Lack of responsiveness to, or interest in, people]
[Failure to cuddle]
[Lack of eye contact and facial responsiveness]
[Indifference or aversion to affection and physical contact]
[Failure to develop cooperative play and peer friendships]

Goals/Objectives
Short-Term Goal
Client will demonstrate trust in one caregiver (as evidenced by facial responsiveness and eye contact) within specified time (depending on severity and chronicity of disorder).

Long-Term Goal
Client will initiate social interactions (physical, verbal, nonverbal) with caregiver by discharge from treatment.

Interventions with *Selected Rationales*
1. Function in a one-to-one relationship with the child. *Consistency of staff-client interaction enhances the establishment of trust.*
2. Provide child with familiar objects (favorite toys, blanket). *These items will offer security during times when the child feels distressed.*
3. Convey a manner of warmth, acceptance, and availability as client attempts to fulfill basic needs. *These characteristics enhance establishment and maintenance of a trusting relationship.*
4. Go slowly. Do not force interactions. Begin with positive reinforcement for eye contact. Gradually introduce touch, smiling, hugging. *The autistic client may feel threatened by an onslaught of stimuli to which he or she is unaccustomed.*
5. Support client with your presence as he or she endeavors to relate to others in the environment. *The presence of an individual with whom a trusting relationship has been established provides a feeling of security.*

Outcome Criteria
1. Client initiates interactions between self and others.
2. Client uses eye contact, facial responsiveness, and other nonverbal behaviors in interactions with others.
3. Client does not withdraw from physical contact.

IMPAIRED VERBAL COMMUNICATION

Definition: *The state in which an individual experiences a decreased or absent ability to use or understand language in human interaction.*

Possible Etiologies ("related to")
[Inability to trust]
[Withdrawal into the self]
[Neurologic changes occurring in response to certain physical conditions, such as neurologic infections, congenital rubella, phenylketonuria, and fragile X syndrome]
[Inadequate parental nurturing]

Defining Characteristics ("evidenced by")
Does not or cannot speak.
[Immature grammatical structure]
[Echolalia]
[Pronoun reversal]
[Inability to name objects]
[Inability to use abstract terms]
[Absence of nonverbal expression (e.g., eye contact, facial responsiveness, gestures)]

Goals/Objectives
Short-Term Goal
Client will establish trust with one caregiver (as evidenced by facial responsiveness and eye contact) by specified time (depending on severity and chronicity of disorder).

Long-Term Goal
Client will have established a means for communicating (verbally or nonverbally) needs and desires to staff by discharge from treatment.

Interventions with *Selected Rationales*
1. Maintain consistency of staff assignment over time. *This facilitates trust and the ability to understand client's actions and communication.*
2. Anticipate and fulfill client's needs until satisfactory communication patterns are established.
3. Use the techniques of CONSENSUAL VALIDATION and SEEKING CLARIFICATION to decode communication patterns. (Examples: "I think you must have meant . . ." or "Did you mean to say that . . . ?") *These techniques work to verify the accuracy of the message received, or to clarify any hid-*

den meanings within the message. Take caution not to "put words into the client's mouth."

4. Use "en face" approach (face-to-face, eye-to-eye) to convey correct nonverbal expressions by example. *Eye contact expresses genuine interest in, and respect for, the individual.*

Outcome Criteria

1. Client is able to communicate in a manner that is understood by others.
2. Client's nonverbal messages are congruent with verbalizations.
3. Client initiates verbal and nonverbal interaction with others.

PERSONAL IDENTITY DISTURBANCE

Definition: Inability to distinguish between self and nonself.

Possible Etiologies ("related to")

[Fixation in presymbiotic phase of development]

[Unfulfilled tasks of trust vs. mistrust]

[Inadequate parental nurturing]

Defining Characteristics ("evidenced by")

[Inability to separate own physiologic and emotional needs from those of others]

[Increased levels of anxiety resulting from contact with others]

[Inability to differentiate own body boundaries from those of others]

[Repeating words he or she hears others say or mimicking movements of others]

Goals/Objectives
Short-Term Goal

Client will name own body parts and body parts of caregiver within specified time (depending on severity and chronicity of disorder).

Long-Term Goal

Client will develop ego identity (evidenced by ability to recognize physical and emotional self as separate from others) by discharge from treatment.

Interventions with *Selected Rationales*
1. Function in a one-to-one relationship with the child. *Consistency of staff-client interaction enhances the establishment of trust.*
2. Assist child to recognize separateness during self-care activities, such as dressing and feeding. *These activities increase child's awareness of self as separate from others.*
3. Point out, and assist child in naming, own body parts. *This activity may increase the child's awareness of self as separate from others.*
4. Gradually increase amount of physical contact, using touch to point out differences between client and nurse. Be cautious with touch until trust is established, *because this gesture may be interpreted by the client as threatening.*
5. Using mirrors and drawings and pictures of the child, reinforce the child's learning of body parts and boundaries.

Outcome Criteria
1. Client is able to differentiate own body parts from those of others.
2. Client communicates ability to separate self from environment by discontinuing use of echolalia (repeating words heard) and echopraxia (imitating movements seen).

DISRUPTIVE BEHAVIOR DISORDERS

ATTENTION-DEFICIT/HYPERACTIVITY DISORDER

Defined

Attention-deficit/hyperactivity disorder (ADHD) is characterized by a persistent pattern of inattention and/or hyperactivity-impulsivity that is more frequent and severe than is typically observed in individuals at a comparable level of development (APA, 1994). The disorder is frequently not diagnosed until the child begins school because, prior to that time, childhood behavior is much more variable than that of older children. ADHD is 4 to 9 times more common in boys than in girls and may occur in as many as 3% to 5% of school-age children. The course can be chronic, persisting into adulthood.

Predisposing Factors

1. **Physiologic**
   a. ***Genetics.*** A number of studies have indicated that hereditary factors may be implicated in the predisposition to ADHD. Siblings of hyperactive children are more likely than normal children to have the disorder.
   b. ***Biochemical.*** A deficit of the neurotransmitters dopamine and norepinephrine has been suggested as a causative factor.
   c. ***Prenatal and Perinatal Factors.*** Some studies link maternal smoking and use of substances with ADHD in their offspring. Premature birth, fetal distress, precipitated or prolonged labor, and perinatal asphyxia have also been implicated.

2. **Psychosocial**
   a. ***Psychodynamic Theory.*** Mahler's (1975) theory suggests that the child with ADHD is fixed in the symbiotic phase of development and has not differentiated self from mother. Ego development is retarded, and impulsive behavior dictated by the id is manifested.
   b. ***Theory of Family Dynamics.*** Bowen (1978) proposes that when a dysfunctional spousal relationship exists, the focus of the disturbance is displaced onto the child, whose behavior in time begins to reflect the patterns of the dysfunctional system.

Symptomatology (Subjective and Objective Data)

The *DSM-IV* (ANA, 1994) identifies the following signs and symptoms of ADHD:

1. **Inattention**
   a. Often fails to give close attention to details or makes careless mistakes in schoolwork, work, or other activities.
   b. Often has difficulty sustaining attention in tasks or play activities.
   c. Often does not seem to listen when spoken to directly.
   d. Often does not follow through on instructions and fails to finish schoolwork, chores, or duties in the workplace (not because of oppositional behavior or failure to understand instructions).

    e. Often has difficulty organizing tasks and activities.

    f. Often avoids, dislikes, or is reluctant to engage in tasks that require sustained mental effort (such as schoolwork or homework).

    g. Often loses things necessary for tasks or activities (e.g., toys, school assignments, pencils, books, or tools).

    h. Is often easily distracted by extraneous stimuli.

    i. Is often forgetful in daily activities.

2. **Hyperactivity**

    a. Often fidgets with hands or feet or squirms in seat.

    b. Often leaves seat in classroom or in other situations in which remaining seated is expected.

    c. Often runs about or climbs excessively in situations in which it is inappropriate (in adolescents or adults, may be limited to subjective feelings of restlessness).

    d. Often has difficulty playing or engaging in leisure activities quietly.

    e. Is often "on the go" or often acts as if "driven by a motor."

    f. Often talks excessively.

3. **Impulsivity**

    a. Often blurts out answers before questions have been completed.

    b. Often has difficulty awaiting turn.

    c. Often interrupts or intrudes on others (e.g., butts into conversations or games).

CONDUCT DISORDER

Defined

The *DSM-IV* describes the essential feature of this disorder as a repetitive and persistent pattern of conduct in which the basic rights of others or major age-appropriate societal norms or rules are violated. The conduct is more serious than the ordinary mischief and pranks of children and adolescents. The disorder is more common in boys than in girls, and the behaviors may continue into adulthood, often meeting the criteria for antisocial personality disorder. Conduct disorder is divided into two subtypes based on the age at onset:

1. **Childhood-Onset Type.** The onset of at least one characteristic of conduct disorder prior to age 10.

2. **Adolescent-Onset Type.** The absence of behaviors associated with conduct disorder prior to age 10.

Predisposing Factors

1. **Physiologic**
   a. ***Birth Temperament.*** Studies (Chess et al, 1970) have been conducted related to differences in temperament of infants at birth. Differences have been observed in relation to attention span, excitability, and adaptability. Additional correlation between these findings and the future development of behavioral disorders remains uncertain.
2. **Psychosocial**
   a. ***Psychodynamic Theory.*** Mahler's (1975) theory suggests that this child is fixed in the separation-individuation phase of development. The child has failed to separate from mother and remains in the dependent position. Fears of abandonment nurture this dependency. The ego remains in an underdeveloped condition.
   b. ***Theory of Family Dynamics.*** The following factors related to family dynamics have been implicated as contributors in the predisposition to this disorder (Clunn, 1991; Popper and Steingard, 1994):

      • Parental rejection
      • Inconsistent management with harsh discipline
      • Early institutional living
      • Frequent shifting of parental figures
      • Large family size
      • Absent father
      • Parents with antisocial personality disorder and/or alcohol dependence
      • Association with a delinquent subgroup

Symptomatology (Subjective and Objective Data)

The *DSM-IV* has identified the following signs and symptoms of conduct disorder:

1. Often bullies, threatens, or intimidates others.
2. Often initiates physical fights.
3. Has used a weapon that can cause serious physical harm to others (e.g., a bat, brick, broken bottle, knife, gun).

4. Has been physically cruel to people.
5. Has been physically cruel to animals.
6. Has stolen while confronting a victim (e.g., mugging, purse snatching, extortion, armed robbery).
7. Has forced someone into sexual activity.
8. Has deliberately engaged in fire setting with the intention of causing serious damage.
9. Has deliberately destroyed others' property (other than by fire setting).
10. Has broken into someone else's house, building, or car.
11. Often lies to obtain goods or favors or to avoid obligations (i.e., "cons" others).
12. Has stolen items of nontrivial value without confronting a victim (e.g., shoplifting, but without breaking and entering; forgery).
13. Often stays out at night despite parental prohibitions, beginning before age 13 years.
14. Has run away from home overnight at least twice while living in parental or parental surrogate home (or once without returning for a lengthy period).
15. Is often truant from school, beginning before age 13 years.

OPPOSITIONAL DEFIANT DISORDER

Defined

The *DSM-IV* defines this disorder as a pattern of negativistic, defiant, disobedient, and hostile behavior toward authority figures that occurs more frequently than is typically observed in individuals of comparable age and developmental level. The disorder typically begins by 8 years of age, and usually not later than early adolescence. The disorder is more prevalent in boys than in girls and is often a developmental antecedent to conduct disorder.

Predisposing Factors

1. **Physiologic**
   a. Refer to this section under Conduct Disorder.
2. **Psychosocial**
   a. *Theory of Family Dynamics.* It is thought that some parents interpret average or increased levels of developmental oppositionalism as hostility and a deliberate effort on the part of the child to be in control. If power and control are issues for parents, or if they

exercise authority for their own needs, a power struggle can be established between the parents and the child that sets the stage for the development of oppositional defiant disorder (Kaplan and Sadock, 1989).

Symptomatology (Subjective and Objective Data)

The *DSM-IV* has identified the following signs and symptoms of oppositional defiant disorder:

1. Often loses temper
2. Often argues with adults
3. Often actively defies or refuses to comply with adult requests or rules
4. Often deliberately annoys people
5. Often blames others for his or her mistakes or misbehavior
6. Is often touchy or easily annoyed by others
7. Is often angry and resentful
8. Is often spiteful or vindictive

Common Nursing Diagnoses and Interventions for Disruptive Behavior Disorders

(Interventions are applicable to various health-care settings, such as inpatient and partial hospitalization, community outpatient clinic, home health, and private practice.)

RISK FOR VIOLENCE: SELF-DIRECTED OR DIRECTED AT OTHERS

Definition: Behaviors in which an individual demonstrates that he/she can be physically, emotionally, and/or sexually harmful either to self or to others.

Related/Risk Factors ("related to")

[Retarded ego development]
[Unsatisfactory parent-child relationship]
[Neurologic alteration related to premature birth, fetal distress, precipitated or prolonged labor]
[Dysfunctional family system]
[Disorganized or chaotic environments]
[Child abuse or neglect]
[Birth temperament]

[Fears of abandonment]
Body language—rigid posture, clenching of fists and jaw, hyperactivity, pacing, breathlessness, and threatening stances.
[History or threats of violence toward self or others or of destruction to the property of others]
Impulsivity
History of cruelty to animals
Suicidal ideation, plan, available means

Goals/Objectives
Short-Term Goal
Client will seek out staff at any time if thoughts of harming self or others should occur.

Long-Term Goal
Client will not harm self or others.

Interventions with *Selected Rationales*
1. Observe client's behavior frequently. Do this through routine activities and interactions to avoid appearing watchful and suspicious. *Clients at high risk for violence require close observation to prevent harm to self or others.*
2. Observe for suicidal behaviors: Verbal statements, such as "I'm going to kill myself," or "Very soon my mother won't have to worry herself about me any longer," or nonverbal behaviors, such as giving away cherished items, and mood swings. *Most clients who attempt suicide have communicated their intent, either verbally or nonverbally.*
3. Determine suicidal intent and available means. Ask, "Do you plan to kill yourself?" and "How do you plan to do it?" *Direct, closed-ended questions are appropriate in this instance. The client who has a usable plan is at higher risk than one who does not.*
4. Obtain verbal or written contract from client agreeing not to harm self and agreeing to seek out staff in the event that such ideation occurs. *Discussion of suicidal feelings with a trusted individual provides a degree of relief to the client. A contract gets the subject out in the open and places some of the responsibility for his or her safety with the client. An attitude of acceptance of the client as a worthwhile individual is conveyed.*
5. Assist client to recognize when anger occurs and to accept those feelings as his or her own. Have client keep an "anger notebook," in which a record of anger expe-

rienced on a 24-hour basis is kept. Information regarding source of anger, behavioral response, and client's perception of the situation should also be noted. Discuss entries with client, suggesting alternative behavioral responses for those which are identified as maladaptive.

6. Act as a role model for appropriate expression of angry feelings, and give positive reinforcement to client for attempting to conform. *It is vital that the client express angry feelings, because suicide and other self-destructive behaviors are often viewed as a result of anger turned inward on the self.*

7. Remove all dangerous objects from client's environment. *The client's physical safety is a nursing priority.*

8. Try to redirect violent behavior with physical outlets for the client's anxiety (e.g., punching bag, jogging, volleyball). *Anxiety and tension can be relieved safely and with benefit to the client in this manner.*

9. Be available to stay with client as anxiety level and tensions begin to rise. *The presence of a trusted individual provides a feeling of security.*

10. Staff should maintain and convey a calm attitude to client. *Anxiety is contagious and can be communicated from staff to client and vice versa. A calm attitude conveys a sense of control and a feeling of security to the client.*

11. Have sufficient staff available to indicate a show of strength to client if it becomes necessary. *This conveys to the client an evidence of control over the situation and provides some physical security for staff.*

12. Administer tranquilizing medications as ordered by physician, or obtain an order if necessary. Monitor medication for effectiveness and for adverse side effects. *Antianxiety medications (e.g., diazepam, chlordiazepoxide, alprazolam) provide relief from the immobilizing effects of anxiety, and facilitate client's cooperation with therapy.*

13. Mechanical restraints or isolation room may be required if less restrictive interventions are unsuccessful. *It is the client's right to expect the use of techniques that ensure safety of the client and others by the least restrictive means.*

Outcome Criteria

1. Anxiety is maintained at a level at which client feels no need for aggression.

2. Client seeks out staff to discuss true feelings.
3. Client recognizes, verbalizes, and accepts possible consequences of own maladaptive behaviors.
4. Client does not harm self or others.

DEFENSIVE COPING

Definition: *The state in which an individual repeatedly projects falsely positive self-evaluation based on a self-protective pattern which defends against underlying perceived threats to positive self-regard.*

Possible Etiologies ("related to")
[Low self-esteem]
[Retarded ego development]
[Negative role models]
[Lack of positive feedback]
[Repeated negative feedback, resulting in feelings of diminished self-worth]
[Unsatisfactory parent-child relationship]
[Disorganized or chaotic environments]
[Child abuse or neglect]
[Dysfunctional family system]
[Neurologic alteration related to premature birth, fetal distress, precipitated or prolonged labor]

Defining Characteristics ("evidenced by")
Denial of obvious problems or weaknesses
Projection of blame or responsibility
Rationalizes failures
Hypersensitive to criticism
Grandiosity
Superior attitude toward others
Difficulty establishing or maintaining relationships
Hostile laughter or ridicule of others
Difficulty in reality testing of perceptions
Lack of follow-through or participation in treatment or therapy

Goals/Objectives
Short-Term Goal
Client will verbalize personal responsibility for difficulties experienced in interpersonal relationships.

Long-Term Goal
Client will demonstrate ability to interact with others without becoming defensive, rationalizing behaviors, or expressing grandiose ideas.

Interventions with *Selected Rationales*
1. Recognize and support basic ego strengths. *Focusing on positive aspects of the personality may help to improve self-concept.*
2. Encourage client to recognize and verbalize feelings of inadequacy and need for acceptance from others, and how these feelings provoke defensive behaviors, such as blaming others for own behaviors. *Recognition of the problem is the first step in the change process toward resolution.*
3. Provide immediate, matter-of-fact, nonthreatening feedback for unacceptable behaviors. *Client may lack knowledge about how he or she is being perceived by others. Providing this information in a nonthreatening manner may help to eliminate these undesirable behaviors.*
4. Help client identify situations that provoke defensiveness and practice through role play more appropriate responses. *Role playing provides confidence to deal with difficult situations when they actually occur.*
5. Provide immediate positive feedback for acceptable behaviors. *Positive feedback enhances self-esteem and encourages repetition of desirable behaviors.*
6. Help client set realistic, concrete goals and determine appropriate actions to meet those goals. *Success increases self-esteem.*
7. With client, evaluate the effectiveness of the new behaviors and discuss any modifications for improvement. *Because of limited problem-solving ability, assistance may be required to reassess and develop new strategies, in the event that certain of the new coping methods prove ineffective.*

Outcome Criteria
1. Client verbalizes and accepts responsibility for own behavior.
2. Client verbalizes correlation between feelings of inadequacy and the need to defend the ego through rationalization and grandiosity.
3. Client does not ridicule or criticize others.
4. Client interacts with others in group situations without taking a defensive stance.

IMPAIRED SOCIAL INTERACTION

Definition: *The state in which an individual participates in an insufficient or excessive quantity or ineffective quality of social exchange.*

Possible Etiologies ("related to")
Self-concept disturbance
[Retarded ego development]
[Neurologic alterations related to premature birth, fetal distress, precipitated or prolonged labor]
[Dysfunctional family system]
[Disorganized or chaotic environments]
[Child abuse or neglect]
[Unsatisfactory parent-child relationship]
[Negative role models]

Defining Characteristics ("evidenced by")
Verbalized or observed discomfort in social situations
Verbalized or observed inability to receive or communicate a satisfying sense of belonging, caring, interest, or shared history
Observed use of unsuccessful social interaction behaviors
Dysfunctional interaction with peers, family, or others
[Behavior unaccepted for appropriate age by dominant cultural group]

Goals/Objectives
Short-Term Goal
Client will interact in age-appropriate manner with nurse in one-to-one relationship within 1 week.

Long-Term Goal
Client will be able to interact with staff and peers, by the time of discharge from treatment, with no indication of discomfort.

Interventions with *Selected Rationales*
1. Develop trusting relationship with client. Be honest; keep all promises; convey acceptance of person, separate from unacceptable behaviors ("It is not YOU, but YOUR BEHAVIOR, that is unacceptable.") *Acceptance of the client increases his or her feelings of self-worth.*
2. Offer to remain with client during initial interactions with others on the unit. *Presence of a trusted individual provides a feeling of security.*

3. Provide constructive criticism and positive reinforcement for efforts. *Positive feedback enhances self-esteem and encourages repetition of desirable behaviors.*
4. Confront client, and withdraw attention, when interactions with others are manipulative or exploitative. *Attention to the unacceptable behavior may reinforce it.*
5. Act as role model for client through appropriate interactions with other clients and staff members.
6. Provide group situations for client. *It is through these group interactions that client will learn socially acceptable behavior, with positive and negative feedback from his or her peers.*

Outcome Criteria
1. Client seeks out staff member for social, as well as therapeutic interaction.
2. Client has formed, and satisfactorily maintained, one interpersonal relationship with another client.
3. Client willingly and appropriately participates in group activities.
4. Client verbalizes reasons for inability to form close interpersonal relationships with others in the past.

INEFFECTIVE INDIVIDUAL COPING

Definition: *The impairment of adaptive behaviors and abilities of a person in meeting life's demands and roles.*

Possible Etiologies ("related to")
Situational crises
Maturational crises
Inadequate support systems
Inadequate coping method
[Negative role models]
[Neurologic alteration related to premature birth, fetal distress, precipitated or prolonged labor]
[Retarded ego development]
[Low self-esteem]
[Dysfunctional family system]
[Disorganized or chaotic environments]
[Child abuse or neglect]

Defining Characteristics ("evidenced by")
Inability to meet [age-appropriate] role expectations
Inability to problem-solve

[Manipulation of others in the environment for purposes of fulfilling own desires]

[Verbal hostility toward staff and peers]

[Hyperactivity, evidenced by excessive motor activity, easily distracted, short attention span]

[Unable to delay gratification]

[Oppositional and defiant responses to adult requests or rules]

Goals/Objectives
Short-Term Goal
Within 7 days, client will demonstrate ability and willingness to follow unit rules.

Long-Term Goal
By discharge from treatment, client will develop, and utilize, age-appropriate, socially acceptable coping skills.

Interventions with *Selected Rationales*
1. If client is hyperactive, make environment safe for continuous large muscle movement. Rearrange furniture and other objects to prevent injury. *Client physical safety is a nursing priority.*
2. Provide large motor activities in which client may participate. Nurse may join in some of these activities *to facilitate relationship development. Tension is released safely and with benefit to the client through physical activities.*
3. Provide frequent, nutritious snacks that client may "eat on the run," *in order to ensure adequate calories to offset client's excessive use of energy.*
4. Set limits on manipulative behavior. ("I understand why you are saying these things [or doing these things] and I will not tolerate these behaviors from you.")
5. Identify for the client the consequences of manipulative behavior. All staff must follow through and be consistent. *Client may try to play one staff member against another, so consistency is vital if intervention is to be successful. Negative consequences may work to decrease unacceptable behaviors.*
6. Do not debate, argue, rationalize, or bargain with the client. *Ignoring these attempts may work to decrease manipulative behaviors.*
7. Caution should be taken to avoid reinforcing manipulative behaviors by providing desired attention.
8. Confront client's use of manipulative behaviors and explore their damaging effects on interpersonal relation-

ships. *Manipulative clients often deny responsibility for their behaviors.*

9. Encourage discussion of angry feelings. Help client identify the true object of the hostility. *Dealing with the feelings honestly and directly will discourage displacement of the anger onto others.*

10. Explore with client alternative ways for handling frustration that would be most suited to his or her lifestyle. Provide support and positive feedback to client as new coping strategies are tried. *Positive feedback encourages use of the acceptable behaviors.*

Outcome Criteria

1. Client is able to delay gratification, without resorting to manipulation of others.
2. Client is able to express anger in socially acceptable manner.
3. Client is able to verbalize alternative, socially acceptable, and lifestyle-appropriate coping skills he or she plans to use in response to frustration.

SELF-ESTEEM DISTURBANCE

Definition: *Negative self-evaluation and feelings about self or self-capabilities, which may be directly or indirectly expressed.*

Possible Etiologies ("related to")

[Retarded ego development]
[Negative role models]
[Lack of positive feedback]
[Repeated negative feedback, resulting in diminished self-worth]
[Unsatisfactory parent-child relationship]
[Disorganized or chaotic environments]
[Child abuse or neglect]
[Dysfunctional family system]

Defining Characteristics ("evidenced by")

[Lack of eye contact]
Self-negating verbalizations
Expressions of shame or guilt
Evaluates self as unable to deal with events
Rationalizes away or rejects positive feedback and exaggerates negative feedback about self

Hesitant to try new things or situations
Denial of problems obvious to others
Projection of blame or responsibility for problems
Rationalization of personal failures
Hypersensitivity to criticism
Grandiosity

Goals/Objectives
Short-Term Goal
Client will independently direct own care and activities of
   daily living within 1 week.

Long-Term Goal
By discharge from treatment, client will exhibit increased
   feelings of self-worth as evidenced by verbal expression
   of positive aspects about self, past accomplishments, and
   future prospects.

Interventions with *Selected Rationales*
1. Ensure that goals are realistic. It is important for client to
   achieve something, so plan for activities in which the possibility for success is likely. *Success enhances self-esteem.*
2. Convey unconditional positive regard for client. *Communication of your acceptance of him or her as a worthwhile human being increases self-esteem.*
3. Spend time with client, both on a one-to-one basis and in
   group activities. *This conveys to client that you feel he
   or she is worth your time.*
4. Assist client in identifying positive aspects of self and in
   developing plans for changing the characteristics he or
   she views as negative.
5. Help client decrease use of denial as a defense mechanism. Give positive reinforcement for problem identification and development of more adaptive coping behaviors.
   *Positive reinforcement enhances self-esteem and in-
   creases client's use of acceptable behaviors.*
6. Encourage and support client in confronting the fear of
   failure by attending therapy activities and undertaking new
   tasks. Offer recognition of successful endeavors and positive reinforcement for attempts made. *Recognition and
   positive reinforcement enhance self-esteem.*

Outcome Criteria
1. Client verbalizes positive perception of self.
2. Client participates in new activities without exhibiting extreme fear of failure.

ANXIETY (MODERATE TO SEVERE)

Definition: *A vague uneasy feeling, the source of which is often nonspecific or unknown to the individual.*

Possible Etiologies ("related to")
Situational and maturational crises
Threat to self-concept [perceived or real]
[Threat (or perceived threat) to physical integrity]
Unmet needs
[Fear of failure]
[Dysfunctional family system]
[Unsatisfactory parent-child relationship]
[Innately, easily agitated temperament since birth]

Defining Characteristics ("evidenced by")
Overexcited
Fearful
Feelings of inadequacy
Fear of unspecific consequences
Restlessness
Insomnia
Poor eye contact
Focus on self
[Continuous attention-seeking behaviors]
[Difficulty concentrating; selective inattention]
[Increased respiratory and heart rates]

Goals/Objectives
Short-Term Goals
Client will be able to verbalize behaviors that become evident as anxiety starts to rise within 7 days.
Client will be able to verbalize strategies to interrupt escalation of anxiety within 7 days.

Long-Term Goal
Client will be able to maintain anxiety below the moderate level, as evidenced by absence of disabling behaviors in response to stress, by discharge from treatment.

Interventions with *Selected Rationales*
1. Establish a trusting relationship with client. Be honest, consistent in responses, and available. Show genuine positive regard. *Honesty, availability and acceptance promote trust in the nurse-client relationship.*
2. Provide activities geared toward reduction of tension and decreasing anxiety (walking or jogging, volleyball, musical exercises, housekeeping chores, group games). *Tension*

and anxiety are released safely and with benefit to the client through physical activities.

3. Encourage client to identify true feelings, and to acknowledge ownership of those feelings. *Anxious clients often deny a relationship between emotional problems and their anxiety. Use of the defense mechanisms of projection and displacement is exaggerated.*

4. The nurse must maintain an atmosphere of calmness; *anxiety is easily transmitted from one person to another.*

5. Offer support during times of elevated anxiety. Reassure client of physical and psychological safety. *Client safety is a nursing priority.*

6. Use of touch is comforting to some clients. However, the nurse must be cautious with its use, *because anxiety may foster suspicion in some individuals who might misinterpret touch as aggression.*

7. As anxiety diminishes, assist client to recognize specific events that preceded its onset. Work on alternative responses to future occurrences. *A plan of action provides the client with a feeling of security for more successfully handling the difficult situation should it recur.*

8. Assist client to recognize signs of escalating anxiety, and explore ways client may intervene before behaviors become disabling.

9. Administer tranquilizing medication, as ordered. Assess for effectiveness, and instruct client regarding possible adverse side effects. *Antianxiety medications (e.g., diazepam, chlordiazepoxide, alprazolam) provide relief from the immobilizing effects of anxiety, and facilitate client's cooperation with therapy.*

Outcome Criteria
1. Client is able to verbalize behaviors that become evident as anxiety starts to rise and actions appropriate to interrupt progression of the condition.
2. Client is able to maintain anxiety at a manageable level.

NONCOMPLIANCE

Definition: *A person's informed decision not to adhere to a therapeutic recommendation.*

Possible Etiologies ("related to")
[Biochemical alteration]

[Neurologic alteration related to premature birth, fetal dis-
   tress, precipitated or prolonged labor]
[Negative temperament]
[Dysfunctional family system]
[Negative role models]
[Retarded ego development]
[Low frustration tolerance and short attention span]
[Denial of problems]

Defining Characteristics ("evidenced by")
Behavior indicative of failure to adhere (to treatment regimen)
[Inability to sit still long enough to complete a task]
[Expression of opposition to requests for participation]
Refusal to follow directions or suggestions of treatment team

Goals/Objectives
Short-Term Goal
Client will participate in and cooperate during therapeutic ac-
   tivities.

Long-Term Goal
Client will complete assigned tasks willingly and independently or with a minimum of assistance.

Interventions with *Selected Rationales*
(For the client with inattention and hyperactivity:)
1. Provide an environment for task efforts that is as free of
   distractions as possible. *Client is highly distractible and
   is unable to perform in the presence of even minimal
   stimulation.*
2. Provide assistance on a one-to-one basis, beginning with
   simple, concrete instructions. *Client lacks the ability to
   assimilate information that is complicated or has abstract meaning.*
3. Ask client to repeat instructions to you *to determine level
   of comprehension.*
4. Establish goals that allow client to complete a part of the
   task, rewarding each step completion with a break for
   physical activity. *Short-term goals are not so overwhelming to one with such a short attention span. The
   positive reinforcement (physical activity) increases
   self-esteem and provides incentive for client to pursue
   the task to completion.*
5. Gradually decrease the amount of assistance given to task
   performance, while assuring the client that assistance is

still available if deemed necessary. *This encourages the client to perform independently while providing a feeling of security with the presence of a trusted individual.*

(For the client with oppositional tendencies:)

6. Set forth a structured plan of therapeutic activities. Start with minimum expectations and increase as client begins to manifest evidence of compliance. *Structure provides security, and one or two activities may not seem as overwhelming as the whole schedule of activities presented at one time.*

7. Establish a system of rewards for compliance with therapy and consequences for noncompliance. Ensure that the rewards and consequences are concepts of value to the client. *Positive and negative reinforcements can contribute to desired changes in behavior.*

8. Convey acceptance of the client separate from the undesirable behaviors being exhibited. ("It is not *you*, but your *behavior*, that is unacceptable.") *Unconditional acceptance enhances self-worth and may contribute to a decrease in the need for passive-aggression toward others.*

Outcome Criteria

1. Client cooperates with staff in an effort to complete assigned tasks.
2. Client complies with treatment by participating in therapies without negativism.
3. Client takes direction from staff without becoming defensive.

TOURETTE'S DISORDER

DEFINED

Tourette's disorder is characterized by the presence of multiple motor tics and one or more vocal tics that may appear simultaneously or at different periods during the illness (APA, 1994). Onset can be as early as age 2, but it occurs most commonly during childhood or early adolescence, with the median age being 7 years. The disorder is more common in boys than in girls. The duration of the disorder is usually lifelong, but the symptoms usually diminish during adolescence and adulthood.

PREDISPOSING FACTORS

1. **Physiologic**
   a. ***Genetics.*** Family studies have shown that Tourette's disorder is more common in relatives of individuals with the disorder than in the general population. Autosomal dominant transmission may be involved (Pauls and Leckman, 1986).
   b. ***Brain Alterations.*** Altered levels of neurotransmitters and dysfunction in the area of the basal ganglia have been implicated in the etiology of Tourette's disorder.
2. **Psychosocial**
   a. It is believed that the genetic predisposition to Tourette's disorder may be reinforced by certain factors in the environment, such as increased prenatal complications, low birth weight, and emotional stress during pregnancy.

SYMPTOMATOLOGY (Subjective and Objective Data)

The *DSM-IV* identifies the following signs and symptoms of Tourette's disorder:

1. The disorder may begin with a single motor tic, such as eye blinking, neck jerking, shoulder shrugging, facial grimacing, or coughing.
2. Complex motor tics may follow, and include touching, squatting, hopping, skipping, deep knee bends, retracing steps, and twirling when walking.
3. Vocal tics include various words or sounds such as clicks, grunts, yelps, barks, sniffs, snorts, coughs, and in about 10% of cases, a complex vocal tic involving the uttering of obscenities.
4. Vocal tics may include repeating certain words or phrases out of context, repeating one's own sounds or words (palilalia), or repeating what others say (echolalia).
5. The movements and vocalizations are experienced as compulsive and irresistible, but they can be suppressed for varying lengths of time.
6. Tics are exacerbated by stress and attenuated during periods in which the individual becomes totally absorbed by an activity.
7. Tics are markedly diminished during sleep.

COMMON NURSING DIAGNOSES AND INTERVENTIONS

(Interventions are applicable to various health-care settings, such as inpatient and partial hospitalization, community outpatient clinic, home health, and private practice.)

RISK FOR VIOLENCE: SELF-DIRECTED OR DIRECTED AT OTHERS

Definition: *Behaviors in which an individual demonstrates that he/she can be physically, emotionally, and/or sexually harmful either to self or to others.*

Related/Risk Factors ("related to")
[Low tolerance for frustration]
[Abnormalities in brain neurotransmitters]
Body language—rigid posture, clenching of fists and jaw, hyperactivity, pacing, breathlessness, and threatening stances
[History or threats of violence toward self or others or of destruction to the property of others]
Impulsivity
Suicidal ideation, plan, available means

Goals/Objectives
Short-Term Goal
Client will seek out staff/support person at any time if thoughts of harming self or others should occur.

Long-Term Goal
Client will not harm self or others.

Interventions with *Selected Rationales*
1. Observe client's behavior frequently through routine activities and interactions. Become aware of behaviors that indicate a rise in agitation. *Stress commonly increases tic behaviors. Recognition of behaviors that precede the onset of aggression may provide the opportunity to intervene before violence occurs.*
2. Monitor for self-destructive behavior and impulses. A staff member may need to stay with the client to prevent self-mutilation. *Client safety is a nursing priority.*
3. Provide hand coverings and other restraints that prevent the client from self-mutilative behaviors. *Provide imme-*

diate external controls against self-aggressive behaviors.

4. Redirect violent behavior with physical outlets for frustration. *Excess energy is released through physical activities and a feeling of relaxation is induced.*

5. Administer medication as ordered by the physician. Several medications have been used to treat Tourette's disorder. The most common ones include the following:

   a. **Haloperidol (Haldol).** Haloperidol has been the drug of choice for Tourette's disorder. Children on this medication must be monitored for adverse effects associated with most antipsychotic medications (see Chapter 20). Because of the potential for adverse effects, haloperidol should be reserved for children with severe symptoms or with symptoms that interfere with their ability to function.

   b. **Pimozide (Orap).** The response rate and side effect profile of pimozide are similar to haloperidol. It is used in the management of severe motor or vocal tics that have failed to respond to more conventional treatment. It is not recommended for children under age 12.

   c. **Clonidine (Catapres).** Clonidine is an antihypertensive medication, the efficacy of which in the treatment of Tourette's disorder has been mixed. Some physicians like it and use it as a drug of first choice because of its relative safety and few side effects.

Outcome Criteria

1. Anxiety is maintained at a level at which client feels no need for aggression.
2. Client seeks out staff or support person for expression of true feelings.
3. Client has not harmed self or others.

IMPAIRED SOCIAL INTERACTION

Definition: *The state in which an individual participates in an insufficient or excessive quantity or ineffective quality of social exchange.*

Possible Etiologies ("related to")
Self-concept disturbance
Low tolerance for frustration

Impulsiveness
Oppositional behavior
Aggressive behavior

Defining Characteristics ("evidenced by")
Verbalized or observed discomfort in social situations
Verbalized or observed inability to receive or communicate a
    satisfying sense of belonging, caring, interest, or shared
    history
Observed use of unsuccessful social interaction behaviors
Dysfunctional interaction with peers, family, or others

Goals/Objectives
Short-Term Goal
Client will develop a one-to-one relationship with a nurse or
    support person within 1 week.

Long-Term Goal
Client will be able to interact with staff and peers using age-
    appropriate, acceptable behaviors.

Interventions with *Selected Rationales*
1. Develop a trusting relationship with the client. Convey acceptance of the person separate from the unacceptable
   behavior. *Unconditional acceptance increases feelings
   of self-worth.*
2. Discuss with client which behaviors are and are not acceptable. Describe in matter-of-fact manner the consequences of unacceptable behavior. Follow through. *Negative reinforcement can alter undesirable behaviors.*
3. Provide group situations for client. *Appropriate social behavior is often learned from the positive and negative
   feedback of peers.*
4. Act as a role model for client through appropriate interactions with others. *Role modeling of a respected individual is one of the strongest forms of learning.*

Outcome Criteria
1. Client seeks out staff or support person for social, as well
   as for therapeutic interaction.
2. Client verbalizes reasons for inability to form close interpersonal relationships with others in the past.
3. Client interacts with others using age-appropriate, acceptable behaviors.

SELF-ESTEEM DISTURBANCE

Definition: *Negative self-evaluation and feelings about self or self-capabilities, which may be directly or indirectly expressed*

Possible Etiologies ("related to")
[Shame associated with tic behaviors]

Defining Characteristics ("evidenced by")
[Lack of eye contact]
Self-negating verbalizations
Expressions of shame or guilt
Hesitant to try new things or situations
[Manipulation of others]

Goals/Objectives
Short-Term Goal
Client will verbalize positive aspects about self not associated
   with tic behaviors.

Long-Term Goal
Client will exhibit increased feeling of self-worth as evidenced by verbal expression of positive aspects about self, past accomplishments, and future prospects.

Interventions with *Selected Rationales*
1. Convey unconditional acceptance and positive regard. *Communication of client as worthwhile human being may increase self-esteem.*
2. Set limits on manipulative behavior. Take caution not to reinforce manipulative behaviors by providing desired attention. Identify the consequences of manipulation. Administer consequences matter-of-factly when manipulation occurs. *Negative consequences may work to decrease unacceptable behaviors.*
3. Help client understand that he or she uses this behavior in order to try to increase own self-esteem. Interventions should reflect other actions to accomplish this goal. *When client feels better about self, the need to manipulate others will diminish.*
4. If client chooses to suppress tics in the presence of others, provide a specified "tic time," during which he or she

"vents" tics, feelings, and behaviors (alone or with staff). *Allows for release of tics and assists in sense of control and management of symptoms (Rosner and Pollice, 1991).*

5. Ensure that client has regular one-to-one time with staff or support person. *Provides opportunity for educating about illness and teaching management tactics. Assists in exploring feelings around illness and incorporating illness into a healthy sense of self (Rosner and Pollice, 1991).*

Outcome Criteria
1. Client verbalizes positive perception of self.
2. Client willingly participates in new activities and situations.

SEPARATION ANXIETY DISORDER

DEFINED

The APA (1994) defines separation anxiety disorder as excessive anxiety concerning separation from the home or from those to whom the person is attached. Onset may occur as early as preschool age, rarely as late as adolescence, but always before age 18, and is more common in girls than in boys.

PREDISPOSING FACTORS

1. **Physiologic**
   a. *Genetics.* The results of studies indicate that a greater number of children with relatives who manifest anxiety problems develop anxiety disorders themselves than do children with no such family patterns.
   b. *Temperament.* Studies have shown that differences in temperamental characteristics at birth may be correlated to the acquisition of fear and anxiety disorders in childhood. This may denote an inherited vulnerability or predisposition toward developing these disorders.
2. **Psychosocial**
   a. *Stressful Life Events.* Studies indicate that children who are predisposed to anxiety disorders may be affected significantly by stressful life events.

b. *Family Influences.* Several theories exist that relate the development of separation anxiety to the following dynamics within the family:

- An overattachment to the mother (primary caregiver)
- Separation conflicts between parent and child
- Enmeshment of members within a family
- Overprotection of the child by the parents
- Transfer of parents' fears and anxieties to the children through role modeling

SYMPTOMATOLOGY (Subjective and Objective Data)

The *DSM-IV* identifies the following signs and symptoms of separation anxiety disorder:

1. Recurrent, excessive distress when separation from home or major attachment figures occurs or is anticipated
2. Persistent and excessive worry about losing, or about possible harm befalling, major attachment figures
3. Persistent and excessive worry that an untoward event will lead to separation from a major attachment figure
4. Persistent reluctance or refusal to go to school or elsewhere because of fear of separation
5. Persistent and excessive fear or reluctance to be alone or without major attachment figures at home or without significant adults in other settings
6. Persistent reluctance or refusal to go to sleep without being near a major attachment figure or to sleep away from home
7. Repeated nightmares involving the theme of separation
8. Repeated complaints of physical symptoms, such as headaches, stomachaches, nausea, or vomiting, when separation from major attachment figures occurs or is anticipated

COMMON NURSING DIAGNOSES AND INTERVENTIONS

(Interventions are applicable to various health-care settings, such as inpatient and partial hospitalization, community outpatient clinic, home health, and private practice.)

ANXIETY (SEVERE)

Definition: *A vague uneasy feeling, the source of which is often nonspecific or unknown to the individual*

Possible Etiologies ("related to")
Family history
Birth temperament
Overattachment to parent
Negative role modeling

Defining Characteristics ("evidenced by")
[Excessive distress when separated from attachment figure]
[Fear of anticipation of separation from attachment figure]
[Fear of being alone or without attachment figure]
[Reluctance or refusal to go to school or anywhere else without attachment figure]
[Nightmares about being separated from attachment figure]
[Somatic symptoms occurring as a result of fear of separation]

Goals/Objectives
Short-Term Goal
Client will discuss fears of separation with trusted individual.

Long-Term Goal
Client will maintain anxiety at no higher than moderate level in the face of events that formerly have precipitated panic.

Interventions with *Selected Rationales*
1. Establish an atmosphere of calmness, trust, and genuine positive regard. *Trust and unconditional acceptance are necessary for satisfactory nurse-client relationship. Calmness is important because anxiety is easily transmitted from one person to another.*
2. Assure client of his or her safety and security. *Symptoms of panic anxiety are very frightening.*
3. Explore the child's or adolescent's fears of separating from the parents. Explore with the parents possible fears they may have of separation from the child. *Some parents may have an underlying fear of separation from the child, of which they are unaware and which they are unconsciously transferring to the child.*
4. Help parents and child initiate realistic goals (e.g., child to stay with sitter for 2 hours with minimal anxiety; or, child

to stay at friend's house without parents until 9:00 PM without experiencing panic anxiety). *Parents may be so frustrated with the child's clinging and demanding behaviors, that assistance with problem-solving may be required.*

5. Give, and encourage parents to give, positive reinforcement for desired behaviors. *Positive reinforcement encourages repetition of desirable behaviors.*

Outcome Criteria
1. Client and parents are able to discuss their fears regarding separation.
2. Client experiences no somatic symptoms from fear of separation.
3. Client maintains anxiety at moderate level when separation occurs or is anticipated.

INEFFECTIVE INDIVIDUAL COPING

Definition: The impairment of adaptive behaviors and abilities of a person in meeting life's demands and roles

Possible Etiologies ("related to")
[Unresolved separation conflicts]
[Inadequate coping skills]

Defining Characteristics ("evidenced by")
[Somatic complaints in response to occurrence or anticipation of separation from attachment figure]

Goals/Objectives
Short-Term Goal
Client will verbalize correlation of somatic symptoms to fear of separation.

Long-Term Goal
Client will demonstrate use of more adaptive coping strategies (than physical symptoms) in response to stressful situations.

Interventions with *Selected Rationales*
1. Encourage child or adolescent to discuss specific situations in life that produce the most distress and describe his or her response to these situations. Include parents in the discussion. *Client and family may be unaware of the correlation between stressful situations and the exacerbation of physical symptoms.*

2. Help the child or adolescent who is perfectionistic to recognize that self-expectations may be unrealistic. Connect times of unmet self-expectations to the exacerbation of physical symptoms. *Recognition of maladaptive patterns is the first step in the change process.*
3. Encourage parents and child to identify more adaptive coping strategies that the child could use in the face of anxiety that feels overwhelming. Practice through role play. *Practice facilitates the use of the desired behavior when the individual is actually faced with the stressful situation.*

Outcome Criteria
1. Client and family verbalize the correlation between separation anxiety and somatic symptoms.
2. Client verbalizes the correlation between unmet self-expectations and somatic symptoms.
3. Client responds to stressful situations without exhibiting physical symptoms.

IMPAIRED SOCIAL INTERACTION

Definition: The state in which an individual participates in an insufficient or excessive quantity or ineffective quality of social exchange

---

Possible Etiologies ("related to")
[Reluctance to be away from attachment figure]

Defining Characteristics ("evidenced by")
[Symptoms of severe anxiety]
Verbalized or observed discomfort in social situations
Verbalized or observed inability to receive or communicate a satisfying sense of belonging, caring, interest, or shared history
Observed use of unsuccessful social interaction behaviors
Dysfunctional interaction with others

Goals/Objectives
Short-Term Goal
Client will spend time with staff or other support person, without presence of attachment figure, without excessive anxiety.

Long-Term Goal
Client will be able to spend time with others (without presence of attachment figure) without excessive anxiety.

Interventions with *Selected Rationales*
1. Develop a trusting relationship with client. *This is the first step in helping the client learn to interact with others.*
2. Attend groups with the child and support efforts to interact with others. Give positive feedback. *Presence of a trusted individual provides security during times of distress. Positive feedback encourages repetition.*
3. Convey to the child the acceptability of his or her not participating in group in the beginning. Gradually encourage small contributions until client is able to participate more fully. *Small successes will gradually increase self-confidence and decrease self-consciousness, so that client will feel less anxious in the group situation.*
4. Help client set small personal goals (e.g., "Today I will speak to one person I don't know"). *Simple, realistic goals provide opportunities for success that increase self-confidence and may encourage the client to attempt more difficult objectives in the future.*

Outcome Criteria
1. Client spends time with others using acceptable, age-appropriate behaviors.
2. Client is able to interact with others away from the attachment figure without excessive anxiety.

Chapter 5

DELIRIUM, DEMENTIA, AND AMNESTIC DISORDERS

BACKGROUND ASSESSMENT DATA

DELIRIUM

Defined

The *DSM-IV* defines delirium as a disturbance of consciousness and a change in cognition that develop rapidly over a short period of time (APA, 1994). The symptoms of delirium usually begin quite abruptly, and the duration is usually brief (e.g., 1 week; rarely more than 1 month). The disorder subsides completely on recovery from the underlying determinant. If the underlying condition persists, the delirium may gradually shift to the syndrome of dementia or progress to coma. The individual then recovers, becomes chronically vegetative, or dies.

Predisposing Factors

The *DSM-IV* differentiates among the disorders of delirium by their etiology, although they share a common symptom presentation. Categories of delirium include the following:

1. **Delirium Due to a General Medical Condition.** Certain medical conditions, such as systemic infections, metabolic disorders, fluid and electrolyte imbalances, liver

or kidney disease, encephalopathy, and head trauma, can cause the symptoms of delirium.

2. **Substance-Induced Delirium.** The symptoms of delirium can be induced by the exposure to a toxin or the ingestion of a medication, such as anticonvulsants, neuroleptics, anxiolytics, antidepressants, cardiovascular medications, antineoplastics, and hormones.
3. **Substance-Intoxication Delirium.** Delirium symptoms can occur in response to taking high doses of cannabis, cocaine, hallucinogens, alcohol, anxiolytics, or narcotics.
4. **Substance-Withdrawal Delirium.** Reduction or termination of long-term, high-dose use of certain substances, such as alcohol, sedatives, hypnotics, or anxiolytics, can result in withdrawal delirium symptoms.
5. **Delirium Due to Multiple Etiologies.** Symptoms of delirium may be related to more than one general medical condition or to the combined effects of a general medical condition and substance use.

Symptomatology (Subjective and Objective Data)

The following symptoms have been identified with the syndrome of delirium:

1. Altered consciousness ranging from hypervigilance to stupor or semicoma.
2. Extreme distractibility with difficulty focusing attention.
3. Disorientation to time and place.
4. Impaired reasoning ability and goal-directed behavior.
5. Disturbance in the sleep-wake cycle.
6. Emotional instability as manifested by fear, anxiety, depression, irritability, anger, euphoria, or apathy.
7. Misperceptions of the environment, including illusions and hallucinations.
8. Autonomic manifestations, such as tachycardia, sweating, flushed face, dilated pupils, and elevated blood pressure.
9. Incoherent speech.
10. Impairment of recent memory.

DEMENTIA

Defined

Dementia is defined as a syndrome of acquired, persistent intellectual impairment with compromised function in multiple spheres of mental activity, such as memory, language, visuospatial skills, emotion or personality, and cognition (Wise and Gray, 1994). The disease usually has a slow, insidious onset and is chronic, progressive, and irreversible.

Predisposing Factors

The *DSM-IV* identifies the following etiologic categories for the syndrome of dementia:

1. **Dementia of the Alzheimer's Type.** The exact cause of Alzheimer's disease is unknown, but several theories have been proposed, such as reduction in brain acetylcholine, accumulation of aluminum in the brain, immune system alterations, head trauma, and genetic factors. Pathologic changes in the brain include atrophy, enlarged ventricles, and the presence of numerous neurofibrillary plaques and tangles. Definitive diagnosis is by biopsy or autopsy examination of brain tissue only.
2. **Vascular Dementia.** This type of dementia is caused by significant cerebrovascular disease. The client suffers the equivalent of small strokes caused by arterial hypertension or cerebral emboli or thrombi, which destroy many areas of the brain. The onset of symptoms is more abrupt than in Alzheimer's disease and runs a highly variable course, progressing in steps rather than as a gradual deterioration.
3. **Dementia Due to HIV Disease.** The immune dysfunction associated with human immunodeficiency virus (HIV) disease can lead to brain infections by other organisms. HIV also appears to cause dementia directly.
4. **Dementia Due to Head Trauma.** The syndrome of symptoms associated with dementia can be brought on by a traumatic brain injury.
5. **Dementia Due to Parkinson's Disease.** Parkinson's disease is caused by a loss of nerve cells in the substantia nigra of the basal ganglia. The symptoms of dementia associated with Parkinson's disease closely resemble those of Alzheimer's disease.
6. **Dementia Due to Huntington's Disease.** This disease is transmitted as a mendelian dominant gene, and damage occurs in the areas of the basal ganglia and the cerebral cortex. A profound dementia occurs within 5 to 10 years of onset.

7. **Dementia Due to Pick's Disease.** Pathology occurs from atrophy in the frontal and temporal lobes of the brain. Symptoms are strikingly similar to those of Alzheimer's disease, and Pick's disease is often misdiagnosed as Alzheimer's.

8. **Dementia Due to Creutzfeldt-Jakob Disease.** This form of dementia is caused by a transmissible virus. The clinical presentation is typical of the syndrome of dementia, and the course is extremely rapid, with progressive deterioration and death within 1 year.

9. **Dementia Due to Other General Medical Conditions.** These include endocrine, hepatic, renal, cardiopulmonary, or neurologic conditions, brain lesions, or system infections.

10. **Substance-Induced Persisting Dementia.** This type of dementia is related to the persisting effects of substances such as alcohol, inhalants, sedatives, hypnotics, anxiolytics, other medications, and environmental toxins. The term "persisting" is used to indicate that the dementia persists long after the effects of substance intoxication or substance withdrawal have subsided.

Symptomatology (Subjective and Objective Data)
The following symptoms have been identified with the syndrome of dementia:

1. Memory impairment (impaired ability to learn new information or to recall previously learned information).
2. Impairment in abstract thinking, judgment, and impulse control.
3. Impairment in language ability, such as difficulty naming objects. In some instances, the individual may not speak at all (aphasia).
4. Personality changes are common.
5. Impaired ability to execute motor activities despite intact motor abilities (apraxia).
6. Disorientation.
7. Wandering.
8. Delusions are common (particularly delusions of persecution).

AMNESTIC DISORDERS

Defined
Amnestic disorders are characterized by an inability to learn new information (short-term memory deficit) despite

normal attention, and an inability to recall previously learned information (long-term memory deficit). No other cognitive deficits exist.

Predisposing Factors

The *DSM-IV* identifies the following categories as etiologies for the syndrome of symptoms known as amnestic disorders:

1. **Amnestic Disorder Due to a General Medical Condition.** The symptoms may be associated with head trauma, cerebrovascular disease, cerebral neoplastic disease, cerebral anoxia, herpes simplex encephalitis, poorly controlled insulin-dependent diabetes, and surgical intervention to the brain (APA, 1994; Wise and Gray, 1994). Transient amnestic syndromes can also occur from epileptic seizures, electroconvulsive therapy, severe migraine, and drug overdose (Wise and Gray, 1994).
2. **Substance-Induced Persisting Amnestic Disorder.** This type of amnestic disorder is related to the persisting effects of substances such as alcohol, sedatives, hypnotics, anxiolytics, other medications, and environmental toxins. The term "persisting" is used to indicate that the symptoms persist long after the effects of substance intoxication or substance withdrawal have subsided.

Symptomatology (Subjective and Objective Data)

The following symptoms have been identified with amnestic disorder:

1. Disorientation to place and time may occur with profound amnesia.
2. There is an inability to recall events from the recent past and events from the remote past. (Events from the very remote past are often more easily recalled than recently occurring ones.)
3. The individual is prone to confabulation. That is, the individual may create imaginary events to fill in the memory gaps.
4. Apathy, lack of initiative, and emotional blandness are common.

COMMON NURSING DIAGNOSES AND INTERVENTIONS FOR DELIRIUM, DEMENTIA, AND AMNESTIC DISORDERS

(Interventions are applicable to various health-care settings, such as inpatient and partial hospitalization, community outpatient clinic, home health, and private practice.)

RISK FOR TRAUMA

Definition: *[The client has] accentuated risk of accidental tissue injury (e.g., wound, burn, fracture)*

Related/Risk Factors ("related to")

[Chronic alteration in structure or function of brain tissue, secondary to the aging process, multiple infarcts, HIV disease, head trauma, chronic substance abuse, or progressively dysfunctional physical condition resulting in the following symptoms:

Disorientation; confusion
Weakness
Muscular incoordination
Seizures
Memory impairment
Poor vision
Extreme psychomotor agitation observed in the late stages of delirium]

[Frequent shuffling of feet and stumbling]
[Falls, caused by muscular incoordination or seizures]
[Bumping into furniture]
[Exposing self to frigid conditions with insufficient protective clothing]
[Cutting self when using sharp instruments]
[History of attempting to light burner or oven and leaving gas on in house]
[Smoking and leaving burning cigarettes in various places; smoking in bed; falling asleep sitting on couch or chair with lighted cigarette in hand]
[Purposeless, thrashing movements; hyperactivity that is out of touch with the environment]

Goals/Objectives
Short-Term Goal
Client will call for assistance when ambulating or carrying out other activities.

Long-Term Goal
Client will not experience physical injury.

Interventions with *Selected Rationales*
1. Assess client's level of disorientation and confusion to determine specific requirements for safety. *Knowledge of client's level of functioning is necessary to formulate appropriate plan of care.*
2. Institute appropriate safety measures, such as the following:
   a. Place furniture in room in an arrangement that best accommodates client's disabilities.
   b. Observe client behaviors frequently; assign staff on one-to-one basis if condition warrants; accompany and assist client when ambulating; use wheelchair for transporting long distances.
   c. Store items that client uses frequently within easy access.
   d. Remove potentially harmful articles from client's room: cigarettes, matches, lighters, sharp objects.
   e. Remain with client while he or she smokes.
   f. Pad side rails and headboard of client with seizure disorder. Institute seizure precautions as described in procedure manual of individual institution.
   Client safety is a nursing priority.
3. Frequently orient client to reality and surroundings. *Disorientation may endanger client safety if he or she unknowingly wanders away from safe environment.*
4. Use tranquilizing medications and soft restraints, as prescribed by physician, for client's protection during periods of excessive hyperactivity. *Use restraints judiciously, because they can increase agitation. They may be required, however, to provide for client safety.*
5. Teach prospective caregivers methods that have been successful in preventing client injury. *These caregivers will be responsible for client's safety after discharge from the hospital. Sharing successful interventions may be helpful.*

Outcome Criteria
1. Client is able to accomplish daily activities within the environment without experiencing injury.
2. Prospective caregivers are able to verbalize means of providing safe environment for client.

RISK FOR VIOLENCE: SELF-DIRECTED OR DIRECTED AT OTHERS

Definition: *Behaviors in which an individual demonstrates that he/she can be physically, emotionally, and/or sexually harmful either to self or to others.*

Related/Risk Factors ("related to")
[Chronic alteration in structure or function of brain tissue, secondary to the aging process, multiple infarcts, HIV disease, head trauma, chronic substance abuse, or progressively dysfunctional physical condition resulting in the following symptoms:

Delusional thinking
Suspiciousness of others
Hallucinations
Illusions
Disorientation or confusion
Impairment of impulse control]

[Inaccurate perception of the environment]
Body language—rigid posture, clenching of fists and jaw, hyperactivity, pacing, breathlessness, and threatening stances.
Suicidal ideation, plan, available means
Cognitive impairment
[Depressed mood]

Goals/Objectives
Short-Term Goal
Client will maintain agitation at manageable level so as not to become violent.

Long-Term Goal
Client will not harm self or others.

Interventions with *Selected Rationales*
1. Assess client's level of anxiety and behaviors that indicate the anxiety is increasing. *Recognizing these behaviors, the nurse may be able to intervene before violence occurs.*
2. Maintain low level of stimuli in client's environment (low lighting, few people, simple decor, low noise level). *Anxiety increases in a highly stimulating environment.*
3. Remove all potentially dangerous objects from client's

environment. *In a disoriented, confused state, the client may use these objects to harm self or others.*

4. Have sufficient staff available to execute a physical confrontation, if necessary. *Assistance may be required from others to provide for physical safety of client or primary nurse or both.*

5. Maintain a calm manner with client. Attempt to prevent frightening the client unnecessarily. Provide continual reassurance and support. *Anxiety is contagious and can be transferred to the client.*

6. Interrupt periods of unreality and reorient. *Client safety is jeopardized during periods of disorientation. Correcting misinterpretations of reality enhances client's feelings of self-worth and personal dignity.*

7. Use tranquilizing medications and soft restraints, as prescribed by physician, for protection of client and others during periods of elevated anxiety. *Use restraints judiciously, because agitation is sometimes increased; however, they may be required to ensure client safety.*

8. Sit with client and provide one-to-one observation if assessed to be actively suicidal. *Client safety is a nursing priority.*

9. Teach relaxation exercises *to intervene in times of increasing anxiety.*

10. Teach prospective caregivers to recognize client behaviors that indicate anxiety is increasing and ways to intervene before violence occurs.

Outcome Criteria
1. Prospective caregivers are able to verbalize behaviors that indicate an increasing anxiety level and ways they may assist client to manage the anxiety before violence occurs.
2. Client is able to control impulse to perform acts of violence against self or others, with assistance from caregivers.

ALTERED THOUGHT PROCESSES

Definition: *A state in which an individual experiences a disruption in cognitive operations and activities.*

Possible Etiologies ("related to")
[Alteration in structure/function of brain tissue, secondary to the following conditions:

- Advanced age
- Vascular disease
- Hypertension
- Cerebral hypoxia
- Long-term abuse of mood- or behavior-altering substances
- Exposure to environmental toxins
- Various other physical disorders that predispose to cerebral abnormalities (see Predisposing Factors)]

Defining Characteristics ("evidenced by")
[Delusional thinking]
Inaccurate interpretation of environment
Memory deficit or problems [and confabulation]
Altered attention span; distractibility
[Disorientation to time, place, person, circumstances, and events]
[Impaired ability to make decisions, problem-solve, reason, abstract or conceptualize, calculate]
[Inappropriate or nonreality-based thinking]

Goals/Objectives
Short-Term Goal
Client will accept explanations of inaccurate interpretations within the environment within 5 days.

Long-Term Goal
With assistance from caregiver, client will be able to interrupt nonreality-based thinking.

Interventions with *Selected Rationales*
1. Frequently orient client to reality and surroundings. Allow client to have familiar objects around him or her. Use other items, such as clock, calendar, and daily schedules, to assist in maintaining reality orientation. *Client safety is jeopardized during periods of disorientation. Maintaining reality orientation enhances client's sense of self-worth and personal dignity.*
2. Teach prospective caregivers how to orient client to time, person, place, and circumstances, as required. *These caregivers will be responsible for client safety after discharge from the hospital. Sharing successful interventions may be helpful.*
3. Give positive feedback when thinking and behavior are appropriate, or when client verbalizes that certain ideas expressed are not based in reality. *Positive feedback in-*

creases self-esteem and enhances desire to repeat ap-propriate behaviors.

4. Use simple explanations and face-to-face interaction when communicating with client. Do not shout message into client's ear. *Speaking slowly and in a face-to-face position is most effective when communicating with an elderly individual experiencing a hearing loss. Visual cues facilitate understanding. Shouting causes distortion of high-pitched sounds and in some instances creates a feeling of discomfort for the client.*

5. Express reasonable doubt if client relays suspicious beliefs in response to delusional thinking. Discuss with client the potential personal negative effects of continued suspiciousness of others. Reinforce accurate perception of people and situations. *Expressions of doubt by a trusted individual may foster similar uncertainties about delusion on the part of the client.*

6. Do not permit rumination of false ideas. When this begins, talk to client about real people and real events. *Reality orientation increases client's sense of self-worth and personal dignity.*

7. Close observation of client's behavior is indicated if delusional thinking reveals an intention for violence. *Client safety is a nursing priority.*

Outcome Criteria

1. With assistance from caregiver, client is able to distinguish between reality-based and nonreality-based thinking.

2. Prospective caregivers are able to verbalize ways in which to orient client to reality, as needed.

SELF-CARE DEFICIT

Definition: *A state in which the individual experiences an impaired ability to perform or complete [activities of daily living (ADL) independently]*

Possible Etiologies ("related to")
[Disorientation]
[Confusion]
[Memory deficits]

Defining Characteristics ("evidenced by")
[Inability to fulfill ADLs]

Goals/Objectives
Short-Term Goal
Client will participate in ADLs with assistance from caregiver.

Long-Term Goal
Client will accomplish ADLs to the best of his or her ability. Unfulfilled needs will be met by caregiver.

Interventions with *Selected Rationales*
1. Provide a simple, structured environment *to minimize confusion:*
   a. Identify self-care deficits and provide assistance as required.
   b. Allow plenty of time for client to perform tasks.
   c. Provide guidance and support for independent actions by talking the client through the task one step at a time.
   d. Provide a structured schedule of activities that does not change from day to day.
   e. ADLs should follow home routine as closely as possible.
   f. Provide for consistency in assignment of daily caregivers.
2. In planning for discharge:
   a. Perform ongoing assessment of client's ability to fulfill nutritional needs, ensure personal safety, follow medication regimen, and communicate need for assistance with those activities that he or she cannot accomplish independently.
   b. Assess prospective caregivers' ability to anticipate and fulfill client's unmet needs. Provide information to assist caregivers with this responsibility. Ensure that caregivers are aware of available community support systems from whom they can seek assistance when required.
   c. National support organizations can provide information:
      National Parkinson Foundation Inc.
      1501 NW 9th Ave.
      Miami, FL 33136
      1-800-327-4545

      Alzheimer's Association
      919 N. Michigan Ave., Suite 1000
      Chicago, IL 60611
      1-800-272-3900

The Centers for Disease Control and Prevention (CDC)
AIDS Hotline
1-800-342-AIDS
(24 hours/day, 7 days/week)

Outcome Criteria
1. Client willingly participates in ADLs.
2. Client accomplishes ADLs to the best of his or her ability.
3. Client's unfulfilled needs are met by caregivers.

SENSORY-PERCEPTUAL ALTERATIONS (Specify)

Definition: A state in which an individual experiences a change in the amount or patterning of oncoming stimuli [either internally or externally initiated] accompanied by a diminished, exaggerated, distorted, or impaired response to such stimuli.

Possible Etiologies ("related to")
[Alteration in structure/function of brain tissue, secondary to the following conditions:
- Advanced age
- Vascular disease
- Hypertension
- Cerebral hypoxia
- Abuse of mood- or behavior-altering substances
- Exposure to environmental toxins
- Various other physical disorders that predispose to cerebral abnormalities (see Predisposing Factors)]

Defining Characteristics ("evidenced by")
[Disorientation to time, place, person, or circumstances]
[Inability to concentrate]
[Visual and auditory distortions]
Inappropriate responses
[Talking and laughing to self]
[Suspiciousness]
Hallucinations

Goals/Objectives
Short-Term Goal
With assistance from caregiver, client will maintain orientation to time, place, person, and circumstances for specified period of time.

Long-Term Goal
Client will demonstrate accurate perception of the environment by responding appropriately to stimuli indigenous to the surroundings.

Interventions with *Selected Rationales*
1. Decrease the amount of stimuli in the client's environment (e.g., low noise level, few people, simple decor). *This decreases the possibility of forming inaccurate sensory perceptions.*
2. Do not reinforce the hallucination. Let client know that you do not share the perception. Maintain reality through reorientation and focus on real situations and people. *Reality orientation decreases false sensory perceptions, and enhances client's sense of self-worth and personal dignity.*
3. Provide reassurance of safety if client responds with fear to inaccurate sensory perception. *Client safety and security is a nursing priority.*
4. Correct client's description of inaccurate perception, and describe the situation as it exists in reality. *Explanation of, and participation in, real situations and real activities interferes with the ability to respond to hallucinations.*
5. Provide a feeling of security and stability in the client's environment by allowing for care to be given by same personnel on a regular basis, if possible.
6. Teach prospective caregivers how to recognize signs and symptoms of client's inaccurate sensory perceptions. Explain techniques they may use to restore reality to the situation.

Outcome Criteria
1. With assistance from caregiver, client is able to recognize when perceptions within the environment are inaccurate.
2. Prospective caregivers are able to verbalize ways in which to correct inaccurate perceptions and restore reality to the situation.

SELF-ESTEEM DISTURBANCE

Definition: Negative self-evaluation or feelings about self or self capabilities, which may be directly or indirectly expressed.

Possible Etiologies ("related to")
[Loss of independent functioning]
[Loss of capacity for remembering]
[Loss of capability for effective verbal communication]

Defining Characteristics ("evidenced by")
[Withdraws into social isolation]
[Lack of eye contact]
[Excessive crying alternating with expressions of anger]
[Refusal to participate in therapies]
[Refusal to participate in own self-care activities]
[Becomes increasingly dependent on others to perform ADLs]
Expressions of shame or guilt

Goals/Objectives
Short-Term Goal
Client will voluntarily spend time with staff and peers in day-room activities within 1 week.

Long-Term Goal
By discharge, client will exhibit increased feelings of self-worth as evidenced by voluntary participation in own self-care and interaction with others.

Interventions with *Selected Rationales*
1. Encourage client to express honest feelings in relation to loss of prior level of functioning. Acknowledge pain of loss. Support client through process of grieving. *Client may be fixed in anger stage of grieving process, which is turned inward on the self, resulting in diminished self-esteem.*
2. Devise methods for assisting client with memory deficit. Examples follow:
   a. Name sign on door identifying client's room.
   b. Identifying sign on outside of dining room door.
   c. Identifying sign on outside of restroom door.
   d. Large clock, with oversized numbers and hands, appropriately placed.
   e. Large calendar, indicating one day at a time, with month, day, and year identified in bold print.
   f. Printed, structured daily schedule, with one copy for client and one posted on unit wall.
   g. "News board" on unit wall where current national and local events may be posted.
   These aids may assist client to function more independently, thereby increasing self-esteem.

3. Encourage client's attempts to communicate. If verbalizations are not understandable, express to client what you think he or she intended to say. It may be necessary to reorient client frequently. *The ability to communicate effectively with others may enhance self-esteem.*
4. Encourage reminiscence and discussion of life review. Also discuss present-day events. Sharing picture albums, if possible, is especially good. *Reminiscence and life review help the client resume progression through the grief process associated with disappointing life events and increase self-esteem as successes are reviewed.*
5. Encourage participation in group activities. Caregiver may need to accompany client at first, until he or she feels secure that the group members will be accepting, regardless of limitations in verbal communication. *Positive feedback from group members will increase self-esteem.*
6. Offer support and empathy when client expresses embarrassment at inability to remember people, events, and places. Focus on accomplishments *to lift self-esteem.*
7. Encourage client to be as independent as possible in self-care activities. Provide written schedule of tasks to be performed. Intervene in areas where client requires assistance. *The ability to perform independently preserves self-esteem.*

Outcome Criteria
1. Client initiates own self-care according to written schedule and willingly accepts assistance as needed.
2. Client interacts with others in group activities, maintaining anxiety at minimal level in response to difficulties with verbal communication.

CAREGIVER ROLE STRAIN

Definition: A caregiver's felt difficulty in performing the family caregiver role.

Possible Etiologies ("related to")
Severity of the care receiver's illness
Duration of the care receiver's illness
Lack of respite and recreation for the caregiver
Caregiver's competing role commitments
Inadequate physical environment for providing care

Family or caregiver isolation
Complexity and amount of caregiving tasks

Defining Characteristics ("evidenced by")
Expressions by caregiver(s) of
Feelings of stress in relationship with care receiver
Feelings of depression and anger
Family conflict around issues of providing care
Feelings that caregiving interferes with other important
roles in their lives

Goals/Objectives
Short-Term Goal
Caregivers will verbalize understanding of ways to facilitate
the caregiver role.

Long-Term Goal
Caregivers will demonstrate effective problem-solving skills
and develop adaptive coping mechanisms to regain equilibrium.

Interventions with *Selected Rationales*
1. Assess caregivers' ability to anticipate and fulfill client's
unmet needs. Provide information to assist caregivers
with this responsibility. *Caregivers may be unaware of
what client will realistically be able to accomplish.
They may be unaware of the progressive nature of the
illness.*
2. Ensure that caregivers are aware of available community
support systems from which they can seek assistance
when required. Examples include adult day-care centers,
housekeeping and homemaker services, respite-care services, or perhaps a local chapter of the Alzheimer's Disease and Related Disorders Association (ADRDA). This organization sponsors a nationwide 24-hour hot line to
provide information and link families who need assistance
with nearby chapters and affiliates. The hot-line number
is 1-800-272-3900. *Caregivers require relief from the
pressures and strain of providing 24-hour care for their
loved one. Studies have shown that elder abuse arises
out of caregiving situations that place overwhelming
stress on the caregivers.*
3. Encourage caregivers to express feelings, particularly anger. *Release of these emotions can serve to prevent
psychopathology, such as depression or psychophysiologic disorders from occurring.*

4. Encourage participation in support groups comprised of members with similar life situations. *Hearing others who are experiencing the same problems discuss ways in which they have coped may help caregiver adopt more adaptive strategies. Individuals who are experiencing similar life situations provide empathy and support for each other.*

Outcome Criteria

1. Caregivers are able to problem solve effectively regarding care of elderly client.
2. Caregivers demonstrate adaptive coping strategies for dealing with stress of caregiver role.
3. Caregivers openly express feelings.
4. Caregivers express desire to join support group of other caregivers.

Chapter 6
SUBSTANCE-RELATED DISORDERS

BACKGROUND ASSESSMENT DATA

The substance-related disorders are composed of two groups: the substance-use disorders (dependence and abuse) and the substance-induced disorders (intoxication and withdrawal). Other substance-induced disorders (delirium, dementia, amnesia, psychosis, mood disorder, anxiety disorder, sexual dysfunction, and sleep disorders) are included in the chapters with which they share symptomatology (e.g., substance-induced mood disorders are included in Chapter 8; substance-induced sexual dysfunction is included in Chapter 12, etc.).

SUBSTANCE-USE DISORDERS

SUBSTANCE ABUSE

Defined
The *DSM-IV* (APA, 1994) defines substance abuse as a maladaptive pattern of substance use manifested by recurrent and significant adverse consequences related to repeated use of the substance. Criteria include the following:

1. Recurrent substance use resulting in a failure to fulfill major role obligations at work, school, or home.
2. Recurrent substance use in situations in which it is physically hazardous.

3. Recurrent substance-related legal problems.
4. Continued substance use despite having persistent or recurrent social or interpersonal problems caused or exacerbated by the effects of the substance.

SUBSTANCE DEPENDENCE

Defined

The *DSM-IV* defines substance dependence by the following criteria:

1. Evidence of tolerance, as identified by either of the following:
    a. A need for increased amounts of the substance to achieve intoxication or the desired effect.
    b. Diminished effect with continued use of the same amount of the substance.
2. Evidence of withdrawal symptoms, as manifested by either of the following:
    a. The characteristic withdrawal syndrome for the substance.
    b. The same (or closely related) substance is taken to relieve or avoid withdrawal symptoms.
3. The substance is often taken in larger amounts or over a longer period than was intended.
4. There is a persistent desire or unsuccessful effort to cut down or control substance use.
5. A great deal of time is spent in activities necessary to obtain, use, or recover from the effects of the substance.

SUBSTANCE-INDUCED DISORDERS

SUBSTANCE INTOXICATION

Defined

The *DSM-IV* defines substance intoxication by the following criteria:

1. The development of a reversible substance-specific syndrome caused by recent ingestion of (or exposure to) a substance.
2. Clinically significant maladaptive behavior or psychologic changes that are caused by the effect of the substance on the central nervous system (CNS) and develop during or shortly after use of the substance.

SUBSTANCE WITHDRAWAL

Defined

The *DSM-IV* defines substance withdrawal by the following criteria:

1. The development of a substance-specific syndrome caused by the cessation of (or reduction in) heavy and prolonged substance use.
2. The substance-specific syndrome causes clinically significant distress or impairment in social, occupational, or other important areas of functioning.

CLASSIFICATION OF SUBSTANCES

ALCOHOL

Even though alcohol is a depressant, it will be considered separately because of the complex effects and widespread nature of its use. Low to moderate consumption produces a feeling of well-being and reduced inhibitions. At higher concentrations, motor and intellectual functioning are impaired, mood becomes very labile, and behaviors characteristic of depression, euphoria, and aggression are exhibited. The only medical use for alcohol (with the exception of its inclusion in a number of pharmacologic concentrates) is as an antidote for methanol consumption.

Examples: Beer, wine, bourbon, scotch, gin, vodka, rum, tequila, liqueurs.

Common substances containing alcohol and used by some dependent individuals to satisfy their need include liquid cough medications, liquid cold preparations, mouthwashes, isopropyl rubbing alcohol, nail polish removers, colognes, aftershave and preshave preparations.

OPIOIDS

Opioids have a medical use as analgesics, antitussives, and antidiarrheals. They produce the effects of analgesia and euphoria by stimulating the opiate receptors in the brain, and thereby mimicking the naturally occurring endorphins.

Examples: Opium, morphine, codeine, heroin, hydromorphone, meperidine, methadone.

Common Street Names: Horse, junk, H (heroin); black stuff, poppy, big O (opium); M, morph (morphine); dollies (methadone); terp (terpin hydrate or cough syrup with codeine).

CNS DEPRESSANTS

CNS depressants have a medical use as antianxiety agents, sedatives, hypnotics, anticonvulsants, and anesthetics. They depress the action of the CNS, resulting in an overall calming, relaxing effect on the individual. At higher dosages they can induce sleep.

Examples: Benzodiazepines, barbiturates, chloral hydrate, methaqualone, ethchlorvynol, meprobamate.

Common Street Names: Peter, Mickey (chloral hydrate); green and whites, roaches (Librium); blues (Valium, 10 mg); yellows (Valium, 5 mg); red birds, red devils (secobarbital); blue birds (Amytal capsules); yellow birds (Nembutal); downers (barbiturates; tranquilizers).

CNS STIMULANTS

CNS stimulants have a medical use in the management of hyperkinesia, narcolepsy, and weight control. They stimulate the action of the central nervous system, resulting in increased alertness, excitation, euphoria, increased pulse rate and blood pressure, insomnia, and loss of appetite.

Examples: Amphetamines, methylphenidate (Ritalin), phenmetrazine (Preludin), cocaine, hydrochloride cocaine, caffeine, tobacco.

Common Street Names: Bennies, wake-ups, uppers, speed (amphetamines); coke, snow, gold dust, girl (cocaine); crack, rock (hydrochloride cocaine); speedball (mixture of heroin and cocaine).

HALLUCINOGENS

Hallucinogens act as sympathomimetic agents, producing effects resembling those resulting from stimulation of the sympathetic nervous system (e.g., excitation, increased energy, distortion of the senses). Therapeutic medical uses for lysergic acid diethylamide (LSD) have been proposed in the treatment of chronic alcoholism and in the reduction of intractable pain, such as terminal malignant disease and phantom limb sensations.

Examples: LSD, mescaline, phencyclidine (PCP).

Common Street Names: Acid, cube, big D, California

sunshine (LSD); angel dust, hog, peace pill, crystal (PCP); cactus, mescal, mesc (mescaline).

CANNABINOLS
Cannabinols depress higher centers in the brain and consequently release lower centers from inhibitory influence. They produce an anxiety-free state of relaxation characterized by a feeling of extreme well-being. Large doses of the drug can produce hallucinations. Marijuana has been used therapeutically in the relief of nausea and vomiting associated with antineoplastic chemotherapy.

Examples: Marijuana, hashish.

Common Street Names: Joints, reefers, pot, grass, Mary Jane (marijuana); hash (hashish).

A profile summary of these psychoactive substances is presented in Table 6–1.

PREDISPOSING FACTORS

1. **Physiologic**
   a. *Genetics.* There is an apparent genetic link involved in the development of substance-related disorders. This is especially evident with alcoholism, less so with other substances. About half of the children of alcoholics become alcoholic, suggesting a possible heredity factor. The statistics are inconclusive regarding abuse of other substances, although children of people who themselves have substance-related disorders are at higher risk for developing these disorders.
   b. *Biochemical.* A second physiologic hypothesis relates to the possibility that alcohol may produce morphinelike substances in the brain that are responsible for alcohol addiction. This occurs when the products of alcohol metabolism react with biologically active amines.
2. **Psychosocial**
   a. *Psychodynamic Theory.* This theory suggests that individuals who abuse substances have underdeveloped egos because of a failure in completing tasks of separation-individuation. The person retains a highly dependent nature, with characteristics of poor impulse control, low frustration tolerance, and low self-esteem. The superego is weak, resulting in ab-

TABLE 6–1 **Psychoactive Substances: A Profile Summary**

Class of Drugs	Symptoms of Use	Therapeutic Uses	Symptoms of Overdose	Trade Names	Common Names
CNS depressants: Alcohol	Relaxation, loss of inhibitions, lack of concentration, drowsiness, slurred speech, sleep	Antidote for methanol consumption; ingredient in many pharmacologic concentrates	Nausea, vomiting; shallow respirations; cold, clammy skin; weak, rapid pulse; coma; possible death	Ethyl alcohol, beer, gin, rum, vodka, bourbon, whiskey, liqueurs, wine, brandy, sherry, champagne	Booze, alcohol, liquor, drinks, cocktails, hiballs, nightcaps, moonshine, white lightening, firewater
Other (barbiturates and nonbarbiturates)	Same as Alcohol	Relief from anxiety and insomnia; as anticonvulsants and anesthetics.	Anxiety, fever, agitation, hallucinations, disorientation, tremors, delirium, convulsions, possible death	Seconal, Nembutal, Amytal Valium, Librium Chloral hydrate Equanil, Miltown	Red birds, yellow birds, blue birds Blues/yellows, green & whites Mickies Downers
CNS Stimulants: Amphetamines and related drugs	Hyperactivity, agitation, euphoria, insomnia, loss of appetite	Management of narcolepsy, hyperkinesia, and weight control	Cardiac arrhythmias, headache, convulsions, hypertension, rapid heart rate, coma, possible death	Dexedrine, Didrex, Tenuate, Preludin, Ritalin, Plegine, Cylert, Ionamin, Sanorex	Uppers, pep pills, wake-ups, bennies, eye-openers, speed, black beauties, sweet A's
Cocaine	Euphoria, hyperactivity, restlessness, talkativeness, increased pulse, dilated pupils	Topical anesthetic	Hallucinations, convulsions, pulmonary edema, respiratory failure, coma, cardiac arrest, possible death	Cocaine hydrochloride	Coke, flake, snow, dust, gold dust, happy dust, girl, cecil, C, toot, blow, crack

Category	Drugs	Effects of Overdose	Medical Uses	Physical/Psychological Effects	Street Names
Opioids	Heroin	Shallow breathing, slowed pulse, clammy skin, pulmonary edema, respiratory arrest, convulsions, coma, possible death	As analgesics; methadone in substitution therapy; heroin has no therapeutic use	Euphoria, lethargy, drowsiness, lack of motivation	Snow, Stuff, H, Harry, Horse
	Morphine				M, Morph, Miss Emma
	Codeine				Schoolboy
	Dilaudid				Lords
	Demerol				Doctors
	Methadone				Dollies
	Percodan				Perkies
	Talwin				T's
	Opium				Big O, black stuff
Hallucinogens	LSD	Agitation, extreme hyperactivity, violence, hallucinations, psychosis, convulsions, possible death	LSD has been proposed in the treatment of chronic alcoholism, and in the reduction of intractable pain.	Visual hallucinations, disorientation, confusion, paranoid delusions, euphoria, anxiety, panic, increased pulse	Acid, cube, big D
	PCP				Angel dust, hog, crystal
	Mescaline				Mesc
	DMT				Businessman's trip
	STP				Serenity and peace
Cannabinols	Cannabis	Fatigue, paranoia, delusions, hallucinations, possible psychosis	Marijuana has been used for relief of nausea and vomiting associated with antineoplastic chemotherapy and to reduce eye pressure in glaucoma patients.	Relaxation, talkativeness, lowered inhibitions, euphoria, mood swings	Marijuana, pot, grass, joint, Mary Jane, MJ
	Hashish				Hash, rope, Sweet Lucy

sence of guilt feelings for their behavior (Freud, 1959).

b. ***Theory of Family Dynamics.*** This theory relates a predisposition to substance-related disorders to the dysfunctional family system. There is often one parent who is absent or who is an overpowering tyrant, and one who is weak and ineffectual. Substance abuse may be evident as the primary method of relieving stress. The child has negative role models and learns to respond to stressful situations in like manner (Leigh, 1985).

COMMON PATTERNS OF USE IN SUBSTANCE-RELATED DISORDERS

SYMPTOMATOLOGY (Subjective and Objective Data)

Alcohol Abuse/Dependence

1. Begins with social drinking that provides feeling of relaxation and well-being. Soon requires more and more to produce the same effects.
2. Drinks in secret; hides bottles of alcohol; drinks first thing in the morning (to "steady my nerves") and at any other opportunity that arises during the day.
3. As the disease progresses, the individual may drink in binges. During a binge, drinking continues until the individual is too intoxicated or too sick to consume any more. Behavior borders on the psychotic, with the individual wavering in and out of reality.
4. Begins to have blackouts. Periods of amnesia occur (in the absence of intoxication or loss of consciousness) during which the individual is unable to remember periods of time or events that have occurred.
5. Chronic use results in multisystem physiologic impairments that include (but are not limited to) the following:
   a. ***Peripheral Neuropathy.*** Numbness, tingling, pain in extremities (caused by thiamine deficiency)
   b. ***Wernicke-Korsakoff Syndrome.*** Mental confusion, agitation, diplopia (caused by thiamine deficiency). Rapid deterioration to coma and death will occur without immediate thiamine replacement.
   c. ***Alcoholic Cardiomyopathy.*** Enlargement of the heart caused by an accumulation of excess lipids in

myocardial cells. Symptoms of tachycardia, dyspnea, and arrhythmias may be evident.
   d. ***Esophagitis.*** Inflammation of, and pain in, the esophagus
   e. ***Esophageal Varices.*** Distended veins in the esophagus, with risk of rupture and subsequent hemorrhage.
   f. ***Gastritis.*** Inflammation of lining of stomach caused by irritation from the alcohol, resulting in pain, nausea, vomiting, and possibility of bleeding because of erosion of blood vessels.
   g. ***Pancreatitis.*** Inflammation of the pancreas, resulting in pain, nausea and vomiting, and abdominal distention. With progressive destruction to the gland, symptoms of diabetes mellitus could occur.
   h. ***Alcoholic Hepatitis.*** Inflammation of the liver, resulting in enlargement, jaundice, right upper quadrant pain, and fever.
   i. ***Cirrhosis of the Liver.*** Fibrous and degenerative changes occurring in response to chronic accumulation of large amounts of fatty acids in the liver. In cirrhosis, symptoms of alcoholic hepatitis progress to include the following:
      • **Portal Hypertension:** Elevation of blood pressure through the portal circulation resulting from defective blood flow through the cirrhotic liver.
      • **Ascites:** An accumulation of serous fluid in the peritoneal cavity.
      • **Hepatic Encephalopathy:** Liver disorder caused by inability of the liver to convert ammonia to urea (the body's natural method of discarding excess ammonia); as serum ammonia levels rise, confusion occurs, accompanied by restlessness, slurred speech, fever, and without intervention, an eventual progression to coma and death.

Alcohol Intoxication

1. Symptoms of alcohol intoxication include disinhibition of sexual or aggressive impulses, mood lability, impaired judgment, impaired social or occupational functioning, slurred speech, incoordination, unsteady gait, nystagmus, and flushed face.
2. Intoxication usually occurs at blood alcohol levels between 100 and 200 mg/dL.

Alcohol Withdrawal

1. Occurs within 4 to 12 hours of cessation of, or reduction in, heavy and prolonged (several days or longer) alcohol use.
2. Symptoms include coarse tremor of hands, tongue, or eyelids; nausea or vomiting; malaise or weakness; tachycardia; sweating, elevated blood pressure; anxiety; depressed mood or irritability; transient hallucinations or illusions; headache; and insomnia.
3. Without aggressive intervention, the individual may progress to *alcohol withdrawal delirium* about the second or third day following cessation of, or reduction in, prolonged, heavy alcohol use. Symptoms include those described under the syndrome of delirium (see Chapter 5).

Amphetamine (or Amphetamine-like) Dependence/Abuse

1. The use of amphetamines is often initiated for their appetite-suppressant effect in an attempt to lose or control weight.
2. Amphetamines are also taken for the initial feeling of well-being and confidence.
3. They are typically taken orally, intravenously, or by nasal inhalation.
4. Chronic daily (or almost daily) use usually results in an increase in dosage over time to produce the desired effect.
5. Episodic use often takes the form of binges, followed by an intense and unpleasant "crash" in which the individual experiences anxiety, irritability, and feelings of fatigue and depression.
6. Continued use appears to be related to a "craving" for the substance, rather than to prevention or alleviation of withdrawal symptoms.

Amphetamine (or Amphetamine-like) Intoxication

1. Amphetamine intoxication usually begins with a "high" feeling, followed by the development of symptoms such as euphoria with enhanced vigor, gregariousness, hyperactivity, restlessness, hypervigilance, interpersonal

sensitivity, talkativeness, anxiety, tension, alertness, grandiosity, stereotypical and repetitive behavior, anger, fighting, and impaired judgment (APA, 1994).
2. Physical signs and symptoms that occur with amphetamine intoxication include tachycardia or bradycardia, pupillary dilation, elevated or lowered blood pressure, perspiration or chills, nausea or vomiting, psychomotor retardation or agitation, muscular weakness, respiratory depression, chest pain or cardiac arrhythmias, confusion, seizures, dyskinesias, dystonias, or coma (APA, 1994).

Amphetamine (or Amphetamine-like) Withdrawal

1. Amphetamine withdrawal symptoms occur after cessation of (or reduction in) amphetamine (or a related substance) use that has been heavy and prolonged.
2. Symptoms of amphetamine withdrawal develop within a few hours to several days and include fatigue; vivid, unpleasant dreams; insomnia or hypersomnia; increased appetite; and psychomotor retardation or agitation.

Cannabis Dependence/Abuse

1. Cannabis preparations are almost always smoked but may also be taken orally.
2. It is commonly regarded incorrectly to be a substance without potential for dependence.
3. Tolerance to the substance may result in increased frequency of its use.
4. Abuse is evidenced by participation in hazardous activities while motor coordination is impaired from cannabis use.

Cannabis Intoxication

1. Cannabis intoxication is characterized by impaired motor coordination, euphoria, anxiety, sensation of slowed time, impaired judgment, and social withdrawal that developed during or shortly after cannabis use (APA, 1994).
2. Physical symptoms of cannabis intoxication include

conjunctival injection, increased appetite, dry mouth, and tachycardia.
3. The impairment of motor skills lasts for 8 to 12 hours.

Cocaine Dependence/Abuse

1. Various forms are smoked, inhaled, injected, or taken orally.
2. Chronic daily (or almost daily) use usually results in an increase in dosage over time to produce the desired effect.
3. Episodic use often takes the form of binges, followed by an intense and unpleasant "crash" in which the individual experiences anxiety, irritability, and feelings of fatigue and depression.
4. The drug user often abuses, or is dependent on, a CNS depressant to relieve the residual effects of cocaine.
5. Cocaine abuse and dependence lead to tolerance of the substance and subsequent use of increasing doses.
6. Continued use appears to be related to a "craving" for the substance, rather than to prevention or alleviation of withdrawal symptoms.

Cocaine Intoxication

1. Symptoms of cocaine intoxication develop during, or shortly after, use of cocaine.
2. Symptoms of cocaine intoxication include euphoria or affective blunting, changes in sociability, hypervigilance, interpersonal sensitivity, anxiety, tension, anger, stereotyped behaviors, impaired judgment, and impaired social or occupational functioning.
3. Physical symptoms of cocaine intoxication include tachycardia or bradycardia, pupillary dilation, elevated or lowered blood pressure, perspiration or chills, nausea or vomiting, psychomotor agitation or retardation, muscular weakness, respiratory depression, chest pain, or cardiac arrhythmias, confusion, seizures, dyskinesias, dystonias, or coma.

Cocaine Withdrawal

1. Symptoms of withdrawal occur after cessation of, or reduction in, cocaine use that has been heavy and prolonged.
2. Symptoms of cocaine withdrawal include dysphoric

mood; fatigue; vivid, unpleasant dreams; insomnia or hypersomnia; increased appetite; psychomotor retardation or agitation.

Hallucinogen Dependence/Abuse

1. Hallucinogenic substances are taken orally.
2. Because the cognitive and perceptual impairment may last for up to 12 hours, use is generally episodic, because the individual must organize time during the daily schedule for its use.
3. Frequent use results in tolerance to the effects of the substance.
4. Dependence is rare, and most people are able to resume their previous lifestyle, following a period of hallucinogen use, without much difficulty.
5. Flashbacks may occur following cessation of hallucinogen use. These episodes consist of visual or auditory misperceptions usually lasting only a few seconds, but sometimes lasting up to several hours.
6. Hallucinogens are highly unpredictable in the effects they may induce each time they are used.

Hallucinogen Intoxication

1. Symptoms of intoxication develop during or shortly after hallucinogen use.
2. Symptoms include marked anxiety or depression, ideas of reference, fear of losing one's mind, paranoid ideation, impaired judgment, and impaired social or occupational functioning.
3. Other symptoms include subjective intensification of perceptions, depersonalization, derealization, illusions, hallucinations, and synesthesias.

Inhalant Dependence/Abuse

1. Effects are induced by inhaling the vapors of volatile substances through the nose or mouth.
2. Examples of substances include glue, gasoline, paint, paint thinners, various cleaning chemicals, typewriter correction fluid.
3. Use of inhalants often begins in childhood, and considerable family dysfunction is characteristic.
4. Use may be daily or episodic, and chronic use may continue into adulthood.

5. Tolerance has been reported among individuals with heavy use, but a withdrawal syndrome from these substances has not been well documented.

Inhalant Intoxication

1. Symptoms of intoxication develop during, or shortly after, use of, or exposure to, volatile inhalants.
2. Symptoms of inhalant intoxication include belligerence, assaultiveness, apathy, impaired judgment, and impaired social or occupational functioning.
3. Physical symptoms of inhalant intoxication include dizziness, nystagmus, incoordination, slurred speech, unsteady gait, lethargy, depressed reflexes, psychomotor retardation, tremor, generalized muscle weakness, blurred vision or diplopia, stupor or coma, and euphoria.

Nicotine Dependence

1. The effects of nicotine are induced through inhaling the smoke of cigarettes, cigars, or pipe tobacco, and orally through the use of snuff or chewing tobacco.
2. Continued use results in a "craving" for the substance.
3. Nicotine is commonly used to relieve or to avoid withdrawal symptoms that occur when the individual has been in a situation where use is restricted.
4. Continued use despite knowledge of medical problems related to smoking is a particularly important health problem.

Nicotine Withdrawal

1. Symptoms of withdrawal develop within 24 hours after abrupt cessation of (or reduction in) nicotine use.
2. Symptoms of nicotine withdrawal include dysphoric or depressed mood, insomnia, irritability, frustration, anger, anxiety, difficulty concentrating, restlessness, decreased heart rate, and increased appetite.

Opioid Dependence/Abuse

1. Various forms are taken orally, intravenously, by nasal inhalation, and by smoking.

2. Dependence occurs after recreational use of the substance "on the street," or after prescribed use of the substance for relief of pain or cough.
3. Chronic use leads to remarkably high levels of tolerance.
4. Once abuse or dependence is established, substance procurement often comes to dominate the person's life.
5. Cessation or decreased consumption results in a "craving" for the substance and produces a specific syndrome of withdrawal.

Opioid Intoxication

1. Symptoms of intoxication develop during or shortly after opioid use.
2. Symptoms of opioid intoxication include euphoria (initially) followed by apathy, dysphoria, psychomotor agitation or retardation, impaired judgment, and impaired social or occupational functioning.
3. Physical symptoms of opioid intoxication include pupillary constriction, drowsiness or coma, slurred speech, and impairment in attention or memory.

Opioid Withdrawal

1. Symptoms of opioid withdrawal occur after cessation of (or reduction in) heavy and prolonged opioid use. Symptoms of withdrawal can also occur after administration of an opioid antagonist after a period of opioid use.
2. Symptoms of opioid withdrawal can occur within minutes to several days following use (or antagonist), and include dysphoric mood, nausea or vomiting, muscle aches, lacrimation or rhinorrhea, pupillary dilation, piloerection, sweating, abdominal cramping, diarrhea, yawning, fever, and insomnia.

Phencyclidine (PCP) Dependence/Abuse

1. Phencyclidine is taken orally, intravenously, or by smoking or inhaling.
2. Use can be on a chronic daily basis, but more often is taken episodically in binges that can last several days.
3. Abuse or dependence can occur after only a short period of occasional use.

4. Unclear if tolerance or withdrawal symptoms develop with use of PCP.

Phencyclidine Intoxication

1. Symptoms of intoxication develop during or shortly after PCP use.
2. Symptoms of PCP intoxication include belligerence, assaultiveness, impulsiveness, unpredictability, psychomotor agitation, impaired judgment, and impaired social or occupational functioning.
3. Physical symptoms occur within an hour or less of PCP use and include vertical or horizontal nystagmus, hypertension or tachycardia, numbness or diminished responsiveness to pain, ataxia, dysarthria, muscle rigidity, seizures or coma, and hyperacusis.

Sedative, Hypnotic, or Anxiolytic Dependence/ Abuse

1. Effects are produced through oral intake of these substances.
2. Dependence can occur following recreational use of the substance "on the street," or after prescribed use of the substance for relief of anxiety or insomnia.
3. Chronic use leads to remarkably high levels of tolerance.
4. Once dependence develops, there is evidence of strong substance-seeking behaviors (obtaining prescriptions from several physicians or resorting to illegal sources to maintain adequate supplies of the substance).
5. Abrupt cessation of these substances can result in life-threatening withdrawal symptoms.

Sedative, Hypnotic or Anxiolytic Intoxication

1. Symptoms of intoxication develop during or shortly after intake of sedatives, hypnotics, or anxiolytics.
2. Symptoms of intoxication include inappropriate sexual or aggressive behavior, mood lability, impaired judgment, and impaired social or occupational functioning.
3. Physical symptoms of sedative, hypnotic, or anxiolytic intoxication include slurred speech, incoordination, unsteady gait, nystagmus, impairment in attention or memory, stupor or coma.

Sedative, Hypnotic or Anxiolytic Withdrawal

1. Withdrawal symptoms occur after cessation of (or reduction in) heavy and prolonged use of sedatives, hypnotics, or anxiolytics.
2. Symptoms of withdrawal occur within several hours to a few days after abrupt cessation or reduction in use of the drug.
3. Symptoms of withdrawal include autonomic hyperactivity (e.g., sweating or pulse rate >100); increased hand tremor; insomnia; nausea or vomiting; transient visual, tactile, or auditory hallucinations or illusions; psychomotor agitation; anxiety; or grand mal seizures.

A summary of symptoms associated with the syndromes of intoxication and withdrawal is presented in Table 6–2.

COMMON NURSING DIAGNOSES AND INTERVENTIONS

(Interventions are applicable to various health-care settings, such as inpatient and partial hospitalization, community outpatient clinic, home health, and private practice.)

RISK FOR INJURY

Definition: *A state in which the individual is at risk of injury as a result of [internal or external] environmental conditions interacting with the individual's adaptive and defensive resources.*

Related/Risk Factors ("related to")
[Substance intoxication]
[Substance withdrawal]
[Disorientation]
[Seizures]
[Hallucinations]
[Psychomotor agitation]
[Unstable vital signs]
[Delirium]
[Flashbacks]
[Panic level of anxiety]

TABLE 6–2   Summary of Symptoms Associated with the Syndromes of Intoxication and Withdrawal

Class of Drugs	Intoxication	Withdrawal	Comments
Alcohol	Aggressiveness, impaired judgment, impaired attention, irritability, euphoria, depression, emotional lability, slurred speech, incoordination, unsteady gait, nystagmus, flushed face	Tremors, nausea/vomiting, malaise, weakness, tachycardia, sweating, elevated blood pressure, anxiety, depressed mood, irritability, hallucinations, headache, insomnia, seizures	Alcohol withdrawal begins within 4–6 hr after last drink. May progress to delirium tremens on 2nd or 3rd d. Use of Librium is common for substitution therapy.
Amphetamines and related substances	Fighting, grandiosity, hypervigilance, psychomotor agitation, impaired judgment, tachycardia, pupillary dilation, elevated blood pressure, perspiration or chills, nausea and vomiting	Anxiety, depressed mood, irritability, craving for the substance, fatigue, insomnia or hypersomnia, psychomotor agitation, paranoid and suicidal ideation	Withdrawal symptoms usually peak within 2–4 d, although depression and irritability may persist for months. Tricyclic antidepressants may be used.
Caffeine	Restlessness, nervousness, excitement, insomnia, flushed face, diuresis, gastrointestinal complaints, muscle twitching, rambling flow of thought and speech, cardiac arrhythmia, periods of inexhaustibility, psychomotor agitation	Headache	Caffeine is contained in coffee, tea, colas, cocoa, chocolate, some over-the-counter analgesics, "cold" preparations, and stimulants.
Cannabis	Euphoria, anxiety, suspiciousness, sensation of slowed time, impaired judgment, social withdrawal, tachycardia, conjunctival redness, increased appetite, hallucinations	Restlessness, irritability, insomnia, loss of appetite	Intoxication occurs immediately and lasts about 3 hr. Oral ingestion is more slowly absorbed and has longer-lasting effects.

Cocaine	Euphoria, fighting, grandiosity, hypervigilance, psychomotor agitation, impaired judgment, tachycardia, elevated blood pressure, pupillary dilation, perspiration or chills, nausea/vomiting, hallucinations, delirium	Depression, anxiety, irritability, fatigue, insomnia or hypersomnia, psychomotor agitation, paranoid or suicidal ideation, apathy, social withdrawal	Large doses of the drug can result in convulsions or death from cardiac arrhythmias or respiratory paralysis.
Inhalants	Belligerence, assaultiveness, apathy, impaired judgment, dizziness, nystagmus, slurred speech, unsteady gait, lethargy, depressed reflexes, tremor, blurred vision, stupor or coma, euphoria, irritation around eyes, throat, and nose		Intoxication occurs within 5 min of inhalation. Symptoms last 60–90 min. Large doses can result in death from CNS depression or cardiac arrhythmia.
Nicotine		Craving for the drug, irritability, anger, frustration, anxiety, difficulty concentrating, restlessness, decreased heart rate, increased appetite, weight gain, tremor, headaches, insomnia	Symptoms begin within 24 hr of last drug use and decrease in intensity over days, weeks, or sometimes longer.
Opioids	Euphoria, lethargy, somnolence, apathy, dysphoria, impaired judgment, pupillary constriction, drowsiness, slurred speech, constipation, nausea, decreased respiratory rate and blood pressure	Craving for the drug, nausea/vomiting, muscle aches, lacrimation or rhinorrhea, pupillary dilation, piloerection or sweating, diarrhea, yawning, fever, insomnia	Withdrawal symptoms appear within 6–8 hr after last dose, reach a peak in the 2nd or 3rd d, and disappear in 7–10 d.

Table continued on following page

133

TABLE 6–2 **Summary of Symptoms Associated with the Syndromes of Intoxication and Withdrawal** (*Continued*)

Class of Drugs	Intoxication	Withdrawal	Comments
Phencyclidine and related substances	Belligerence, assaultiveness, impulsiveness, psychomotor agitation, impaired judgment, nystagmus, increased heart rate and blood pressure, diminished pain response, ataxia, dysarthria, muscle rigidity, seizures, hyperacusis, delirium		Delirium can occur within 24 hr after use of phencyclidine, or may occur up to a week following recovery from an overdose of the drug.
Sedatives, hypnotics, anxiolytics	Disinhibition of sexual or aggressive impulses, mood lability, impaired judgment, slurred speech, incoordination, unsteady gait, impairment in attention or memory, disorientation, confusion	Nausea/vomiting, malaise, weakness, tachycardia, sweating, anxiety, irritability, orthostatic hypotension, tremor, insomnia, seizures	Withdrawal may progress to delirium, usually within 1 wk of last use. Long-acting barbiturates or benzodiazepines may be used in withdrawal substitution therapy.

From Townsend, 1996, pp. 382–383, with permission.

Goals/Objectives
Short-Term Goal
Client's condition will stabilize within 72 hours.

Long-Term Goal
Client will not experience physical injury.

Interventions with *Selected Rationales*
1. Assess client's level of disorientation to determine specific requirements for safety. *Knowledge of client's level of functioning is necessary to formulate appropriate plan of care.*
2. Obtain a drug history, if possible, to determine
   a. Type of substance(s) used.
   b. Time of last ingestion and amount consumed.
   c. Length and frequency of consumption.
   d. Amount consumed on a daily basis.
3. Obtain urine sample for laboratory analysis of substance content. *Subjective history is often not accurate. Knowledge regarding substance ingestion is important for accurate assessment of client condition.*
4. Place client in quiet, private room. *Excessive stimuli increase client agitation.*
5. Institute necessary safety precautions:
   a. Observe client behaviors frequently; assign staff on one-to-one basis if condition is warranted; accompany and assist client when ambulating; use wheelchair for transporting long distances.
   b. Be sure that side rails are up when client is in bed.
   c. Pad headboard and side rails of bed with thick towels to protect client in case of seizure.
   d. Use mechanical restraints as necessary to protect client if excessive hyperactivity accompanies the disorientation.
   Client safety is a nursing priority.
6. Ensure that smoking materials and other potentially harmful objects are stored outside client's access. *Client may harm self or others in disoriented, confused state.*
7. Frequently orient client to reality and surroundings. *Disorientation may endanger client safety if he or she unknowingly wanders away from safe environment.*
8. Monitor vital signs every 15 minutes initially and less frequently as acute symptoms subside. *Vital signs provide the most reliable information regarding client condition and need for medication during acute detoxification period.*

9. Follow medication regimen, as ordered by physician. Common medical intervention for detoxification from the following substances includes:
   a. **Alcohol.** Chlordiazepoxide (Librium) is given orally every 4 to 8 hours in decreasing doses until withdrawal is complete. In clients with liver disease, accumulation of the longer-acting agents, such as chlordiazepoxide (Librium), may be problematic, and the use of the shorter-acting benzodiazepine, oxazepam (Serax), is more appropriate. Some physicians may order anticonvulsant medication to be used prophylactically; however, this is not a universal intervention. Multivitamin therapy, in combination with daily thiamine (either orally or by injection), is common protocol.
   b. **Narcotics.** Narcotic antagonists, such as naloxone (Narcan), nalorphine (Nalline), or levallorphan (Lorfan), are administered intravenously for narcotic overdose. Withdrawal is managed with rest and nutritional therapy. Substitution therapy may be instituted to decrease withdrawal symptoms using propoxyphene (Darvon) for weaker effects or methadone (Dolophine) for longer effects.
   c. **Depressants.** Substitution therapy may be instituted to decrease withdrawal symptoms using a long-acting barbiturate, such as phenobarbital (Luminal). Some physicians prescribe oxazepam (Serax) as needed for objective symptoms, gradually decreasing the dosage until the drug is discontinued.
   d. **Stimulants.** Treatment of overdose is geared toward stabilization of vital signs. Intravenous antihypertensives may be used, along with IV diazepam (Valium) to control seizures. Chlordiazepoxide may be administered orally for the first few days while the client is "crashing."
   e. **Hallucinogens and Cannabinols.** Medications are normally not prescribed for withdrawal from these substances. However, in the event of overdose, diazepam (Valium) or chlordiazepoxide (Librium) may be given as needed to decrease agitation.

Outcome Criteria
1. Client is no longer exhibiting any signs or symptoms of substance intoxication or withdrawal.
2. Client shows no evidence of physical injury obtained during substance intoxication or withdrawal.

INEFFECTIVE DENIAL

Definition: *The state of a conscious or unconscious attempt to disavow the knowledge or meaning of an event to reduce anxiety or fear to the detriment of health.*

Possible Etiologies ("related to")
[Weak, underdeveloped ego]
[Underlying fears and anxieties]
[Low self-esteem]
[Fixation in early level of development]

Defining Characteristics ("evidenced by")
[Denies substance abuse or dependence]
[Denies that substance use creates problems in his or her life]
[Continues to use substance, knowing it contributes to impairment in functioning or exacerbation of physical symptoms]
[Uses substance(s) in physically hazardous situations]
[Use of rationalization and projection to explain maladaptive behaviors]
Unable to admit impact of disease on life pattern

Goals/Objectives
Short-Term Goal
Client will divert attention away from external issues and focus on behavioral outcomes associated with substance use.

Long-Term Goal
Client will verbalize acceptance of responsibility for own behavior and acknowledge association between substance use and personal problems.

Interventions with *Selected Rationales*
1. Begin by working to develop a trusting nurse-client relationship. Be honest. Keep all promises. *Trust is the basis of a therapeutic relationship.*
2. Convey an attitude of acceptance to the client. Ensure that he or she understands, "It is not *you* but your *behavior* that is unacceptable." *An attitude of acceptance promotes feelings of dignity and self-worth.*
3. Provide information to correct misconceptions about substance abuse. Client may rationalize his or her behavior with statements such as, "I'm not an alcoholic. I can stop

drinking any time I want. Besides, I only drink beer." or "I only smoke pot to relax before class. So what? I know lots of people who do. Besides, you can't get hooked on pot." *Many myths abound regarding use of specific substances. Factual information presented in a matter-of-fact, nonjudgmental way explaining what behaviors constitute substance-related disorders may help the client focus on his or her own behaviors as an illness that requires help.*

4. Identify recent maladaptive behaviors or situations that have occurred in the client's life, and discuss how use of substances may have been a contributing factor. *The first step in decreasing use of denial is for client to see the relationship between substance use and personal problems.*

5. Use confrontation with caring. Do not allow client to fantasize about his or her lifestyle. (Examples: "It is my understanding that the last time you drank alcohol, you . . ." or "The lab report shows that you were under the influence of alcohol when you had the accident that injured three people.") *Confrontation interferes with client's ability to use denial; a caring attitude preserves self-esteem and avoids putting the client on the defensive.*

6. Do not accept the use of rationalization or projection as client attempts to make excuses for, or blame his or her behavior on, other people or situations. *Rationalization and projection prolong the stage of denial that problems exist in the client's life because of substance use.*

7. Encourage participation in group activities. *Peer feedback is often more accepted than feedback from authority figures. Peer pressure can be a strong factor, as well as the association with individuals who are experiencing or who have experienced similar problems.*

8. Offer immediate positive recognition of client's expressions of insight gained regarding illness and acceptance of responsibility for own behavior. *Positive reinforcement enhances self-esteem and encourages repetition of desirable behaviors.*

Outcome Criteria

1. Client verbalizes understanding of the relationship between personal problems and the use of substances.

2. Client verbalizes acceptance of responsibility for own behavior.

3. Client verbalizes understanding of substance dependence and abuse as an illness requiring ongoing support and treatment.

INEFFECTIVE INDIVIDUAL COPING

Definition: The impairment of adaptive behaviors and abilities of a person in meeting life's demands and roles.

Possible Etiologies ("related to")
[Inadequate support systems]
[Inadequate coping skills]
[Underdeveloped ego]
[Possible hereditary factor]
[Dysfunctional family system]
[Negative role modeling]
Personal vulnerability

Defining Characteristics ("evidenced by")
[Low self-esteem]
[Chronic anxiety]
[Chronic depression]
Inability to meet role expectations
Alteration in societal participation
Inability to meet basic needs
Inappropriate use of defense mechanisms
[Substance abuse]
[Low frustration tolerance]
[Need for immediate gratification]
[Manipulative behavior]

Goals/Objectives
Short-Term Goal
Client will express true feelings associated with use of substances as a method of coping with stress.

Long-Term Goal
Client will be able to verbalize adaptive coping mechanisms to use, instead of substance abuse, in response to stress.

Interventions with *Selected Rationales*
1. Establish trusting relationship with client (be honest; keep appointments; be available to spend time). *The therapeutic nurse-client relationship is built on trust.*
2. Set limits on manipulative behavior. Be sure that the client knows what is acceptable, what is not, and the consequences for violating the limits set. Ensure that all staff maintain consistency with this intervention. *Client is unable to establish own limits, so you must do so for him or her. Unless administration of consequences for vi-*

olation of limits is consistent, manipulative behavior will not be eliminated.

3. Encourage client to verbalize feelings, fears, anxieties. Answer any questions he or she may have regarding the disorder. *Verbalization of feelings in a nonthreatening environment may help client come to terms with long-unresolved issues.*

4. Explain the effects of substance abuse on the body. Emphasize that prognosis is closely related to abstinence. *Many clients lack knowledge regarding the deleterious effects of substance abuse on the body.*

5. Explore with client the options available to assist with stressful situations rather than resorting to substance abuse (e.g., contacting various members of Alcoholics Anonymous or Narcotics Anonymous; physical exercise; relaxation techniques; meditation). *Client may have persistently resorted to chemical abuse, and thus may possess little or no knowledge of adaptive responses to stress.*

6. Provide positive reinforcement for evidence of gratification delayed appropriately. *Positive reinforcement enhances self-esteem and encourages client to repeat acceptable behaviors.*

7. Encourage client to be as independent as possible in own self-care. Provide positive feedback for independent decision-making and effective use of problem-solving skills.

Outcome Criteria
1. Client is able to verbalize adaptive coping strategies for use as alternatives to substance use in response to stress.
2. Client is able to verbalize the names of support people from whom he or she may seek help when the desire for substance use is intense.

ALTERED NUTRITION: LESS THAN BODY REQUIREMENTS

Definition: *The state in which an individual experiences an intake of nutrients insufficient to meet metabolic needs.*

Possible Etiologies ("related to")
[Drinking alcohol instead of eating nourishing food]
[Eating only "junk food"]
[Eating nothing (or very little) while on a "binge"]

[No money for food (having spent what is available on substances)]

[Problems with malabsorption caused by chronic alcohol abuse]

Defining Characteristics ("evidenced by")
Loss of weight
Pale conjunctiva and mucous membranes
Poor muscle tone
[Poor skin turgor]
[Edema of extremities]
[Electrolyte imbalances]
[Cheilosis (cracks at corners of mouth)]
[Scaley dermatitis]
[Weakness]
[Neuropathies]
[Anemias]
[Ascites]

Goals/Objectives
Short-Term Goals
Client will gain 2 lb during next 7 days.
Client's electrolytes will be restored to normal within 1 week.

Long-Term Goal
Client will exhibit no signs or symptoms of malnutrition by discharge. (This would not be a realistic goal for a chronic alcoholic in the end stages of the disease. For such a client, it would be more appropriate to establish short-term goals, as realistic step objectives, to use in the evaluation of care given.)

Interventions with *Selected Rationales*
1. In collaboration with dietitian, determine number of calories required to provide adequate nutrition and realistic (according to body structure and height) weight gain.
2. Strict documentation of intake, output, and calorie count. *This information is necessary to make an accurate nutritional assessment and maintain client safety.*
3. Weigh daily. *Weight loss or gain is important assessment information.*
4. Determine client's likes and dislikes and collaborate with dietitian to provide favorite foods. *Client is more likely to eat foods that he or she particularly enjoys.*
5. Ensure that client receives small, frequent feedings, including a bedtime snack, rather than three larger meals.

Large amounts of food may be objectionable, or even intolerable, to the client.

6. Administer vitamin and mineral supplements, as ordered by physician, *to improve nutritional state.*
7. If appropriate, ask family members or significant others to bring in special foods that client particularly enjoys.
8. Monitor laboratory work, and report significant changes to physician.
9. Explain the importance of adequate nutrition. *Client may have inadequate or inaccurate knowledge regarding the contribution of good nutrition to overall wellness.*

Outcome Criteria

1. Client has achieved and maintained at least 90% of normal body weight.
2. Vital signs, blood pressure, and laboratory serum studies are within normal limits.
3. Client is able to verbalize importance of adequate nutrition.

SELF-ESTEEM DISTURBANCE

Definition: *Negative self-evaluation and feelings about self or self-capabilities, which may be directly or indirectly expressed.*

Possible Etiologies ("related to")

[Retarded ego development]
[Dysfunctional family system]
[Lack of positive feedback]
[Perceived failures]

Defining Characteristics ("evidenced by")

[Difficulty accepting positive reinforcement]
[Failure to take responsibility for self-care]
[Self-destructive behavior (substance abuse)]
[Lack of eye contact]
[Withdraws into social isolation]
[Highly critical and judgmental of self and others]
[Sense of worthlessness]
[Fear of failure]
[Unable to recognize own accomplishments]
[Setting self up for failure by establishing unrealistic goals]
[Unsatisfactory interpersonal relationships]
[Negative or pessimistic outlook]
Denial of problems obvious to others

Projection of blame or responsibility for problems
Rationalizing personal failures
Hypersensitivity to slight criticism
Grandiosity

Goals/Objectives
Short-Term Goal
Client will accept responsibility for personal failures and verbalize the role substances played in those failures.

Long-Term Goal
By discharge, client will exhibit increased feelings of self-worth as evidenced by verbal expression of positive aspects about self, past accomplishments, and future prospects.

Interventions with *Selected Rationales*
1. Be accepting of client and his or her negativism. *An attitude of acceptance enhances feelings of self-worth.*
2. Spend time with client *to convey acceptance and contribute toward feelings of self-worth.*
3. Help client to recognize and focus on strengths and accomplishments. Discuss past (real or perceived) failures, but minimize amount of attention devoted to them beyond client's need to accept responsibility for them. *Client must accept responsibility for own behavior before change in behavior can occur. Minimizing attention to past failures may help to eliminate negative ruminations and increase client's sense of self-worth.*
4. Encourage participation in group activities *from which client may receive positive feedback and support from peers.*
5. Help client identify areas he or she would like to change about self and assist with problem solving toward this effort. *Low self-worth may interfere with client's perception of own problem-solving ability. Assistance may be required.*
6. Assure that client is not becoming increasingly dependent and that he or she is accepting responsibility for own behaviors. *Client must be able to function independently if he or she is to be successful within the less-structured community environment.*
7. Ensure that therapy groups offer client simple methods of achievement. Offer recognition and positive feedback for actual accomplishments. *Successes and recognition increase self-esteem.*

8. Provide instruction in assertiveness techniques: the ability to recognize the difference between passive, assertive, and aggressive behaviors; the importance of respecting the human rights of others while protecting one's own basic human rights. *Self-esteem is enhanced by the ability to interact with others in an assertive manner.*
9. Teach effective communication techniques, such as the use of "I" messages and placing emphasis on ways to avoid making judgmental statements.

Outcome Criteria
1. Client is able to verbalize positive aspects about self.
2. Client is able to communicate assertively with others.
3. Client expresses an optimistic outlook for the future.

KNOWLEDGE DEFICIT (Effects of Substance Abuse on the Body)

Definition: *Absence or deficiency of cognitive information related to [the effects of substance abuse on the body and its interference with achievement and maintenance of optimal wellness].*

Possible Etiologies ("related to")
Lack of interest in learning
[Low self-esteem]
[Denial of need for information]
[Denial of risks involved with substance abuse]
Unfamiliarity with information resources

Defining Characteristics ("evidenced by")
[Abuse of substances]
[Statement of lack of knowledge]
[Statement of misconception]
[Request for information]
Verbalization of the problem

Goals/Objectives
Short-Term Goal
Client will be able to verbalize effects of [substance used] on the body following implementation of teaching plan.

Long-Term Goal
Client will verbalize the importance of abstaining from use of [substance] in order to maintain optimal wellness.

Interventions with *Selected Rationales*

1. Assess client's level of knowledge regarding effects of [substance] on body. *Baseline assessment of knowledge is required in order to develop appropriate teaching plan for client.*
2. Assess client's level of anxiety and readiness to learn. *Learning does not take place beyond moderate level of anxiety.*
3. Determine method of learning most appropriate for client (e.g., discussion, question and answer, use of audio or visual aids, oral or written method). *Level of education and development are important considerations as to methodology selected.*
4. Develop teaching plan, including measurable objectives for the learner. *Measurable objectives provide criteria on which to base evaluation of the teaching experience.*
5. Include significant others, if possible. *Lifestyle changes often affect all family members.*
6. Implement teaching plan at a time that facilitates, and in a place that is conducive to, optimal learning (e.g., in the evening when family members visit, in an empty, quiet classroom or group therapy room). *Learning is enhanced by an environment with few distractions.*
7. Begin with simple concepts and progress to the more complex. *Retention is increased if introductory material presented is easy to understand.*
8. Include information on physical effects of [substance], its capacity for physiologic and psychological dependence, its effects on family functioning, its effects on a fetus (and the importance of contraceptive use until abstinence has been achieved), and the importance of regular participation in an appropriate treatment program.
9. Provide activities for client and significant others in which to actively participate during the learning exercise. *Active participation increases retention.*
10. Ask client and significant others to demonstrate knowledge gained by verbalizing information presented. *Verbalization of knowledge gained is a measurable method of evaluating the teaching experience.*
11. Provide positive feedback for participation, as well as for accurate demonstration of knowledge gained. *Positive feedback enhances self-esteem and encourages repetition of acceptable behaviors.*
12. Evaluate teaching plan. Identify strengths and weak-

nesses, and any changes that may enhance the effectiveness of the plan.

Outcome Criteria

1. Client is able to verbalize effects of [substance] on the body.
2. Client verbalizes understanding of risks involved in use of [substance].
3. Client is able to verbalize community resources for obtaining knowledge and support with substance-related problems.

Chapter 7

SCHIZOPHRENIA AND OTHER PSYCHOTIC DISORDERS

BACKGROUND ASSESSMENT DATA

The syndrome of symptoms associated with schizophrenia and other psychotic disorders reveals alterations in content and organization of thoughts, perception of sensory input, affect or emotional tone, sense of identity, volition, psychomotor behavior, and ability to establish satisfactory interpersonal relationships.

CATEGORIES

Paranoid Schizophrenia
Paranoid schizophrenia is characterized by extreme suspiciousness of others and by delusions and hallucinations of a persecutory or grandiose nature. The individual is often tense and guarded and may be argumentative, hostile, and aggressive.

Disorganized Schizophrenia
In disorganized schizophrenia, behavior is typically regressive and primitive. Affect is inappropriate, with common characteristics being silliness, incongruous giggling, facial grimaces, and extreme social withdrawal. Communication is consistently incoherent.

Catatonic Schizophrenia

Catatonic schizophrenia manifests itself in the form of *stupor* (marked psychomotor retardation, mutism, waxy flexibility [posturing], negativism, and rigidity) or *excitement* (extreme psychomotor agitation, leading to exhaustion or the possibility of hurting self or others if not curtailed).

Undifferentiated Schizophrenia

Undifferentiated schizophrenia is characterized by disorganized behaviors and psychotic symptoms (e.g., delusions, hallucinations, incoherence, and grossly disorganized behavior) that may appear in more than one category.

Residual Schizophrenia

Behavior in residual schizophrenia is eccentric, but psychotic symptoms, if present at all, are not prominent. Social withdrawal and inappropriate affect are characteristic. The patient has a history of at least one episode of schizophrenia in which psychotic symptoms were prominent.

Schizoaffective Disorder

Schizoaffective disorder refers to behaviors characteristic of schizophrenia, in addition to those indicative of disorders of mood, such as depression or mania.

Brief Psychotic Disorder

The essential features of brief psychotic disorder include a sudden onset of psychotic symptoms in response to a severe psychosocial stressor. The symptoms last at least 1 day but less than 1 month with a virtual return to the premorbid level of functioning. The diagnosis is further specified by whether or not it follows a severe identifiable stressor or if the onset occurs within 4 weeks postpartum.

Schizophreniform Disorder

The essential features of schizophreniform disorder are identical to those of schizophrenia, with the exception that the duration is at least 1 month but less than 6 months. The diagnosis is termed "provisional" if a diagnosis must be made prior to recovery.

Delusional Disorder

Delusional disorder is characterized by the presence of one or more nonbizarre delusions that persist for at least 1 month. Hallucinatory activity is not prominent. Apart from the delusions, behavior is not bizarre. The following types are based on the predominant delusional theme (AMA, 1994):

1. **Persecutory Type.** Delusions that one is being malevolently treated in some way.
2. **Jealous Type.** Delusions that one's sexual partner is unfaithful.
3. **Erotomanic Type.** Delusions that another person of higher status is in love with him or her.
4. **Somatic Type.** Delusions that the person has some physical defect, disorder, or disease.
5. **Grandiose Type.** Delusions of inflated worth, power, knowledge, special identity, or special relationship to a deity or famous person.

Shared Psychotic Disorder (Folie à Deux)

In shared psychotic disorder, a delusional system develops in the context of a close relationship with another person who already has a psychotic disorder with prominent delusions.

Psychotic Disorder Due to a General Medical Condition

The *DSM-IV* identifies the essential features of this disorder as prominent hallucinations and delusions that can be directly attributed to a general medical condition. Examples of general medical conditions that may cause psychotic symptoms include neurologic conditions (e.g., neoplasms, Huntington's disease, CNS infections); endocrine conditions (e.g., hyperthyroidism, hypothyroidism, hypoadrenocorticism); metabolic conditions (e.g., hypoxia, hypercarbia, hypoglycemia); autoimmune disorders (e.g., systemic lupus erythematosus); and others (e.g., fluid or electrolyte imbalances, hepatic or renal diseases).

Substance-Induced Psychotic Disorder

The essential features of this disorder are the presence of prominent hallucinations and delusions that are judged to be directly attributable to the physiologic effects of a substance (i.e., a drug of abuse, a medication, or toxin exposure) (APA, 1994).

PREDISPOSING FACTORS

1. **Physiologic**
   a. ***Genetics.*** Studies (Heston, 1977; Gottesman, 1978) have indicated that certain genetic factors may be involved in the development of a psychotic disorder. Results have shown that individuals are at higher risk for the disorder if there is a familial pattern of involvement (parents, siblings, other relatives).
   b. ***Histologic Changes.*** Scheibel (1991) has suggested that schizophrenic disorders may in fact be a birth defect, occurring in the hippocampus region of the brain, and related to an influenza virus encountered by the mother during the second trimester of pregnancy. The studies have shown a "disordering" of the pyramidal cells in the brains of schizophrenics, but the cells in the brains of nonschizophrenic individuals appeared to be arranged in an orderly fashion. Further research is required to determine the possible link between this birth defect and the development of schizophrenia.
   c. ***The Dopamine Hypothesis.*** A biochemical theory suggests the involvement of elevated levels of the neurotransmitter dopamine, which is thought to produce the symptoms of overactivity and fragmentation of associations that are commonly observed in psychoses (Hollandsworth, 1990).

2. **Psychosocial**
   a. ***Family Systems Theory.*** Bowen (1978) describes the development of schizophrenia as it evolves out of a dysfunctional family system. Conflict between spouses drives one parent to attach to the child. This overinvestment in the child redirects the focus of anxiety in the family, and a more stable condition results. A symbiotic relationship develops between parent and child; the child remains totally dependent on the parent into adulthood and is unable to respond to the demands of adult functioning.
   b. ***Interpersonal Theory.*** Sullivan (1953) relates that the psychotic person is the product of a parent-child relationship fraught with intense anxiety. The child receives confusing and conflicting messages from the

parent and is unable to establish trust. High levels of anxiety are maintained, and the child's concept of self is one of ambiguity. Psychosis offers relief from anxiety and security from intimate relatedness.

c. ***Psychodynamic Theory.*** Birchwood and coworkers (1989) assert that psychosis is the result of a weak ego, development of which has been inhibited by a cold, overprotective, and domineering mother. *Double-blind communication* may also be a factor in this theory of causation. Double-blind communication occurs when a verbal statement is made accompanied by a nonverbal expression that is incongruent. These incompatible communications may also interfere with ego development, thereby causing the individual to generate false ideas and exhibit extreme mistrust of all communications. Because of weak ego development, the adolescent or young adult is unable to deal with the demands of adult living and retreats into a form of thinking from early childhood.

Credibility of the psychosocial theories is currently being challenged. Schizophrenia is commonly considered to be a brain disorder.

SYMPTOMATOLOGY (Subjective/Objective Data)

1. **Autism.** There is a focus inward. The individual may create his or her own world. Words and events may take on special meaning to the psychotic person, meaning of a highly symbolic nature that only the individual can understand.
2. **Emotional Ambivalence.** Powerful emotions of love, hate, and fear produce much conflict within the individual. Each tends to balance the other until an emotional neutralization occurs, and the individual experiences apathy or indifference.
3. **Inappropriate Affect.** The affect is blunted or flat, and often inappropriate (e.g., person who laughs when told of the death of a parent).
4. **Associative Looseness.** This term describes the very disorganized thoughts and verbalizations of the psychotic person. Ideas shift from one unrelated subject to another. When the condition is severe, speech may be incoherent.
5. **Echolalia.** The psychotic person often repeats words he or she hears.

6. **Echopraxia.** The psychotic person often repeats movements he or she sees in others. (Echolalia and echopraxia are products of the person's very weak ego boundaries.)

7. **Neologisms.** Words that are invented by the psychotic person that are meaningless to others, but have symbolic meaning to the individual.

8. **Concrete Thinking.** The psychotic person has difficulty thinking on the abstract level and may use literal translations concerning aspects of the environment.

9. **Clang Associations.** The individual uses rhyming words in a nonsensical pattern.

10. **Word Salad.** The psychotic person may put together a random jumble of words without any logical connection.

11. **Mutism.** Psychotic individuals may refuse or be unable to speak.

12. **Circumstantiality.** Circumstantiality refers to a psychotic person's delay in reaching the point of a communication because of unnecessary and tedious details.

13. **Tangentiality.** Tangentiality differs from circumstantiality in that the person never really gets to the point of the communication. Unrelated topics are introduced, and the original discussion is lost.

14. **Perseveration.** The individual who exhibits perseveration persistently repeats the same word or idea in response to different questions.

15. **Delusions.** False ideas or beliefs. Types of delusions include the following:
    a. *Grandeur.* The person has an exaggerated feeling of importance or power.
    b. *Persecution.* The person feels threatened and believes others intend harm or persecution toward him or her in some way.
    c. *Reference.* All events within the environment are referred by the psychotic person to himself or herself.
    d. *Control or Influence.* The individual believes certain objects or people have control over his or her behavior.

16. **Hallucinations.** Hallucinations are false sensory perceptions that may involve any of the five senses. Auditory and visual hallucinations are most common, although olfactory, tactile, and gustatory hallucinations can occur.

17. **Regression.** A primary ego defense mechanism used in psychoses. Childlike mannerisms and comfort techniques are employed. Socially inappropriate behavior may be evident.
18. **Religiosity.** The psychotic person becomes preoccupied with religious ideas, a defense mechanism thought to be used in an attempt to provide stability and structure to disorganized thoughts and behaviors.

COMMON NURSING DIAGNOSES AND INTERVENTIONS
(Interventions are applicable to various health-care settings, such as inpatient and partial hospitalization, community outpatient clinic, home health, and private practice.)

RISK FOR VIOLENCE: SELF-DIRECTED OR DIRECTED AT OTHERS

Definition: *Behaviors in which an individual demonstrates that he/she can be physically, emotionally, and/or sexually harmful either to self or to others.*

Related/Risk Factors ("related to")
[Lack of trust (suspiciousness of others)]
[Panic level of anxiety]
[Catatonic excitement]
[Negative role modeling]
[Rage reactions]
[Command hallucinations]
[Delusional thinking]
Body language—rigid posture, clenching of fists and jaw, hyperactivity, pacing, breathlessness, and threatening stances.
[History or threats of violence toward self or others or of destruction to the property of others]
Impulsivity
Suicidal ideation, plan, available means
[Perception of the environment as threatening]
[Receiving auditory or visual "suggestions" of a threatening nature]

Goals/Objectives
Short-Term Goal
Within [a specified time], client will recognize signs of increasing anxiety and agitation and report to staff for assistance with intervention.

Long-Term Goal
Client will not harm self or others.

Interventions with *Selected Rationales*

1. Maintain low level of stimuli in client's environment (low lighting, few people, simple decor, low noise level). *Anxiety level rises in a stimulating environment. A suspicious, agitated client may perceive individuals as threatening.*
2. Observe client's behavior frequently (every 15 minutes). Do this in a manner of carrying out routine activities, *so as to avoid creating suspiciousness in the individual. Close observation is necessary so that intervention can occur if required to ensure client (and others') safety.*
3. Remove all dangerous objects from client's environment, *so that in his or her agitated, confused state, client may not use them to harm self or others.*
4. Try to redirect the violent behavior with physical outlets for the client's anxiety (e.g., punching bag). *Physical exercise is a safe and effective way of relieving pent-up tension.*
5. Staff should maintain and convey a calm attitude toward client. *Anxiety is contagious and can be transmitted from staff to client.*
6. Have sufficient staff available to indicate a show of strength to client if it becomes necessary. *This shows the client evidence of control over the situation and provides some physical security for staff.*
7. Administer tranquilizing medications as ordered by physician. Monitor medication for its effectiveness and for any adverse side effects. *The avenue of the "least restrictive alternative" must be selected when planning interventions for a psychiatric client.*
8. If client is not calmed by "talking down" or by medication, use of mechanical restraints may be necessary. Be sure to have sufficient staff available to assist. Follow protocol established by the institution. Most states require that the physician reevaluate and issue a new order for restraints every 3 hours, except between midnight

and 8:00 AM. If the client has previously refused medication, administer after restraints have been applied. Most states consider this intervention appropriate in emergency situations or in the event that a client would likely harm self or others.

9. Observe the client in restraints every 15 minutes (or according to institutional policy). Ensure that circulation to extremities is not compromised (check temperature, color, pulses). Assist client with needs related to nutrition, hydration, and elimination. Position client so that comfort is facilitated and aspiration can be prevented. *Client safety is a nursing priority.*

10. As agitation decreases, assess client's readiness for restraint removal or reduction. Remove one restraint at a time, while assessing client's response. *This minimizes risk of injury to client and staff.*

Outcome Criteria

1. Anxiety is maintained at a level at which client feels no need for aggression.
2. Client demonstrates trust of others in his or her environment.
3. Client maintains reality orientation.

SOCIAL ISOLATION

Definition: *Condition of aloneness experienced by the individual and perceived as imposed by others and as a negative or threatened state.*

Possible Etiologies ("related to")

[Lack of trust]
[Panic level of anxiety]
[Regression to earlier level of development]
[Delusional thinking]
[Past experiences of difficulty in interactions with others]
[Weak ego development]
[Repressed fears]

Defining Characteristics ("evidenced by")

[Staying alone in room]
Uncommunicative, withdrawn, no eye contact, [mutism, autism]
Sad, dull affect
[Lying on bed in fetal position with back to door]

Inappropriate or immature interests and activities for developmental age or stage

Preoccupation with own thoughts; repetitive, meaningless
actions

[Approaching staff for interaction, then refusing to respond
to staff's acknowledgment]

Expression of feelings of rejection or of aloneness imposed
by others

Goals/Objectives
Short-Term Goal
Client will willingly attend therapy activities accompanied by
trusted staff member within 1 week.

Long-Term Goal
Client will voluntarily spend time with other clients and staff
members in group activities on the unit by discharge.

Interventions with *Selected Rationales*
1. Convey an accepting attitude by making brief, frequent
contacts. *An accepting attitude increases feelings of
self-worth and facilitates trust.*
2. Show unconditional positive regard. *This conveys your
belief in the client as a worthwhile human being.*
3. Be with the client to offer support during group activities
that may be frightening or difficult for him or her. *The
presence of a trusted individual provides emotional
security for the client.*
4. Be honest and keep all promises. *Honesty and dependability promote a trusting relationship.*
5. Orient client to time, person, and place, as necessary.
6. Be cautious with touch. Allow client extra space and an
avenue for exit if he or she becomes too anxious. *A suspicious client may perceive touch as a threatening gesture.*
7. Administer tranquilizing medications as ordered by physician. Monitor for effectiveness and for adverse side effects. *Antipsychotic medications help to reduce psychotic symptoms in some individuals, thereby
facilitating interactions with others.*
8. Discuss with client the signs of increasing anxiety and
techniques to interrupt the response (e.g., relaxation exercises, thought stopping). *Maladaptive behaviors such
as withdrawal and suspiciousness are manifested during times of increased anxiety.*

9. Give recognition and positive reinforcement for client's voluntary interactions with others. *Positive reinforcement enhances self-esteem and encourages repetition of acceptable behaviors.*

Outcome Criteria
1. Client demonstrates willingness and desire to socialize with others.
2. Client voluntarily attends group activities.
3. Client approaches others in appropriate manner for one-to-one interaction.

INEFFECTIVE INDIVIDUAL COPING

Definition: Impairment of adaptive behaviors and abilities of a person in meeting life's demands and roles.

Possible Etiologies ("related to")
[Inability to trust]
[Panic level of anxiety]
Personal vulnerability
[Low self-esteem]
[Inadequate support systems]
[Negative role model]
[Repressed fears]
[Underdeveloped ego]
[Possible hereditary factor]
[Dysfunctional family system]

Defining Characteristics ("evidenced by")
[Suspiciousness of others, resulting in:]
  • Alteration in societal participation
  • Inability to meet basic needs
  • Inappropriate use of defense mechanisms

Goals/Objectives
Short-Term Goal
Client will develop trust in at least one staff member within 1 week.

Long-Term Goal
Client will demonstrate use of more adaptive coping skills as evidenced by appropriateness of interactions and willingness to participate in the therapeutic community.

Interventions with *Selected Rationales*

1. Encourage same staff to work with client as much as possible *in order to promote development of trusting relationship.*
2. Avoid physical contact. *Suspicious clients may perceive touch as a threatening gesture.*
3. Avoid laughing, whispering, or talking quietly where client can see but not hear what is being said. *Suspicious clients often believe others are discussing them, and secretive behaviors reinforce the paranoid feelings.*
4. Be honest and keep all promises. *Honesty and dependability promote a trusting relationship.*
5. A creative approach may have to be used to encourage food intake (e.g., canned food and own can opener or family-style meals). *Suspicious clients may believe they are being poisoned and refuse to eat food from the individually prepared tray.*
6. Mouth checks may be necessary following medication administration *to verify if client is swallowing the tablets or capsules. Suspicious clients may believe they are being poisoned with their medication and attempt to discard the pills.*
7. Activities should never include anything competitive. Activities that encourage a one-to-one relationship with the nurse or therapist are best. *Competitive activities are very threatening to suspicious clients.*
8. Encourage client to verbalize true feelings. The nurse should avoid becoming defensive when angry feelings are directed at him or her. *Verbalization of feelings in a nonthreatening environment may help client come to terms with long-unresolved issues.*
9. An assertive, matter-of-fact, yet genuine approach will be least threatening to the suspicious person. *The suspicious client does not have the capacity to relate to an overly friendly, overly cheerful attitude.*

Outcome Criteria

1. Client is able to appraise situations realistically and refrain from projecting own feelings onto the environment.
2. Client is able to recognize and clarify possible misinterpretations of the behaviors and verbalizations of others.
3. Client eats food from tray and takes medications without evidence of mistrust.
4. Client appropriately interacts and cooperates with staff and peers in therapeutic community setting.

SENSORY-PERCEPTUAL ALTERATION: AUDITORY/VISUAL

Definition: *A state in which an individual experiences a change in the amount or patterning of oncoming stimuli [either internally or externally initiated] accompanied by a diminished, exaggerated, distorted, or impaired response to such stimuli.*

Possible Etiologies ("related to")
[Panic level of anxiety]
[Withdrawal into the self]
[Stress sufficiently severe to threaten an already weak ego]

Defining Characteristics ("evidenced by")
[Talking and laughing to self]
[Listening pose (tilting head to one side as if listening)]
[Stops talking in middle of sentence to listen]
[Disorientation]
[Poor concentration]
[Rapid mood swings]
[Disordered thought sequencing]
Inappropriate responses

Goals/Objectives
Short-Term Goal
Client will discuss content of hallucinations with nurse or therapist within 1 week.

Long-Term Goal
Client will be able to define and test reality, eliminating the occurrence of hallucinations.
(This goal may not be realistic for the individual with chronic illness who has experienced auditory hallucinations for many years.) A more realistic goal may be:
Client will verbalize understanding that the voices are a result of his or her illness and demonstrate ways to interrupt the hallucination.

Interventions with *Selected Rationales*
1. Observe client for signs of hallucinations (listening pose, laughing or talking to self, stopping in midsentence). *Early intervention may prevent aggressive responses to command hallucinations.*

2. Avoid touching the client before warning him or her that you are about to do so. *Client may perceive touch as threatening and respond in an aggressive manner.*

3. An attitude of acceptance will encourage the client to share the content of the hallucination with you. *This is important in order to prevent possible injury to the client or others from command hallucinations.*

4. Do not reinforce the hallucination. Use "the voices" instead of words like "they," which imply validation. Let client know that you do not share the perception. Say, "Even though I realize that the voices are real to you, I do not hear any voices speaking." *The nurse must be honest with the client so that he or she may realize that the hallucinations are not real.*

5. Try to connect the times of the hallucinations to times of increased anxiety. Help the client to understand this connection. *If client can learn to interrupt escalating anxiety, hallucinations may be prevented.*

6. Try to distract the client away from the hallucination. *Involvement in interpersonal activities and explanation of the actual situation will help bring the client back to reality.*

7. For some clients, auditory hallucinations persist after the acute psychotic episode has subsided. Listening to the radio or watching television helps distract some clients from attention to the voices. Others have benefitted from an intervention called *voice dismissal.* With this technique, the client is taught to say loudly, "Go away!" or "Leave me alone!", thereby exerting some conscious control over the behavior.

Outcome Criteria

1. Client is able to recognize that hallucinations occur at times of extreme anxiety.

2. Client is able to recognize signs of increasing anxiety and employ techniques to interrupt the response.

ALTERED THOUGHT PROCESSES

Definition: A state in which an individual experiences a disruption in cognitive operations and activities.

Possible Etiologies ("related to")
[Inability to trust]
[Panic level of anxiety]

[Repressed fears]
[Stress sufficiently severe to threaten an already weak ego]
[Possible hereditary factor]

Defining Characteristics ("evidenced by")
[Delusional thinking (false ideas)]
[Inability to concentrate]
Hypervigilance
[Altered attention span]—distractibility
Inaccurate interpretation of the environment
[Impaired ability to make decisions, problem-solve, reason, abstract or conceptualize, calculate]
[Inappropriate social behavior (reflecting inaccurate thinking)]

Goals/Objectives
Short-Term Goal
By the end of 2 weeks, client will recognize and verbalize that false ideas occur at times of increased anxiety.

Long-Term Goal
Depending on chronicity of disease process, choose the most realistic long-term goal for the client:
1. By discharge from treatment, client will experience (verbalize evidence of) no delusional thoughts.
2. By discharge from treatment, client will be able to differentiate between delusional thinking and reality.

Interventions with *Selected Rationales*
1. Convey your acceptance of client's need for the false belief, while letting him or her know that you do not share the belief. *It is important to communicate to the client that you do not accept the delusion as reality.*
2. Do not argue or deny the belief. Use *reasonable doubt* as a therapeutic technique: "I find that hard to believe." *Arguing with the client or denying the belief serves no useful purpose, because delusional ideas are not eliminated by this approach, and the development of a trusting relationship may be impeded.*
3. Help client try to connect the false beliefs to times of increased anxiety. Discuss techniques that could be used to control anxiety (e.g., deep breathing exercises, other relaxation exercises, thought stopping techniques). *If the client can learn to interrupt escalating anxiety, delusional thinking may be prevented.*
4. Reinforce and focus on reality. Discourage long ruminations about the irrational thinking. Talk about real events and real people. *Discussions that focus on the false*

ideas are purposeless and useless, and may even aggravate the psychosis.

5. Assist and support client in his or her attempt to verbalize feelings of anxiety, fear, or insecurity. *Verbalization of feelings in a nonthreatening environment may help client come to terms with long-unresolved issues.*

Outcome Criteria
1. Verbalizations reflect thinking processes oriented in reality.
2. Client is able to maintain activities of daily living to his or her maximal ability.
3. Client is able to refrain from responding to delusional thoughts, should they occur.

IMPAIRED VERBAL COMMUNICATION

Definition: *The state in which an individual experiences a decreased or absent ability to use or understand language in human interaction*

Possible Etiologies ("related to")
[Inability to trust]
[Panic level of anxiety]
[Regression to earlier level of development]
[Withdrawal into the self]
[Disordered, unrealistic thinking]

Defining Characteristics ("evidenced by")
[Loose association of ideas]
[Use of words that are symbolic to the individual (neologisms)]
[Use of words in a meaningless, disconnected manner (word salad)]
[Use of words that rhyme in a nonsensical fashion (clang association)]
[Repetition of words that are heard (echolalia)]
[Does not speak (mutism)]
[Verbalizations reflect concrete thinking (inability to think in abstract terms)]
[Poor eye contact (either no eye contact or continuous staring into the other person's eyes)]

Goals/Objectives
Short-Term Goal
Client will demonstrate ability to remain on one topic, using appropriate, intermittent eye contact for 5 minutes with nurse or therapist.

Long-Term Goal
By discharge from treatment, client will demonstrate ability to carry on a verbal communication in a socially acceptable manner with staff and peers.

Interventions with *Selected Rationales*
1. Use the techniques of *consensual validation* and *seeking clarification* to decode communication patterns. (Examples: "Is it that you mean . . . ?" or "I don't understand what you mean by that. Would you please explain it to me?") *These techniques reveal to the client how he or she is being perceived by others, while the responsibility for not understanding is accepted by the nurse.*
2. Maintain consistency of staff assignment over time, *to facilitate trust and the ability to understand client's actions and communication.*
3. In a nonthreatening manner, explain to client how his or her behavior and verbalizations are viewed by, and may alienate, others.
4. If client is unable or unwilling to speak (mutism), use of the technique of *verbalizing the implied* is therapeutic. (Example: "That must have been very difficult for you when . . .") *This may help to convey empathy, develop trust, and eventually encourage client to discuss painful issues.*
5. Anticipate and fulfill client's needs until satisfactory communication patterns return. *Client comfort and safety are nursing priorities.*

Outcome Criteria
1. Client is able to communicate in a manner that is understood by others.
2. Client's nonverbal messages are congruent with verbalizations.
3. Client is able to recognize that disorganized thinking and impaired verbal communication occur at times of increased anxiety, and intervene to interrupt the process.

SELF-CARE DEFICIT (Identify Specific Area)

Definition: *A state in which the individual experiences an impaired ability to perform or complete [activities of daily living].*

Possible Etiologies ("related to")
[Withdrawal into the self]
[Regression to an earlier level of development]
[Panic level of anxiety]
Perceptual or cognitive impairment
[Inability to trust]

Defining Characteristics ("evidenced by")
[Difficulty bringing or] inability to bring food from receptacle to mouth.
Inability [or refusal] to wash body or body parts.
[Impaired ability or lack of interest in selecting appropriate clothing to wear, dressing, grooming, or maintaining appearance at a satisfactory level.]
[Inability or unwillingness to carry out toileting procedures without assistance.]

Goals/Objectives
Short-Term Goal
Client will verbalize a desire to perform activities of daily living by end of 1 week.

Long-Term Goal
Client will be able to perform activities of daily living in an independent manner and demonstrate a willingness to do so by discharge from treatment.

Interventions with *Selected Rationales*
1. Encourage client to perform normal activities of daily living to his or her level of ability. *Successful performance of independent activities enhances self-esteem.*
2. Encourage independence, but intervene when client is unable to perform. *Client comfort and safety are nursing priorities.*
3. Offer recognition and positive reinforcement for independent accomplishments. (Example: "Mrs. J., I see you have put on a clean dress and combed your hair.") *Positive reinforcement enhances self-esteem and encourages repetition of desirable behaviors.*
4. Show client, on concrete level, how to perform activities

with which he or she is having difficulty. (Example: If client is not eating, place spoon in his or her hand, scoop some food into it, and say, "Now, eat a bite of mashed potatoes (or other food)." *Because concrete thinking prevails, explanations must be provided at the client's concrete level of comprehension.*

5. Keep strict records of food and fluid intake. *This information is necessary to acquire an accurate nutritional assessment.*

6. Offer nutritious snacks and fluids between meals. *Client may be unable to tolerate large amounts of food at mealtimes and may therefore require additional nourishment at other times during the day to receive adequate nutrition.*

7. If client is not eating because of suspiciousness and fears of being poisoned, provide canned foods and allow client to open them. Or, if possible, suggest that food be served family-style, *so that client may see everyone eating from the same servings.*

8. If client is soiling self, establish routine schedule for toileting needs. Assist client to bathroom on hourly or bi-hourly schedule, as need is determined, until he or she is able to fulfill this need without assistance.

Outcome Criteria
1. Client feeds self without assistance.
2. Client selects appropriate clothing, dresses and grooms self daily without assistance.
3. Client maintains optimal level of personal hygiene by bathing daily and carrying out essential toileting procedures without assistance.

SLEEP PATTERN DISTURBANCE

Definition: Disruption of sleep time, which causes client discomfort or interferes with the client's desired lifestyle.

Possible Etiologies ("related to")
[Panic level of anxiety]
[Repressed fears]
[Hallucinations]
[Delusional thinking]

Defining Characteristics ("evidenced by")
[Difficulty falling asleep]

[Awakening very early in the morning]

[Pacing; other signs of increasing irritability caused by lack of sleep]

Frequent yawning, [nodding off to sleep]

Goals/Objectives
Short-Term Goal

Within first week of treatment, client will fall asleep within 30 minutes of retiring and sleep 5 hours without awakening, with use of sedative if needed.

Long-Term Goal

By discharge from treatment, client will be able to fall asleep within 30 minutes of retiring and sleep 6 to 8 hours without a sleeping aid.

Interventions with *Selected Rationales*

1. Keep strict records of sleeping patterns. *Accurate baseline data are important in planning care to assist client with this problem.*
2. Discourage sleep during the day *to promote more restful sleep at night.*
3. Administer antipsychotic medication at bedtime *so client does not become drowsy during the day.*
4. Assist with measures that promote sleep, such as warm, nonstimulating drinks, light snacks, warm baths, and back rubs.
5. Performing relaxation exercises to soft music may be helpful prior to sleep.
6. Limit intake of caffeinated drinks such as tea, coffee, and colas. *Caffeine is a CNS stimulant and may interfere with the client's achievement of rest and sleep.*

Outcome Criteria

1. Client is able to fall asleep within 30 minutes after retiring.
2. Client sleeps at least 6 consecutive hours without awakening.
3. Client does not require a sedative to fall asleep.

Chapter 8
MOOD DISORDERS

BACKGROUND ASSESSMENT DATA

Mood is defined as an individual's sustained emotional tone, which significantly influences behavior, personality, and perception. A disturbance in mood is the predominant feature of the mood disorders (APA, 1994). Mood disorders are classified as depressive or bipolar.

DEPRESSIVE DISORDERS

Major Depressive Disorder
Major depressive disorder is described as a disturbance of mood involving depression or loss of interest or pleasure in the usual activities and pastimes. There is evidence of interference in social and occupational functioning for at least 2 weeks. There is no history of manic behavior and the symptoms cannot be attributed to use of substances or a general medical condition. The following specifiers may be used to further describe the depressive episode:

1. **Single Episode or Recurrent.** This specifier identifies whether or not the individual has experienced prior episodes of depression.
2. **Mild, Moderate, or Severe.** These categories are identified by the number and severity of symptoms.
3. **With Psychotic Features.** Impairment of reality testing, such as the presence of hallucinations or delusions, is evident.
4. **With Melancholic Features.** This is a typically severe form of major depressive episode. Symptoms are exag-

gerated. There is a loss of interest in all activities. Depression is regularly worse in the morning. There is a history of major depressive episodes that have responded well to somatic antidepressant therapy.

5. **Chronic.** This classification applies when the current episode of depressed mood has been evident continuously for at least the past 2 years.

6. **With Seasonal Pattern.** This diagnosis indicates the presence of depressive symptoms during the fall or winter months. This diagnosis is made when the number of seasonal depressive episodes substantially outnumber the nonseasonal depressive episodes that have occurred over the individual's lifetime (APA, 1994). This disorder has previously been identified in the literature as seasonal affective disorder (SAD).

7. **With Postpartum Onset.** This specifier is used when symptoms of major depression occur within 4 weeks postpartum.

Dysthymic Disorder

A mood disturbance with characteristics similar to, if somewhat milder than, those ascribed to major depressive disorder. There is no evidence of psychotic symptoms.

BIPOLAR DISORDERS

These disorders are characterized by mood swings from profound depression to extreme euphoria (mania), with intervening periods of normalcy.

During an episode of *mania*, the mood is elevated, expansive, or irritable. Motor activity is excessive and frenzied. Psychotic features may be present. A somewhat milder form is called *hypomania*. It is usually not severe enough to require hospitalization, and it does not include psychotic features.

The diagnostic picture for *bipolar depression* is identical to that described for major depressive disorder, with one addition. The client must have a history of one or more manic episodes.

When the symptom presentation includes rapidly alternating moods (sadness, irritability, euphoria) accompanied by symptoms associated with both depression and mania, the individual is given a diagnosis of *bipolar disorder, mixed*.

Bipolar I Disorder

Bipolar I disorder is the diagnosis given to an individual who is experiencing, or has experienced, a full syndrome of manic or mixed symptoms. The client may also have experienced episodes of depression.

Bipolar II Disorder

Bipolar II disorder is characterized by recurrent bouts of major depression with the episodic occurrence of hypomania. This individual has never experienced a full syndrome of manic or mixed symptoms.

Cyclothymic Disorder

The essential feature is a chronic mood disturbance of at least 2 years' duration, involving numerous periods of depression and hypomania, but not of sufficient severity and duration to meet the criteria for either bipolar I or II disorder. There is an absence of psychotic features.

MOOD DISORDER DUE TO GENERAL MEDICAL CONDITION

This disorder is characterized by a prominent and persistent disturbance in mood (either depression or mania) that is judged to be the direct result of the physiologic effects of a general medical condition (APA, 1994).

SUBSTANCE-INDUCED MOOD DISORDER

The disturbance of mood (depression or mania) associated with this disorder is considered to be the direct result of the physiologic effects of a substance (e.g., use or abuse of a drug or a medication, or toxin exposure).

MAJOR DEPRESSIVE DISORDER; DYSTHYMIC DISORDER

PREDISPOSING FACTORS

1. **Physiologic**
   a. *Genetic.* Numerous studies have been conducted that support the involvement of heredity in depressive illness. The disorder is 1.5 to 3 times more com-

mon among first-degree relatives of individuals with
the disorder than among the general population.

b. ***Biochemical.*** A biochemical theory implicates the
biogenic amines norepinephrine, dopamine, and serotonin. The levels of these chemicals have been
found to be deficient in individuals with depressive
illness (Janowsky et al, 1988).

c. ***Neuroendocrine Disturbances.*** Elevated levels of
serum cortisol and decreased levels of thyroid stimulating hormone have been associated with depressed mood in some individuals.

d. ***Medication Side Effects.*** A number of drugs can produce a depressive syndrome as a side effect. Common ones include anxiolytics, antipsychotics, and
sedative-hypnotics. Antihypertensive medications
such as propranolol and reserpine have been known
to produce depressive symptoms.

e. ***Other Physiologic Conditions.*** Depressive symptoms may occur in the presence of electrolyte disturbances, nutritional deficiencies, and with certain
physical disorders, such as cardiovascular accident,
systemic lupus erythematosus, hepatitis, and diabetes mellitus.

2. **Psychosocial**

a. ***Psychoanalytic.*** This theory (Klein, 1934) implicates
an unsatisfactory, early mother-infant relationship as
a predisposition to depressive illness. The infant's
needs go unfulfilled, a condition that is viewed as a
loss. The grief response goes unresolved, and rage
and hostility are turned inward on the self. The ego
remains weak, while the supergo expands and becomes punitive.

b. ***Cognitive.*** These theorists (Beck et al, 1979) believe
that depressive illness occurs as a result of impaired
cognition. Disturbed thought processes foster a negative evaluation of self by the individual. The perceptions are of inadequacy and worthlessness. Outlook for the future is one of pessimism and
hopelessness.

c. ***Learning Theory.*** This theory (Seligman, 1973) proposes that depressive illness is predisposed by the
individual's belief that there is a lack of control over
his or her life situations. It is thought that this belief
arises out of experiences which result in failure (either perceived or real). Following numerous failures,

the individual feels helpless to succeed at any endeavor and therefore gives up trying. This "learned helplessness" is viewed as a predisposition to depressive illness.

d. *Object Loss Theory.* This theory (Bowlby, 1973) suggests that depressive illness occurs if the person is separated from, or abandoned by, a significant other during the first 6 months of life. The bonding process is interrupted, and the child withdraws from people and the environment.

SYMPTOMATOLOGY (Subjective and Objective Data)

1. The affect of a depressed person is one of sadness, dejection, helplessness, and hopelessness. The outlook is gloomy and pessimistic. A feeling of worthlessness prevails.

2. Thoughts are slowed and concentration is difficult. Obsessive ideas and rumination of negative thoughts is common. In severe depression (major depressive disorder or bipolar depression), psychotic features such as hallucinations and delusions may be evident, reflecting misinterpretations of the environment.

3. Physically, there is evidence of weakness and fatigue—very little energy to carry on activities of daily living. The individual may express an exaggerated concern over bodily functioning, seemingly experiencing heightened sensitivity to somatic sensations.

   Some individuals may be inclined toward excessive eating and drinking, while others may experience anorexia and weight loss.

   In response to a general slowdown of the body, digestion is often sluggish, constipation is common, and urinary retention is possible.

   Sleep disturbances are common, either insomnia or hypersomnia. At the less severe level (dysthymic disorder), individuals tend to feel their best early in the morning, then continually feel worse as the day progresses. The opposite is true of persons experiencing severe depression. The exact cause of this phenomenon is unknown, but it is thought to be related to the circadian rhythm of the hormones and their effects on the body.

4. A general slowdown of motor activity commonly accompanies depression (psychomotor retardation). En-

ergy level is depleted, movements are lethargic, and performance of daily activities is extremely difficult. Regression is common, evidenced by withdrawal into the self and retreat to the fetal position.

Severely depressed persons may manifest psychomotor activity through symptoms of agitation. These are constant, rapid, purposeless movements, out of touch with the environment.

5. Verbalizations are limited. When depressed persons do speak, the content may be either ruminations regarding their own life regrets or, in psychotic clients, a reflection of their delusional thinking.

6. Social participation is diminished. The depressed client has an inclination toward egocentrism and narcissism—an intense focus on the self. This discourages others from pursuing a relationship with the individual, which increases his or her feelings of worthlessness and penchant for isolation.

COMMON NURSING DIAGNOSES AND INTERVENTIONS FOR DEPRESSION

(Interventions are applicable to various health-care settings, such as inpatient and partial hospitalization, community outpatient clinic, home health, and private practice.)

RISK FOR SELF-DIRECTED VIOLENCE

Definition: *Behaviors in which an individual demonstrates that he/she can be physically, emotionally, and/or sexually harmful to self.*

Related/Risk Factors ("related to")
[Depressed mood]
[Feelings of worthlessness]
[Anger turned inward]
[Punitive superego and irrational feelings of guilt]
[Numerous failures (learned helplessness)]
[Feelings of abandonment by significant other]
[Hopelessness]
[Misinterpretations of reality]
[Making direct or indirect statements indicating a desire to commit suicide]

[History of previous suicide attempts]
[Has suicide plan and means to carry it out]
[Putting business affairs in order; writing a will; giving away prized possessions]
[Hallucinations]
[Delusional thinking]
[Statements regarding hopelessness for improvement of life situation]
Suicidal ideation, plan, available means

Goals/Objectives
Short-Term Goals
1. Client will seek out staff when feeling urge to harm self.
2. Client will make short-term verbal (or written) contract with nurse not to harm self.

Long-Term Goal
Client will not harm self.

Interventions with *Selected Rationales*
1. Ask client directly: "Have you thought about killing yourself? If so, what do you plan to do? Do you have the means to carry out this plan?" *The risk of suicide is greatly increased if the client has developed a plan and particularly if means exist for the client to execute the plan.*
2. Create a safe environment for the client. Remove all potentially harmful objects from client's access (sharp objects, straps, belts, ties, glass items). *Client safety is a nursing priority.*
3. Formulate a short-term verbal contract with the client that he or she will not harm self during specific time period. When that contract expires, make another, and so forth. *Discussion of suicidal feelings with a trusted individual provides a degree of relief to the client. A contract gets the subject out in the open and places some of the responsibility for the client's safety with the client. An attitude of acceptance of the client as a worthwhile individual is conveyed.*
4. Secure promise from client that he or she will seek out a staff member or support person if thoughts of suicide emerge. *Suicidal clients are often very ambivalent about their feelings. Discussion of feelings with a trusted individual may provide assistance before the client experiences a crisis situation.*
5. Encourage verbalizations of honest feelings. Through exploration and discussion, help client to identify symbols of hope in his or her life.

6. Encourage client to express angry feelings within appropriate limits. Provide safe method of hostility release. Help client to identify true source of anger and to work on adaptive coping skills for use outside the hospital. *Depression and suicidal behaviors may be viewed as anger turned inward on the self. If this anger can be verbalized in a nonthreatening environment, the client may be able to resolve these feelings, regardless of the discomfort involved.*

7. Identify community resources that client may use as support system and from whom he or she may request help if feeling suicidal. *Having a concrete plan for seeking assistance during a crisis may discourage or prevent self-destructive behaviors.*

8. Orient client to reality, as required. Point out sensory misperceptions or misinterpretations of the environment. Take care not to belittle client's fears or indicate disapproval of verbal expressions.

9. Most important, spend time with client. *This provides a feeling of safety and security, while also conveying the message, "I want to spend time with you because I think you are a worthwhile person."*

Outcome Criteria

1. Client verbalizes no thoughts of suicide.
2. Client commits no acts of self-violence.
3. Client is able to verbalize names of resources outside the hospital from whom he or she may request help if feeling suicidal.

DYSFUNCTIONAL GRIEVING

Definition: Extended, unsuccessful use of intellectual and emotional responses by which individuals (families, communities) attempt to work through the process of modifying self-concept based upon the perception of [actual or] potential loss.

Possible Etiologies ("related to")

[Real or perceived loss of any concept of value to the individual]

[Bereavement overload (cumulative grief from multiple unresolved losses)]

[Thwarted grieving response to a loss]

[Absence of anticipatory grieving]
[Feelings of guilt generated by ambivalent relationship with lost concept]

Defining Characteristics ("evidenced by")
Idealization of lost [concept]
Denial of loss
[Excessive anger, expressed inappropriately]
[Obsessions with past experiences]
[Ruminations of guilt feelings, excessive and exaggerated out of proportion to the situation]
Developmental regression
Difficulty in expressing loss
Repetitive use of ineffectual behaviors associated with attempts to reinvest in relationships
Reliving of past experiences with little or no reduction of intensity of the grief
Prolonged interference with life functioning, with onset or exacerbation of somatic or psychosomatic responses
Labile affect
Alterations in eating habits, sleep patterns, dream patterns, activity level, libido

Goals/Objectives
Short-Term Goal
Client will express anger toward lost concept.

Long-Term Goal
Client will be able to verbalize behaviors associated with the normal stages of grief. Client will be able to recognize own position in grief process as he or she progresses at own pace toward resolution.

Interventions with *Selected Rationales*
1. Determine stage of grief in which client is fixed. Identify behaviors associated with this stage. *Accurate baseline assessment data are necessary to effectively plan care for the grieving client.*
2. Develop trusting relationship with client. Show empathy and caring. Be honest and keep all promises. *Trust is the basis for a therapeutic relationship.*
3. Convey an accepting attitude and enable the client to express feelings openly. *An accepting attitude conveys to the client that you believe he or she is a worthwhile person. Trust is enhanced.*
4. Encourage client to express anger. Do not become defensive if initial expression of anger is displaced on nurse

or therapist. Assist client to explore angry feelings so that they may be directed toward the intended object or person. *Verbalization of feelings in a nonthreatening environment may help client come to terms with unresolved issues.*

5. Assist client to discharge pent-up anger through participation in large motor activities (e.g., brisk walks, jogging, physical exercises, volleyball, punching bag, exercise bike). *Physical exercise provides a safe and effective method for discharging pent-up tension.*

6. Teach the normal stages of grief and behaviors associated with each stage. Help client to understand that feelings such as guilt and anger toward the lost concept are appropriate and acceptable during the grief process. *Knowledge of acceptability of the feelings associated with normal grieving may help to relieve some of the guilt that these responses generate.*

7. Encourage client to review relationship with the lost concept. With support and sensitivity, point out reality of the situation in areas where misrepresentations are expressed. *Client must give up an idealized perception and be able to accept both positive and negative aspects about the lost concept before the grief process is complete.*

8. Communicate to client that crying is acceptable. Use of touch is therapeutic and appropriate with most clients. Knowledge of cultural influences specific to the client is important before using this technique.

9. Assist client in problem solving as he or she attempts to determine methods for more adaptive coping with the experienced loss. Provide positive feedback for strategies identified and decisions made. *Positive feedback increases self-esteem and encourages repetition of desirable behaviors.*

10. Encourage client to reach out for spiritual support during this time in whatever form is desirable to him or her. Assess spiritual needs of client and assist as necessary in the fulfillment of those needs.

Outcome Criteria
1. Client is able to verbalize normal stages of the grief process and behaviors associated with each stage.
2. Client is able to identify own position within the grief process and express honest feelings related to the lost concept.

3. Client is no longer manifesting exaggerated emotions and behaviors related to dysfunctional grieving and is able to carry out activities of daily living independently.

SELF-ESTEEM DISTURBANCE

Definition: *Negative self-evaluation and feelings about self or self-capabilities, which may be directly or indirectly expressed.*

Possible Etiologies ("related to")
[Lack of positive feedback]
[Feelings of abandonment by significant other]
[Numerous failures (learned helplessness)]
[Underdeveloped ego and punitive superego]
[Impaired cognition fostering negative view of self]

Defining Characteristics ("evidenced by")
[Difficulty accepting positive reinforcement]
[Withdrawal into social isolation]
[Being highly critical and judgmental of self and others]
[Expressions of worthlessness]
[Fear of failure]
[Inability to recognize own accomplishments]
[Setting self up for failure by establishing unrealistic goals]
[Unsatisfactory interpersonal relationships]
[Negative, pessimistic outlook]
Hypersensitive to slight or criticism
Grandiosity

Goals/Objectives
Short-Term Goals
1. Within reasonable time period, client will discuss fear of failure with nurse.
2. Within reasonable time period, client will verbalize things he or she likes about self.

Long-Term Goals
1. By discharge from treatment, client will exhibit increased feelings of self-worth as evidenced by verbal expression of positive aspects about self, past accomplishments, and future prospects.
2. By discharge from treatment, client will exhibit increased feelings of self-worth by setting realistic goals and trying

to reach them, thereby demonstrating a decrease in fear of failure.

Interventions with *Selected Rationales*

1. Be accepting of client and his or her negativism. *An attitude of acceptance enhances feelings of self-worth.*
2. Spend time with client *to convey acceptance and contribute toward feelings of self-worth.*
3. Help client to recognize and focus on strengths and accomplishments. Minimize attention given to past (real or perceived) failures. *Lack of attention may help to eliminate negative ruminations.*
4. Encourage participation in group activities *from which client may receive positive feedback and support from peers.*
5. Help client identify areas he or she would like to change about self, and assist with problem solving toward this effort. *Low self-worth may interfere with client's perception of own problem-solving ability. Assistance may be required.*
6. Ensure that client is not becoming increasingly dependent and that he or she is accepting responsibility for own behaviors. *Client must be able to function independently if he or she is to be successful within the less-structured community environment.*
7. Ensure that therapy groups offer client simple methods of achievement. Offer recognition and positive feedback for actual accomplishments. *Successes and recognition increase self-esteem.*
8. Teach assertiveness techniques: the ability to recognize the differences among passive, assertive, and aggressive behaviors, and the importance of respecting the human rights of others while protecting one's own basic human rights. *Self-esteem is enhanced by the ability to interact with others in an assertive manner.*
9. Teach effective communication techniques, such as the use of "I" messages. Emphasize ways to avoid making judgmental statements.
10. Assist client to perform aspects of self-care when required. Offer positive feedback for tasks performed independently. *Positive feedback enhances self-esteem and encourages repetition of desirable behaviors.*

Outcome Criteria

1. Client is able to verbalize positive aspects about self.
2. Client is able to communicate assertively with others.
3. Client expresses some optimism and hope for the future.

4. Client sets realistic goals for self and demonstrates willing attempt to reach them.

SOCIAL ISOLATION/IMPAIRED SOCIAL INTERACTION

Definition: *Social isolation is the condition of aloneness experienced by the individual and perceived as imposed by others and as a negative or threatened state; impaired social interaction is the state in which an individual participates in an insufficient or excessive quantity or ineffective quality of social exchange.*

Possible Etiologies ("related to")
[Developmental regression]
[Egocentric behaviors (which offend others and discourage relationships)]
Altered thought processes [delusional thinking]
[Fear of rejection or failure of the interaction]
[Impaired cognition fostering negative view of self]
[Unresolved grief]
Absence of available significant others or peers

Defining Characteristics ("evidenced by")
Sad, dull affect
Being uncommunicative, withdrawn; lacking eye contact
Preoccupation with own thoughts; performance of repetitive, meaningless actions
Seeking to be alone
[Assuming fetal position]
Expression of feelings of aloneness or rejection
Verbalization or observation of discomfort in social situations
Dysfunctional interaction with peers, family, and others

Goals/Objectives
Short-Term Goal
Client will develop trusting relationship with nurse or counselor within reasonable period of time.

Long-Term Goals
1. Client will voluntarily spend time with other clients and nurse or therapist in group activities by discharge from treatment.
2. Client will refrain from using egocentric behaviors that offend others and discourage relationships by discharge from treatment.

Interventions with *Selected Rationales*
1. Spend time with client. This may mean just sitting in silence for a while. *Your presence may help improve client's perception of self as a worthwhile person.*
2. Develop a therapeutic nurse-client relationship through frequent, brief contacts and an accepting attitude. Show unconditional positive regard. *Your presence, acceptance, and conveyance of positive regard enhance the client's feelings of self-worth.*
3. After client feels comfortable in a one-to-one relationship, encourage attendance in group activities. May need to attend with client the first few times to offer support. Accept client's decision to remove self from group situation if anxiety becomes too great. *The presence of a trusted individual provides emotional security for the client.*
4. Verbally acknowledge client's absence from any group activities. *Knowledge that his or her absence was noticed may reinforce the client's feelings of self-worth.*
5. Teach assertiveness techniques. Interactions with others may be discouraged by client's use of passive or aggressive behaviors. *Knowledge of the use of assertive techniques could improve client's relationships with others.*
6. Provide direct feedback about client's interactions with others. Do this in a nonjudgmental manner. Help client learn how to respond more appropriately in interactions with others. Teach client skills which may be used to approach others in a more socially acceptable manner. Practice these skills through role play. *Client may not realize how he or she is being perceived by others. Direct feedback from a trusted individual may help to alter these behaviors in a positive manner. Having practiced these skills in role play facilitates their use in real situations.*
7. The depressed client must have lots of structure in his or her life due to the impairment in decision-making and problem-solving ability. Devise a plan of therapeutic activities and provide client with a written time schedule. *Remember:* The client who is moderately depressed feels best early in the day, whereas later in the day is a better time for the severely depressed individual to participate in activities.
8. Provide positive reinforcement for client's voluntary interactions with others. *Positive reinforcement enhances*

self-esteem and encourages repetition of desirable behaviors.

Outcome Criteria

1. Client demonstrates willingness and desire to socialize with others.
2. Client voluntarily attends group activities.
3. Client approaches others in appropriate manner for one-to-one interaction.

POWERLESSNESS

Definition: *The perception of the individual that his or her own action will not significantly affect an outcome; a perceived lack of control over a current situation or immediate happening.*

Possible Etiologies ("related to")

Lifestyle of helplessness
Health-care environment
[Dysfunctional grieving process]
[Lack of positive feedback]
[Consistent negative feedback]

Defining Characteristics ("evidenced by")

Verbal expressions of having no control or influence over situation, outcome, or self-care
Nonparticipation in care or decision making when opportunities are provided
Expression of doubt regarding role performance
Reluctance to express true feelings, fearing alienation from caregivers
Apathy
Dependence on others that may result in irritability, resentment, anger, and guilt
Passivity

Goals/Objectives
Short-Term Goal

Client will participate in decision making regarding own care within 5 days.

Long-Term Goal
Client will be able to effectively problem-solve ways to take control of his or her life situation by discharge from treatment, thereby decreasing feelings of powerlessness.

Interventions with *Selected Rationales*
1. Encourage client to take as much responsibility as possible for own self-care practices. *Providing client with choices will increase his or her feelings of control.* Examples:
   a. Include client in setting the goals of care he or she wishes to achieve.
   b. Allow client to establish own schedule for self-care activities.
   c. Provide client with privacy as need is determined.
   d. Provide positive feedback for decisions made. Respect client's right to make those decisions independently, and refrain from attempting to influence him or her toward those which may seem more logical.
2. Assist client to set realistic goals. *Unrealistic goals set the client up for failure and reinforce feelings of powerlessness.*
3. Help client identify areas of life situation that he or she can control. *Client's emotional condition interferes with his or her ability to solve problems. Assistance is required to perceive the benefits and consequences of available alternatives accurately.*
4. Help client identify areas of life situation that are not within his or her ability to control. Encourage verbalization of feelings related to this inability *in an effort to deal with unresolved issues and accept what cannot be changed.*
5. Identify ways in which client can achieve. Encourage participation in these activities, and provide positive reinforcement for participation, as well as for achievement. *Positive reinforcement enhances self-esteem and encourages repetition of desirable behaviors.*

Outcome Criteria
1. Client verbalizes choices made in a plan to maintain control over his or her life situation.
2. Client verbalizes honest feelings about life situations over which he or she has no control.
3. Client is able to verbalize system for problem solving as required for adequate role performance.

ALTERED THOUGHT PROCESSES

Definition: *A state in which an individual experiences a disruption in cognitive operations and activities.*

Possible Etiologies ("related to")
[Withdrawal into the self]
[Underdeveloped ego; punitive superego]
[Impaired cognition fostering negative perception of self and
   the environment]

Defining Characteristics ("evidenced by")
Inaccurate interpretation of environment
[Delusional thinking]
Hypovigilance
[Altered attention span]—distractibility
Egocentricity
[Impaired ability to make decisions, problem-solve, reason]
[Negative ruminations]

Goals/Objectives
Short-Term Goal
Client will recognize and verbalize when interpretations of the
   environment are inaccurate within 1 week.

Long-Term Goal
Client will experience no delusional or distorted thinking by
   discharge from treatment.

Interventions with *Selected Rationales*
1. Convey your acceptance of client's need for the false belief, while letting him or her know that you do not share the delusion. *A positive response would convey to the client that you accept the delusion as reality.*
2. Do not argue or deny the belief. Use *reasonable doubt* as a therapeutic technique: "I find that hard to believe." *Arguing with the client or denying the belief serves no useful purpose, as delusional ideas are not eliminated by this approach, and the development of a trusting relationship may be impeded.*
3. Use the techniques of *consensual validation* and *seeking clarification* when communication reflects alteration in thinking. (Examples: "Is it that you mean . . . ?" or "I don't understand what you mean by that. Would you please ex-

plain?'') *These techniques reveal to the client how he or she is being perceived by others, while the responsibility for not understanding is accepted by the nurse.*
4. Reinforce and focus on reality. Talk about real events and real people. Use real situations and events to divert client away from long, purposeless, repetitive verbalizations of false ideas.
5. Give positive reinforcement as client is able to differentiate between reality-based and nonreality-based thinking. *Positive reinforcement enhances self-esteem and encourages repetition of desirable behaviors.*
6. Teach client to intervene, using thought-stopping techniques, when irrational or negative thoughts prevail. *Thought stopping* involves using the command ''stop!'' or a loud noise (such as hand clapping) to interrupt unwanted thoughts. *This noise or command distracts the individual from the undesirable thinking that often precedes undesirable emotions or behaviors.*
7. Use touch cautiously, particularly if thoughts reveal ideas of persecution. *Clients who are suspicious may perceive touch as threatening and may respond with aggression.*

Outcome Criteria
1. Client's thinking processes reflect accurate interpretation of the environment.
2. Client is able to recognize negative or irrational thoughts and intervene to ''stop'' their progression.

ALTERED NUTRITION, LESS THAN BODY REQUIREMENTS

Definition: *The state in which an individual experiences an intake of nutrients insufficient to meet metabolic needs.*

Possible Etiologies ("related to")
Inability to ingest food because of:
[Depressed mood]
[Loss of appetite]
[Energy level too low to meet own nutritional needs]
[Regression to lower level of development]
[Ideas of self-destruction]
Lack of interest in food

Defining Characteristics ("evidenced by")
Loss of weight
Pale conjunctiva and mucous membranes
Poor muscle tone
[Amenorrhea]
[Poor skin turgor]
[Edema of extremities]
[Electrolyte imbalances]
[Weakness]
[Constipation]
[Anemias]

Goals/Objectives
Short-Term Goal
Client will gain 2 lb per week for the next 3 weeks.

Long-Term Goal
Client will exhibit no signs or symptoms of malnutrition by discharge from treatment (e.g., electrolytes and blood counts will be within normal limits; a steady weight gain will be demonstrated; constipation will be corrected; client will exhibit increased energy in participation of activities).

Interventions with *Selected Rationales*
1. In collaboration with dietitian, determine number of calories required to provide adequate nutrition and realistic (according to body structure and height) weight gain.
2. To prevent constipation, ensure that diet includes foods high in fiber content. Encourage client to increase fluid consumption and physical exercise to promote normal bowel functioning. *Depressed clients are particularly vulnerable to constipation because of psychomotor retardation. Constipation is also a common side effect of many antidepressant medications.*
3. Keep strict documentation of intake, output, and calorie count. *This information is necessary to make an accurate nutritional assessment and maintain client safety.*
4. Weigh client daily. *Weight loss or gain is important assessment information.*
5. Determine client's likes and dislikes and collaborate with dietitian to provide favorite foods. *Client is more likely to eat foods that he or she particularly enjoys.*
6. Ensure that client receives small, frequent feedings, including a bedtime snack, rather than three larger meals. *Large amounts of food may be objectionable, or even intolerable, to the client.*

7. Administer vitamin and mineral supplements and stool softeners or bulk extenders, as ordered by physician.
8. If appropriate, ask family members or significant others to bring in special foods that client particularly enjoys.
9. Stay with client during meals *to assist as needed and to offer support and encouragement.*
10. Monitor laboratory values, and report significant changes to physician. *Laboratory values provide objective data regarding nutritional status.*
11. Explain the importance of adequate nutrition and fluid intake. *Client may have inadequate or inaccurate knowledge regarding the contribution of good nutrition to overall wellness.*

Outcome Criteria
1. Client has shown a slow, progressive weight gain during hospitalization.
2. Vital signs, blood pressure, and laboratory serum studies are within normal limits.
3. Client is able to verbalize importance of adequate nutrition and fluid intake.

SLEEP PATTERN DISTURBANCE

Definition: *Disruption of sleep time that causes client discomfort or interferes with desired lifestyle.*

Possible Etiologies ("related to")
[Depressed mood]
[Repressed fears]
[Feelings of hopelessness]
[Fear of failure]
[Anxiety, moderate to severe]
[Hallucinations]
[Delusional thinking]

Defining Characteristics ("evidenced by")
Verbal complaints of difficulty falling asleep
Awakening earlier or later than desired
Interrupted sleep
Verbal complaints of not feeling well rested
[Remaining awake 30 minutes after going to bed]
[Awakening very early in the morning and being unable to go back to sleep]
[Excessive yawning and desire to nap during the day]
[Hypersomnia; using sleep as an escape]

Goals/Objectives
Short-Term Goal
Client will be able to sleep 4 to 6 hours with the aid of a sleeping medication within 5 days.

Long-Term Goal
Client will be able to fall asleep within 30 minutes of retiring, and obtain 6 to 8 hours of uninterrupted sleep each night without medication by discharge from treatment.

Interventions with *Selected Rationales*
1. Keep strict records of sleeping patterns. *Accurate baseline data are important in planning care to assist client with this problem.*
2. Discourage sleep during the day *to promote more restful sleep at night.*
3. Administer antidepressant medication at bedtime *so client does not become drowsy during the day.*
4. Assist with measures that may promote sleep, such as warm, nonstimulating drinks, light snacks, warm baths, back rubs.
5. Performing relaxation exercises to soft music may be helpful prior to sleep.
6. Limit intake of caffeinated drinks, such as tea, coffee, and colas. *Caffeine is a CNS stimulant that may interfere with the client's achievement of rest and sleep.*
7. Administer sedative medications, as ordered, *to assist client to achieve sleep until normal sleep pattern is restored.*
8. For client experiencing hypersomnia, set limits on time spent in room. Plan stimulating diversionary activities on a structured, daily schedule. Explore fears and feelings that sleep is helping to suppress.

Outcome Criteria
1. Client is sleeping 6 to 8 hours per night without medication.
2. Client is able to fall asleep within 30 minutes of retiring.
3. Client is dealing with fears and feelings rather than escaping from them through excessive sleep.

BIPOLAR DISORDER, MANIA

PREDISPOSING FACTORS
1. **Physiologic**
   a. ***Genetics.*** Studies indicate that there is an increased incidence of bipolar disorder in first-degree relatives

of individuals with the disorder than in the general population. If one identical twin has bipolar disorder, the possibility is as high as 80% that the other will also develop the disorder (Kolata, 1987). Bipolar disorder appears to be equally common in men and women (APA, 1994). Increasing evidence continues to support the role of genetics in the predisposition to bipolar disorder.

b. ***Biochemical.*** Just as there is an indication of lowered levels of norepinephrine and dopamine during an episode of depression, the opposite appears to be true of an individual experiencing a manic episode (Kaplan and Sadock, 1989). Thus, the behavioral responses of elation and euphoria may be caused by an excess of these biogenic amines in the brain. It has also been suggested that manic individuals have increased intracellular sodium and calcium. These electrolyte imbalances may be related to abnormalities in cellular membrane function in bipolar disorder.

2. **Psychosocial**

(NOTE: The credibility of psychosocial theories has declined in recent years. Conditions such as schizophrenia and bipolar disorder are being viewed by many as disorders of the brain with biologic etiologies. The etiology of these illnesses remains unclear, however, and it is possible that both biologic and psychosocial factors are influential. For this reason, a discussion of the psychoanalytic theory of bipolar disorder is included.)

a. ***Psychoanalytic Theory.*** This theory suggests that the mother (or primary caregiver) receives great pleasure from the early dependence of the infant (Haber et al, 1987). As the child matures and seeks increasing autonomy and independence, the mother begins to feel threatened. She labels the child "bad" as behaviors that assert independence continue. The child learns the necessity of fulfilling parental expectations in order to gain affection, even at the expense of negating his or her own needs and desires. This creates ambivalent feelings in the child, who comes to resent the demands made by the parents, while yet strongly desiring to please them. The dynamics of bipolar disorder arise out of this love-hate relationship with the parents. Ego development is disrupted, giving way to a punitive superego (anger turned inward—depression). When the depression subsides, the ego may yet be too weak to control the impulsive, excessive behavior dominated by the id (the manifestations of mania). In this psychoanalytic model, mania is viewed as the mirror image of depression— a "denial of inner depression" (Kaplan and Sadock, 1989).

SYMPTOMATOLOGY (Subjective and Objective Data)

1. The affect of a manic individual is one of elation and euphoria—a continuous "high." However, the affect is very labile and may change quickly to hostility, particularly in response to attempts at limit setting, or to sadness, ruminating about past failures.
2. Alterations in thought processes and communication patterns are manifested by the following:
   a. *Flight of Ideas.* There is a continuous, rapid shift from one topic to another.
   b. *Loquaciousness.* The pressure of the speech is so forceful and strong that it is difficult to interrupt maladaptive thought processes.
   c. *Delusions of Grandeur.* The individual believes he or she is all important, all powerful, with feelings of greatness and magnificence.
   d. *Delusions of Persecution.* The individual believes someone or something desires to harm or violate him or her in some way.
3. Motor activity is constant. The individual is literally moving at all times.
4. Dress is often inappropriate: bright colors that do not match; clothing inappropriate for age or stature; excessive makeup and jewelry.
5. The individual has a meager appetite, despite excessive activity level. He or she is unable or unwilling to stop moving in order to eat.
6. Sleep patterns are disturbed. Client becomes oblivious to feelings of fatigue, and rest and sleep are abandoned for days or weeks.
7. Spending sprees are common. Individual spends large amounts of money, which is not available, on numerous items, which are not needed.
8. Usual inhibitions are discarded in favor of sexual and behavioral indiscretions.

9. Manipulative behavior and limit testing are common in the attempt to fulfill personal desires. Verbal or physical hostility may follow his or her failure in these attempts.
10. Projection is a major defense mechanism. The individual refuses to accept responsibility for the negative consequences of personal behavior.
11. There is an inability to concentrate because of a limited attention span. The individual is easily distracted by even the slightest stimulus in the environment.
12. Alterations in sensory perception may occur, and the individual may experience hallucinations.
13. As agitation increases, symptoms intensify. Unless the client is placed in a protective environment, death can occur from exhaustion or injury.

COMMON NURSING DIAGNOSES AND INTERVENTIONS FOR MANIA
(Interventions are applicable to various health-care settings, such as inpatient and partial hospitalization, community outpatient clinic, home health, and private practice.)

RISK FOR INJURY

Definition: *A state in which the individual is at risk of injury as a result of environmental conditions interacting with the individual's adaptive and defensive resources.*

Related/Risk Factors ("related to")
[Extreme hyperactivity]
[Destructive behaviors]
[Anger directed at the environment]
[Hitting head (hand, arm, foot, etc.) against wall when angry]
[Temper tantrums—becomes destructive of inanimate objects]
[Increased agitation and lack of control over purposeless, and potentially injurious, movements]

Goals/Objectives
Short-Term Goal
Client will no longer exhibit potentially injurious movements after 24 hours with administration of tranquilizing medication.

Long-Term Goal
Client will experience no physical injury.

Interventions with *Selected Rationales*
1. Reduce environmental stimuli. Assign private room, if possible, with soft lighting, low noise level, and simple room decor. *In hyperactive state, client is extremely distractible, and responses to even the slightest stimuli are exaggerated.*
2. Assign to quiet unit, if possible. *Milieu unit may be too distracting.*
3. Limit group activities. Help client try to establish one or two close relationships. *Client's ability to interact with others is impaired. He or she feels more secure in a one-to-one relationship that is consistent over time.*
4. Remove hazardous objects and substances from client's environment (including smoking materials). *Client's rationality is impaired, and he or she may harm self inadvertently. Client safety is a nursing priority.*
5. Stay with the client *to offer support and provide a feeling of security* as agitation grows and hyperactivity increases.
6. Provide structured schedule of activities that includes established rest periods throughout the day. *A structured schedule provides a feeling of security for the client.*
7. Provide physical activities as a substitution for purposeless hyperactivity. (Examples: brisk walks, housekeeping chores, dance therapy, aerobics.) *Physical exercise provides a safe and effective means of relieving pent-up tension.*
8. Administer tranquilizing medication, as ordered by physician. Antipsychotic drugs, such as chlorpromazine (Thorazine) or haloperidol (Haldol), are commonly prescribed for rapid relief of agitation and hyperactivity. Observe for effectiveness and evidence of adverse side effects.

Outcome Criteria
1. Client is no longer exhibiting signs of physical agitation.
2. Client exhibits no evidence of physical injury obtained while experiencing hyperactive behavior.

RISK FOR VIOLENCE: SELF-DIRECTED OR DIRECTED AT OTHERS

Definition: *Behaviors in which an individual demonstrates that he/she can be physically, emotionally, and/or sexually harmful either to self or to others.*

Related/Risk Factors ("related to")
Manic excitement
[Dysfunctional grieving—denial of depression]
[Hereditary factors]
[Biochemical alterations]
[Threat to self-concept]
[Suspicion of others]
[Paranoid ideation]
[Delusions]
[Hallucinations]
[Rage reactions]
Body language—rigid posture, clenching of fists and jaw, hyperactivity, pacing, breathlessness, and threatening stances
[History or threats of violence toward self or others or of destruction to the property of others]
Impulsivity
Suicidal ideation, plan, available means
Repetition of verbalizations (continuous complaints, requests, and demands)

Goals/Objectives
Short-Term Goal
Client's agitation will be maintained at manageable level with the administration of tranquilizing medication during first week of treatment (decreasing risk of violence to self or others).

Long-Term Goal
Client will not harm self or others.

Interventions with *Selected Rationales*
1. Maintain low level of stimuli in client's environment (low lighting, few people, simple decor, low noise level). *Anxiety and agitation rise in a stimulating environment. Individuals may be perceived as threatening by a suspicious, agitated client.*

2. Observe client's behavior frequently (every 15 minutes). *Close observation is required so that intervention can occur if required to ensure client's (and others') safety.*

3. Remove all dangerous objects from client's environment (sharp objects, glass or mirrored items, belts, ties, smoking materials) *so that in his or her agitated, hyperactive state, client may not use them to harm self or others.*

4. Try to redirect the violent behavior with physical outlets for the client's hostility (e.g., punching bag). *Physical exercise is a safe and effective way of relieving pent-up tension.*

5. Staff should maintain and convey a calm attitude to the client. Respond matter-of-factly to verbal hostility. *Anxiety is contagious and can be transmitted from staff to client.*

6. Have sufficient staff available to indicate a show of strength to client if necessary. *This conveys to the client evidence of control over the situation and provides some physical security for staff.*

7. Administer tranquilizing medications as ordered by physician. Monitor medication for effectiveness and for adverse side effects.

8. If the client is not calmed by "talking down" or by medication, use mechanical restraints as necessary. Be sure to have sufficient staff available to assist. Follow protocol established by the institution. Most states require that the physician reevaluate and issue a new order for restraints every 3 hours, except between midnight and 8:00 AM. If the client has refused medication, administer after restraints have been applied. Most states consider this intervention appropriate in emergency situations or in the event that a client would likely harm self or others.

9. Observe the client in restraints every 15 minutes (or according to institutional policy). Ensure that circulation to extremities is not compromised (check temperature, color, pulses). Assist client with needs related to nutrition, hydration, and elimination. Position client so that comfort is facilitated and aspiration can be prevented. *Client safety is a nursing priority.*

10. As agitation decreases, assess client's readiness for restraint removal or reduction. Remove one restraint at a time, while assessing client's response. *This procedure minimizes the risk of injury to client and staff.*

Outcome Criteria
1. Client is able to verbalize anger in an appropriate manner.
2. There is no evidence of violent behavior to self or others.
3. Client is no longer exhibiting hyperactive behaviors.

ALTERED NUTRITION, LESS THAN BODY REQUIREMENTS

Definition: *The state in which an individual experiences an intake of nutrients insufficient to meet metabolic needs.*

Possible Etiologies ("related to")
[Refusal or inability to sit still long enough to eat meals]
[Lack of appetite]
[Excessive physical agitation]
[Physical exertion in excess of energy produced through caloric intake]
Lack of interest in food

Defining Characteristics ("evidenced by")
Loss of weight
Pale conjunctiva and mucous membranes
Poor muscle tone
[Amenorrhea]
[Poor skin turgor]
[Anemias]
[Electrolyte imbalances]

Goals/Objectives
Short-Term Goal
Client will consume sufficient finger foods and between-meal snacks to meet recommended daily allowances of nutrients.

Long-Term Goal
Client will exhibit no signs or symptoms of malnutrition.

Interventions with *Selected Rationales*
1. In collaboration with dietitian, determine number of calories required to provide adequate nutrition for maintenance or realistic (according to body structure and height) weight gain.

2. Provide client with high-protein, high-calorie, nutritious finger foods and drinks that can be consumed "on the run." *Because of hyperactive state, client has difficulty sitting still long enough to eat a meal. The likelihood is greater that he or she will consume food and drinks that can be carried around and eaten with little effort.*

3. Have juice and snacks available on the unit at all times. *Nutritious intake is required on a regular basis to compensate for increased caloric requirements due to hyperactivity.*

4. Maintain accurate record of intake, output, and calorie count. *This information is necessary to make an accurate nutritional assessment and maintain client's safety.*

5. Weigh client daily. *Weight loss or gain is important nutritional assessment information.*

6. Determine client's likes and dislikes, and collaborate with dietitian to provide favorite foods. *Client is more likely to eat foods that he or she particularly enjoys.*

7. Administer vitamin and mineral supplements, as ordered by physician, *to improve nutritional state.*

8. Pace or walk with client as finger foods are taken. As agitation subsides, sit with client during meals. Offer support and encouragement. Assess and record amount consumed. *Presence of a trusted individual may provide feeling of security and decrease agitation. Encouragement and positive reinforcement increase self-esteem and foster repetition of desired behaviors.*

9. Monitor laboratory values, and report significant changes to physician. *Laboratory values provide objective nutritional assessment data.*

10. Explain the importance of adequate nutrition and fluid intake. *Client may have inadequate or inaccurate knowledge regarding the contribution of good nutrition to overall wellness.*

Outcome Criteria

1. Client has gained (maintained) weight during hospitalization.

2. Vital signs, blood pressure, and laboratory serum studies are within normal limits.

3. Client is able to verbalize importance of adequate nutrition and fluid intake.

ALTERED THOUGHT PROCESSES

Definition: *A state in which an individual experiences a disruption in cognitive operations and activities.*

Possible Etiologies ("related to")
[Hereditary factors]
[Biochemical alterations]
[Unmet dependency needs]
[Unresolved grief—denial of depression]

Defining Characteristics ("evidenced by")
Inaccurate interpretation of environment
Hypervigilance
[Altered attention span]—distractibility
Egocentricity
[Decreased ability to grasp ideas]
[Inability to follow]
[Impaired ability to make decisions, problem-solve, reason]
[Delusions of grandeur]
[Delusions of persecution]
[Suspiciousness]

Goals/Objectives
Short-Term Goal
Within 1 week, client will be able to recognize and verbalize
  when thinking is nonreality-based.

Long-Term Goal
Client will experience no delusional thinking by discharge
  from treatment.

Interventions with *Selected Rationales*
1. Convey your acceptance of client's need for the false belief, while letting him or her know that you do not share the delusion. *A positive response would convey to the client that you accept the delusion as reality.*
2. Do not argue or deny the belief. Use *reasonable doubt* as a therapeutic technique: "I find that hard to believe." *Arguing with the client or denying the belief serves no useful purpose, because delusional ideas are not eliminated by this approach, and the development of a trusting relationship may be impeded.*
3. Use the techniques of *consensual validation* and *seeking clarification* when communication reflects alteration in thinking. (Examples: "Is it that you mean . . . ?" or "I don't

understand what you mean by that. Would you please explain?'') *These techniques reveal to the client how he or she is being perceived by others, and the responsibility for not understanding is accepted by the nurse.*

4. Reinforce and focus on reality. Talk about real events and real people. Use real situations and events to divert client away from long, tedious, repetitive verbalizations of false ideas.

5. Give positive reinforcement as client is able to differentiate between reality-based and nonreality-based thinking. *Positive reinforcement enhances self-esteem and encourages repetition of desirable behaviors.*

6. Teach client to intervene, using thought-stopping techniques, when irrational thoughts prevail. Thought stopping involves using the command ''Stop!'' or a loud noise (such as hand clapping) to interrupt unwanted thoughts. *This noise or command distracts the individual from the undesirable thinking, which often precedes undesirable emotions or behaviors.*

7. Use touch cautiously, particularly if thoughts reveal ideas of persecution. *Clients who are suspicious may perceive touch as threatening and may respond with aggression.*

Outcome Criteria
1. Thought processes reflect an accurate interpretation of environment.
2. Client is able to recognize thoughts that are not based in reality, and intervene to stop their progression.

SENSORY-PERCEPTUAL ALTERATION

Definition: A state in which an individual experiences a change in the amount or patterning of oncoming stimuli [either internally or externally initiated] accompanied by a diminished, exaggerated, distorted or impaired response to such stimuli.

Possible Etiologies (''related to'')
[Hereditary factors]
[Biochemical alterations]
[Unmet dependency needs]
[Unresolved grief—denial of depression]
[Sleep deprivation]

Defining Characteristics ("evidenced by")
Change in usual response to stimuli
Hallucinations
Disorientation
Inappropriate responses
[Rapid mood swings]
[Exaggerated emotional responses]
[Visual and auditory distortions]
[Talking and laughing to self]
[Listening pose (tilting head to one side as if listening)]
[Stops talking in middle of sentence to listen]

Goals/Objectives
Short-Term Goal
Client will be able to recognize and verbalize when he or she
is interpreting the environment inaccurately.

Long-Term Goal
Client will be able to define and test reality, eliminating the
occurrence of sensory misperceptions.

Interventions with *Selected Rationales*
1. Observe client for signs of hallucinations (listening pose,
laughing or talking to self, stopping in midsentence). *Early
intervention may prevent aggressive responses to
command hallucinations.*
2. Avoid touching the client before warning him or her that
you are about to do so. *Client may perceive touch as
threatening and respond in an aggressive manner.*
3. An attitude of acceptance will encourage the client to
share the content of the hallucination with you. *This is
important in order to prevent possible injury to the client or others from command hallucinations.*
4. Do not reinforce the hallucination. Use "the voices" in-
stead of words like "they" that imply validation. Let the
client know that you do not share the perception. Say,
"Even though I realize that the voices are real to you, I do
not hear any voices speaking." *The nurse must be honest with the client so that he or she may realize that
the hallucinations are not real.*
5. Try to connect the times of the misperceptions to times
of increased anxiety. Help client to understand this connection. *If client can learn to interrupt the escalating
anxiety, reality orientation may be maintained.*
6. Try to distract the client away from the misperception.
*Involvement in interpersonal activities and explana-
tion of the actual situation may bring the client back to
reality.*

Outcome Criteria

1. Client is able to differentiate between reality and unrealistic events or situations.
2. Client is able to refrain from responding to false sensory perceptions.

IMPAIRED SOCIAL INTERACTION

Definition: *The state in which an individual participates in an insufficient or excessive quantity or ineffective quality of social exchange.*

Possible Etiologies ("related to")

Altered thought processes
[Strong dependency needs]
[Delusions of grandeur]
[Delusions of persecution]
[Underdeveloped ego]
[Low self-esteem]

Defining Characteristics ("evidenced by")

Verbalized or observed discomfort in social situations
Verbalized or observed inability to receive or communicate a satisfying sense of belonging, caring, interest, or shared history
Observed use of unsuccessful social interaction behaviors
Dysfunctional interaction with peers, family and others
[Excessive use of projection—does not accept responsibility for own behavior]
[Verbal manipulation]
[Inability to delay gratification]

Goals/Objectives
Short-Term Goal
Client will verbalize which of his or her interaction behaviors are appropriate and which are inappropriate within 1 week.

Long-Term Goal
Client will demonstrate use of appropriate interaction skills as evidenced by lack of, or marked decrease in, manipulation of others to fulfill own desires.

Interventions with *Selected Rationales*

1. Recognize the purpose these behaviors serve for the client: to reduce feelings of insecurity by increasing feelings of power and control. *Understanding the motivation be-*

hind the manipulation may facilitate acceptance of the individual and his or her behavior.

2. Set limits on manipulative behaviors. Explain to client what you expect and what the consequences are if the limits are violated. Limits must be agreed upon by all staff who will be working with the client. *Client is unable to establish own limits, so this must be done for him or her. Unless administration of consequences for violation of limits is consistent, manipulative behavior will not be eliminated.*

3. Do not argue, bargain, or try to reason with the client. Merely state what the limits are and what is expected. Be sure to follow through with consequences if limits are violated. *Consistency is essential for success of this intervention.* Do not let this "charmer" talk you out of it. *Ignoring these attempts may work to decrease manipulative behaviors.*

4. Provide positive reinforcement for nonmanipulative behaviors. Explore feelings, and help the client seek more appropriate ways of dealing with them. *Positive reinforcement enhances self-esteem and promotes repetition of desirable behaviors.*

5. Help client recognize consequences of own behaviors and refrain from attributing them to others. *Client must accept responsibility for own behaviors before adaptive change can occur.*

6. Help client identify positive aspects about self, recognize accomplishments, and feel good about them. *As self-esteem is increased, client will feel less need to manipulate others for own gratification.*

Outcome Criteria
1. Client is able to verbalize positive aspects about self.
2. Client accepts responsibility for own behaviors.
3. Client does not manipulate others for gratification of own needs.

SLEEP PATTERN DISTURBANCE

Definition: *Disruption of sleep time, which causes client discomfort or interferes with desired lifestyle.*

Possible Etiologies ("related to")
[Excessive hyperactivity]
[Agitation]
[Biochemical alterations]

Defining Characteristics ("evidenced by")
[Pacing in hall during sleeping hours]
[Remaining awake 45 minutes after retiring]
[Sleeping only short periods at a time]
[Numerous periods of wakefulness during the night]
[Awakening and rising extremely early in the morning; exhibiting signs of restlessness]

Goals/Objectives
Short-Term Goal
With the aid of a sleeping medication, within 3 days, client will sleep 4 to 6 hours without awakening.

Long-Term Goal
By discharge from treatment, client will be able to acquire 6 to 8 hours of uninterrupted sleep without medication.

Interventions with *Selected Rationales*
1. Provide a quiet environment, with a low level of stimulation. *Hyperactivity increases and ability to achieve sleep and rest are hindered in a stimulating environment.*
2. Monitor sleep patterns. Provide structured schedule of activities that includes established times for naps or rest. *Accurate baseline data are important in planning care to assist client with this problem. A structured schedule, including time for naps, will help the hyperactive client achieve much-needed rest.*
3. Assess client's activity level. Client may ignore or be unaware of feelings of fatigue. Observe for signs such as increasing restlessness; fine tremors; slurred speech; and puffy, dark circles under eyes. *Client can collapse from exhaustion if hyperactivity is uninterrupted and rest is not achieved.*
4. Before bedtime, provide nursing measures that promote sleep, such as back rub; warm bath; warm, nonstimulating drinks; soft music; and relaxation exercises.
5. Prohibit intake of caffeinated drinks, such as tea, coffee, and colas. *Caffeine is a CNS stimulant and may interfere with the client's achievement of rest and sleep.*
6. Administer sedative medications, as ordered, to assist client achieve sleep until normal sleep pattern is restored.

Outcome Criteria
1. Client is sleeping 6 to 8 hours per night without medication.
2. Within 30 minutes of retiring, client is able to fall asleep.
3. Client is dealing openly with fears and feelings rather than manifesting denial of them through hyperactivity.

Chapter 9
ANXIETY DISORDERS

BACKGROUND ASSESSMENT DATA

The characteristic features of this group of disorders are symptoms of anxiety and avoidance behavior. Anxiety disorders are categorized in the following manner:

PANIC DISORDER (With or Without Agoraphobia)
Panic disorder is characterized by recurrent panic attacks, the onset of which are unpredictable, and manifested by intense apprehension, fear, or terror, often associated with feelings of impending doom, and accompanied by intense physical discomfort. The attacks usually last minutes or, more rarely, hours. If accompanied by agoraphobia, there is a fear of being in places or situations from which escape might be difficult or in which help might not be available in the event of a panic attack (APA, 1994). Common agoraphobic situations include being outside the home alone; being in a crowd or standing in a line; being on a bridge; and traveling in a bus, train, or car.

AGORAPHOBIA WITHOUT HISTORY OF PANIC DISORDER
The *DSM-IV* identifies the essential feature of this disorder as fear of being in places or situations from which escape might be difficult, or in which help might not be available in the event of suddenly developing a symptom(s) that could be incapacitating or extremely embarrassing. Travel

is restricted, or the individual needs a companion when away from home, or else endures agoraphobic situations despite intense anxiety.

SOCIAL PHOBIA

Social phobia is characterized by a persistent fear of behaving or performing in the presence of others in a way that will be humiliating or embarrassing to the individual. The individual has extreme concerns about being exposed to possible scrutiny by others and fears social or performance situations in which embarrassment may occur (APA, 1994). Exposure to the phobic situation is avoided, or endured with intense anxiety. Common social phobias include speaking or writing in front of a group of people, eating in the presence of others, and using public restrooms.

SPECIFIC PHOBIA

Formerly called simple phobia, this disorder is characterized by persistent fears of specific objects or situations. These phobias are fairly widespread among the general population, the most common being fear of animals (zoophobia), fear of closed places (claustrophobia), and fear of heights (acrophobia). Exposure to the phobic stimulus is avoided or endured with intense anxiety.

OBSESSIVE-COMPULSIVE DISORDER

This disorder is characterized by involuntary recurring thoughts or images which the individual is unable to ignore, and recurring impulse to perform a seemingly purposeless activity. These obsessions and compulsions serve to prevent extreme anxiety on the part of the individual.

POSTTRAUMATIC STRESS DISORDER

Posttraumatic stress disorder (PTSD) is characterized by the development of physiologic and behavioral symptoms following a psychologically traumatic event that is generally outside the range of usual human experience. The stressor, which would be considered markedly distressing to almost anyone, has usually been experienced with intense fear, terror, and helplessness. If duration of the symptoms is 3 months or more, the diagnosis is specified as "chronic." If there is a delay of 6 months or more in the onset of symptoms, the diagnosis is specified as "delayed onset."

GENERALIZED ANXIETY DISORDER

This disorder is characterized by chronic, unrealistic, and excessive anxiety and worry. The symptoms must have occurred more days than not for at least 6 months and must cause clinically significant distress or impairment in social, occupational, or other important areas of functioning. Symptoms include restlessness, feeling "on edge," easily fatigued, difficulty concentrating, and irritability.

ANXIETY DISORDER DUE TO A GENERAL MEDICAL CONDITION

The symptoms of this disorder are judged to be the direct physiologic consequence of a general medical condition. Symptoms may include prominent generalized anxiety symptoms, panic attacks, or obsessions or compulsions (APA, 1994). Medical conditions that have been known to cause anxiety disorders include endocrine, cardiovascular, respiratory, metabolic, and neurologic conditions.

SUBSTANCE-INDUCED ANXIETY DISORDER

The *DSM-IV* (APA, 1994) describes the essential features of this disorder as prominent anxiety symptoms that are judged to be caused by the direct physiologic effects of a substance (i.e., a drug of abuse, a medication, or toxin exposure). The symptoms may occur during substance intoxication or withdrawal, and may involve prominent anxiety, panic attacks, phobias, or obsessions or compulsions.

PREDISPOSING FACTORS

1. **Physiologic**
   a. *Biochemical.* Although biochemical and neurophysiologic influences in the etiology of these disorders has been investigated, no definitive relationship has yet been established. Increased levels of norepinephrine have been noted in panic and generalized anx-

iety disorders. Decreased levels of serotonin have been implicated in the etiology of obsessive-compulsive disorder.

b. *Genetic.* Studies suggest that anxiety disorders are prevalent within the general population. It has been shown that they are more common among first-degree biologic relatives of people with the disorders than among the general population (APA, 1994).

c. *Medical or Substance-Induced.* Anxiety disorders may be caused by a variety of medical conditions or the ingestion of various substances. (Refer to previous section on categories of anxiety disorders.)

2. **Psychosocial**

a. *Psychodynamic.* This theory (Erikson, 1963) suggests a predisposition to anxiety disorders when tasks assigned to earlier developmental stages go unresolved. In response to stress, behaviors associated with these earlier stages appear, as the individual regresses to, or is fixated in, the earlier level of development.

b. *Interpersonal.* Sullivan (1953) attributes the anxiety response to difficulty in interpersonal relationships that stem from the early mother (primary caregiver)-child relationship. The child does not receive the unconditional love and nurturing he or she requires. Futile attempts to "earn" this love result in a fragile ego and the persistent fear of disapproval from others throughout life.

c. *Sociocultural.* Horney (1939) suggests that anxiety disorders are predisposed by a multitude of contradictions occurring within our society that contribute to feelings of insecurity and helplessness. (Example: Teaching that "all men are created equal," as the child grows up observing numerous inequalities.)

SYMPTOMATOLOGY (Subjective and Objective Data)

An individual may experience a panic attack under any of the following conditions:

- As the predominant disturbance, with no apparent precipitant
- When exposed to a phobic stimulus
- When attempts are made to curtail ritualistic behavior
- Following a psychologically traumatic event

Symptoms include the following (APA, 1994):

- Palpitations, pounding heart, or accelerated heart rate
- Sweating
- Trembling or shaking
- Sensations of shortness of breath or smothering
- Feeling of choking
- Chest pain or discomfort
- Nausea or abdominal distress
- Feeling dizzy, unsteady, lightheaded, or faint
- Derealization (feelings of unreality) or depersonalization (being detached from oneself)
- Fear of losing control or going crazy
- Fear of dying
- Paresthesias (numbness or tingling sensations)
- Chills or hot flashes

Other symptoms of anxiety disorders include the following:

1. Restlessness, feeling "on edge," excessive worry, being easily fatigued, difficulty concentrating, irritability, muscle tension, and sleep disturbances (generalized anxiety disorder).
2. Recurrent and intrusive recollections or dreams about the traumatic event, feeling of reliving the trauma (flashback episodes), difficulty feeling emotion (a "numbing" affect), insomnia, irritability or outbursts of anger (PTSD).
3. Repetitive, obsessive thoughts, common ones being related to violence, contamination, and doubt; repetitive, compulsive performance of purposeless activity, such as handwashing, counting, checking, touching (obsessive-compulsive disorder).
4. Marked and persistent fears of specific objects or situations (specific phobia), social or performance situations (social phobia), or being in a situation from which one has difficulty escaping (agoraphobia).

COMMON NURSING DIAGNOSES AND INTERVENTIONS
(Interventions are applicable to various health-care settings, such as inpatient and partial hospitalization, community outpatient clinic, home health, and private practice.)

ANXIETY (PANIC)

Definition: *A vague uneasy feeling, the source of which is often nonspecific or unknown to the individual.*

Possible Etiologies ("related to")
Unconscious conflict about essential values and goals of life
Situational and maturational crises
[Real or perceived] threat to self-concept
[Real or perceived] threat of death
Unmet needs
[Fixation in earlier level of development]
[Being exposed to a phobic stimulus]
[Attempts at interference with ritualistic behaviors]
[Traumatic experience]

Defining Characteristics ("evidenced by")
[Dyspnea]
[Palpitations]
[Chest pain or discomfort]
[Choking or smothering sensations]
[Dizziness, vertigo, or unsteady feelings]
[Feelings of unreality]
[Paresthesias]
[Hot and cold flashes]
[Sweating]
[Faintness]
[Trembling or shaking]
[Fear of dying, going crazy, or doing something uncontrolled
   during an attack]
Restlessness
Insomnia
[Nausea or abdominal distress]
[Nightmares or visual perceptions of traumatic event]

Goals/Objectives
Short-Term Goal
Client will verbalize ways to intervene in escalating anxiety
   within 1 week.

Long-Term Goal
Client will be able to recognize symptoms of onset of anxiety
   and intervene before reaching panic stage by discharge
   from treatment.

Interventions with *Selected Rationales*

1. Maintain a calm, nonthreatening manner while working with client. *Anxiety is contagious and may be transferred from staff to client or vice versa. Client develops feeling of security in presence of calm staff person.*

2. Reassure client of his or her safety and security. This can be conveyed by physical presence of nurse. Do not leave client alone at this time. *Client may fear for his or her life. Presence of a trusted individual provides client with feeling of security and assurance of personal safety.*

3. Use simple words and brief messages, spoken calmly and clearly, to explain hospital experiences to client. *In an intensely anxious situation, client is unable to comprehend anything but the most elemental communication.*

4. Keep immediate surroundings low in stimuli (dim lighting, few people, simple decor). *A stimulating environment may increase level of anxiety.*

5. Administer tranquilizing medication, as ordered by physician. Assess medication for effectiveness and for adverse side effects.

6. When level of anxiety has been reduced, explore with client possible reasons for occurrence. *Recognition of precipitating factor(s) is the first step in teaching the client to interrupt escalation of the anxiety.*

7. Encourage client to talk about traumatic experience under nonthreatening conditions. Help client work through feelings of guilt related to the traumatic event. Help client understand that this was an event to which most people would have responded in like manner. Support client during flashbacks of the experience. *Verbalization of feelings in a nonthreatening environment may help client come to terms with unresolved issues.*

8. Teach signs and symptoms of escalating anxiety, and ways to interrupt its progression (e.g., relaxation techniques, deep-breathing exercises, physical exercises, brisk walks, jogging, meditation).

Outcome Criteria

1. Client is able to maintain anxiety at level in which problem solving can be accomplished.

2. Client is able to verbalize signs and symptoms of escalating anxiety.

3. Client is able to demonstrate techniques for interrupting the progression of anxiety to the panic level.

FEAR

Definition: *A feeling of dread related to an identifiable source which the person validates.*

Possible Etiologies ("related to")
[Specific phobias]
[Being in place or situation from which escape might be difficult]
[Causing embarrassment to self in front of others]

Defining Characteristics ("evidenced by")
[Refuses to leave own home alone]
[Refuses to eat in public]
[Refuses to speak or perform in public]
[Refuses to expose self to (specify phobic object or situation)]
Subjective ability to identify fearful object or situation
Symptoms of apprehension or sympathetic stimulation in presence of phobic object or situation

Goals/Objectives
Short-Term Goal
Client will discuss phobic object or situation with nurse or therapist within 5 days.

Long-Term Goal
Client will be able to function in presence of phobic object or situation without experiencing panic anxiety by discharge from treatment.

Interventions with *Selected Rationales*
1. Reassure client of his or her safety and security. *At panic level of anxiety, client may fear for own life.*
2. Explore client's perception of threat to physical integrity or threat to self-concept. *It is important to understand the client's perception of the phobic object or situation in order to assist with the desensitization process.*
3. Discuss reality of the situation with client in order to recognize aspects that can be changed and those that cannot. *Client must accept the reality of the situation (aspects that cannot change) before the work of reducing the fear can progress.*
4. Include client in making decisions related to selection of alternative coping strategies. (Example: Client may choose either to avoid the phobic stimulus or attempt to eliminate the fear associated with it.) *Allowing the client*

choices provides a measure of control and serves to increase feelings of self-worth.

5. If the client elects to work on elimination of the fear, techniques of desensitization may be employed. This is a systematic plan of behavior modification, designed to expose the individual gradually to the situation or object (either in reality or through fantasizing) until the fear is no longer experienced. This is also sometimes accomplished through implosion therapy, in which the individual is "flooded" with stimuli related to the phobic situation or object (rather than in gradual steps) until anxiety is no longer experienced in relation to the object or situation. *Fear is decreased as the physical and psychological sensations diminish in response to repeated exposure to the phobic stimulus under nonthreatening conditions.*

6. Encourage client to explore underlying feelings that may be contributing to irrational fears. Help client to understand how facing these feelings, rather than suppressing them, can result in more adaptive coping abilities. *Verbalization of feelings in a nonthreatening environment may help client come to terms with unresolved issues.*

Outcome Criteria

1. Client does not experience disabling fear when exposed to phobic object or situation, *or*
2. Client verbalizes ways in which he or she will be able to avoid the phobic object or situation with minimal change in lifestyle.
3. Client is able to demonstrate adaptive coping techniques that may be used to maintain anxiety at a tolerable level.

INEFFECTIVE INDIVIDUAL COPING

Definition: *The impairment of adaptive behaviors and abilities of a person in meeting life's demands.*

Possible Etiologies ("related to")

[Fixation in earlier level of development]
[Underdeveloped ego; punitive superego]
[Fear of failure]
[Unmet dependency needs]
Situational crises

Personal vulnerability
[Inadequate support systems]
Maturational crises

Defining Characteristics ("evidenced by")
[Ritualistic behavior]
[Obsessive thoughts]
Inability to meet basic needs
Inability to meet role expectations
Inability to problem-solve
Alteration in societal participation

Goals/Objectives
Short-Term Goal
Within 1 week, client will decrease participation in ritualistic
    behavior to half of time being spent in ritualistic behavior
    on admission.

Long-Term Goal
By discharge from treatment, client will demonstrate ability
    to cope effectively without resorting to obsessive-compul-
    sive behaviors or increased dependency.

Interventions with *Selected Rationales*
1. Assess client's level of anxiety. Try to determine the types
   of situations that increase anxiety and result in ritualistic
   behaviors. *Recognition of precipitating factors is the
   first step in teaching the client to interrupt the escalating anxiety.*
2. Initially meet client's dependency needs as required. Encourage independence and give positive reinforcement
   for independent behaviors. *Sudden and complete elimination of all avenues for dependency would create intense anxiety on the part of the client. Positive reinforcement enhances self-esteem and encourages
   repetition of desired behaviors.*
3. In the beginning of treatment allow plenty of time for rituals. Do not be judgmental or verbalize disapproval of the
   behavior. *To deny client this activity may precipitate
   panic level of anxiety.*
4. Support client's efforts to explore the meaning and purpose of the behavior. *Client may be unaware of the relationship between emotional problems and compulsive behaviors. Recognition is important before
   change can occur.*

5. Provide structured schedule of activities for the client, including adequate time for completion of rituals. *Structure provides a feeling of security for the anxious client.*
6. Gradually begin to limit amount of time alloted for ritualistic behavior as client becomes more involved in unit activities. *Anxiety is minimized when client is able to replace ritualistic behaviors with more adaptive ones.*
7. Give positive reinforcement for nonritualistic behaviors. *Positive reinforcement enhances self-esteem and encourages repetition of desired behaviors.*
8. Encourage recognition of situations that provoke obsessive thoughts or ritualistic behaviors. Explain ways of interrupting these thoughts and patterns of behavior (e.g., thought-stopping techniques, relaxation techniques, physical exercise, or other constructive activity with which client feels comfortable).

Outcome Criteria
1. Client is able to verbalize signs and symptoms of increasing anxiety and intervene to maintain anxiety at manageable level.
2. Client demonstrates ability to interrupt obsessive thoughts and refrain from ritualistic behaviors in response to stressful situations.

POWERLESSNESS

Definition: The perception that one's own action will not significantly affect an outcome; a perceived lack of control over a current situation or immediate happening.

Possible Etiologies ("related to")
Lifestyle of helplessness
[Fear of disapproval from others]
[Fixation in earlier level of development]
[Unmet dependency needs]
[Lack of positive feedback]
[Consistent negative feedback]

Defining Characteristics ("evidenced by")
Verbal expressions of having no control or influence over situation, outcome, or self-care

Nonparticipation in care or decision making when opportunities are provided

Expression of doubt regarding role performance

Reluctance to express true feelings, fearing alienation from caregivers

Apathy

Dependence on others that may result in irritability, resentment, anger, and guilt

Passivity

Goals/Objectives
Short-Term Goal

Client will participate in decision making regarding own care within 5 days.

Long-Term Goal

Client will be able to effectively problem-solve ways to take control of his or her life situation by discharge, thereby decreasing feelings of powerlessness.

Interventions with *Selected Rationales*

1. Allow client to take as much responsibility as possible for own self-care practices. *Providing client with choices will increase his or her feelings of control.* Examples are as follows:
   a. Include client in setting the goals of care he or she wishes to achieve.
   b. Allow client to establish own schedule for self-care activities.
   c. Provide client with privacy as need is determined.
   d. Provide positive feedback for decisions made. Respect client's right to make those decisions independently, and refrain from attempting to influence him or her toward those that may seem more logical.
2. Assist client to set realistic goals. *Unrealistic goals set the client up for failure and reinforce feelings of powerlessness.*
3. Help identify areas of life situation that client can control. *Client's emotional condition interferes with his or her ability to solve problems. Assistance is required to perceive the benefits and consequences of available alternatives accurately.*
4. Help client identify areas of life situation that are not within his or her ability to control. Encourage verbalization of feelings related to this inability *in an effort to deal with unresolved issues and accept what cannot be changed.*

5. Identify ways in which client can achieve. Encourage participation in these activities, and provide positive reinforcement for participation, as well as for achievement.
*Positive reinforcement enhances self-esteem and
encourages repetition of desirable behaviors.*

Outcome Criteria
1. Client verbalizes choices made in a plan to maintain control over his or her life situation.
2. Client verbalizes honest feelings about life situations over
which he or she has no control.
3. Client is able to verbalize system for problem solving as
required for adequate role performance.

SOCIAL ISOLATION

Definition: *Condition of aloneness experienced by the individual and perceived as imposed by others and as a negative
or threatened state.*

Possible Etiologies ("related to")
[Panic level of anxiety]
[Regression to earlier level of development]
[Past experiences of difficulty in interactions with others]
[Need to engage in ritualistic behavior in order to keep anxiety
    under control]
[Repressed fears]

Defining Characteristics ("evidenced by")
[Stays alone in room]
Inability to communicate, withdrawal, lack of eye contact
Inappropriate or immature interests and activities for devel-
    opmental age or stage
Preoccupation with own thoughts; repetitive, meaningless
    actions
Expression of feelings of rejection or of aloneness imposed
    by others
Experiencing feelings of difference from others
Insecurity in public

Goals/Objectives
Short-Term Goal
Client will willingly attend therapy activities accompanied by trusted support person within 1 week.

Long-Term Goal
Client will voluntarily spend time with other clients and staff members in group activities by discharge from treatment.

Interventions with *Selected Rationales*
1. Convey an accepting attitude by making brief, frequent contacts. *An accepting attitude increases feelings of self-worth and facilitates trust.*
2. Show unconditional positive regard. *Conveys your belief in the client as a worthwhile human being.*
3. Be with the client to offer support during group activities that may be frightening or difficult for him or her. *The presence of a trusted individual provides emotional security for the client.*
4. Be honest and keep all promises. *Honesty and dependability promote a trusting relationship.*
5. Be cautious with touch. Allow client extra space and an avenue for exit if he or she becomes too anxious. *A person in panic anxiety may perceive touch as a threatening gesture.*
6. Administer tranquilizing medications as ordered by physician. Monitor for effectiveness, as well as for adverse side effects. *Antianxiety medications such as diazepam, chlordiazepoxide, or alprazolam, help to reduce level of anxiety in most individuals, thereby facilitating interactions with others.*
7. Discuss with client the signs of increasing anxiety and techniques to interrupt the response (e.g., relaxation exercises, thought stopping). *Maladaptive behaviors, such as withdrawal and suspiciousness, are manifested during times of increased anxiety.*
8. Give recognition and positive reinforcement for client's voluntary interactions with others. *Positive reinforcement enhances self-esteem and encourages repetition of acceptable behaviors.*

Outcome Criteria
1. Client demonstrates willingness or desire to socialize with others.
2. Client voluntarily attends group activities.
3. Client approaches others in appropriate manner for one-to-one interaction.

SELF-CARE DEFICIT (IDENTIFY SPECIFIC AREA)

Definition: *A state in which the individual experiences an impaired ability to perform or complete [activities of daily living (ADL) independently].*

Possible Etiologies ("related to")
[Regression to an earlier level of development]
[Withdrawal; isolation from others]
[Unmet dependency needs]
[Excessive ritualistic behavior]
[Disabling anxiety]
[Irrational fears]

Defining Characteristics ("evidenced by")
[Unwillingness to bathe regularly]
[Uncombed hair; dirty clothes; offensive body and breath odor; disheveled appearance]
[Eating only a few bites of food off meal tray]
[Lack of interest in selecting appropriate clothing to wear, dressing, grooming, or maintaining appearance at a satisfactory level]
[Incontinence]

Goals/Objectives
Short-Term Goal
Client will verbalize desire to take control of self-care activities within 5 days.

Long-Term Goal
Client will be able to take care of own ADL and demonstrate a willingness to do so by discharge from treatment.

Interventions with *Selected Rationales*
1. Urge client to perform normal ADL to his or her level of ability. *Successful performance of independent activities enhances self-esteem.*
2. Encourage independence, but intervene when client is unable to perform. *Client comfort and safety are nursing priorities.*
3. Offer recognition and positive reinforcement for independent accomplishments. (Example: "Mrs. J., I see you have put on a clean dress and combed your hair.") *Positive reinforcement enhances self-esteem and encourages repetition of desired behaviors.*

4. Show client how to perform activities with which he or she is having difficulty. *When anxiety is high, client may require simple, concrete demonstrations of activities that would be performed without difficulty under normal conditions.*
5. Keep strict records of food and fluid intake. *This information is necessary to formulate an accurate nutritional assessment.*
6. Offer nutritious snacks and fluids between meals. *Client may be unable to tolerate large amounts of food at mealtimes and may therefore require additional nourishment at other times during the day to receive adequate nutrition.*
7. If client is incontinent, establish routine schedule for toileting needs. Assist client to bathroom on hourly or bi-hourly schedule, as need is determined, until he or she is able to fulfill this need without assistance.

Outcome Criteria
1. Client feeds self, leaving no more than a few bites of food on food tray.
2. Client selects appropriate clothing and dresses and grooms self daily.
3. Client maintains optimal level of personal hygiene by bathing daily and carrying out essential toileting procedures without assistance.

Chapter 10

SOMATOFORM AND SLEEP DISORDERS

BACKGROUND ASSESSMENT DATA

Somatoform disorders are identified by the presence of physical symptoms for which there are no demonstrable organic findings or known physiologic mechanisms and for which there is evidence, or a strong presumption, that the symptoms are linked to psychological factors or conflicts. Disordered sleep is a problem that identifies abnormalities in the amount, quality, or timing of sleep and abnormal behavioral or physiologic events occurring in association with sleep, specific sleep stages, or sleep-wake transitions. The *DSM-IV* (APA, 1994) identifies the following categories of somatoform and sleep disorders:

SOMATIZATION DISORDER
Somatization disorder is a chronic syndrome of multiple somatic symptoms that cannot be explained medically and are associated with psychosocial distress and long-term seeking of assistance from health-care professionals. Symptoms can represent virtually any organ system but commonly are expressed as neurologic, gastrointestinal, psychosexual, or cardiopulmonary disorders. Onset of the disorder is usually in adolescence or early adulthood and is more common in women than in men. The disorder usually runs a fluctuating course, with periods of remission and exacerbation.

PAIN DISORDER

The essential feature of pain disorder is severe and prolonged pain that causes clinically significant distress or impairment in social, occupational, or other important areas of functioning (APA, 1994). This diagnosis is made when psychological factors have been judged to have a major role in the onset, severity, exacerbation, or maintenance of the pain, even when the physical examination reveals pathology that is associated with the pain.

HYPOCHONDRIASIS

Hypochondriasis is an unrealistic preoccupation with the fear of having a serious illness. The *DSM-IV* suggests that this fear arises out of an unrealistic interpretation of physical signs and sensations. Occasionally medical disease may be present, but in the hypochondriacal individual, the symptoms are grossly disproportionate to the degree of pathology (Barsky, 1989). Individuals with hypochondriasis often have a long history of "doctor shopping" and are convinced that they are not receiving the proper care.

CONVERSION DISORDER

Conversion disorder is a loss of or change in body function resulting from a psychological conflict, the physical symptoms of which cannot be explained by any known medical disorder or pathophysiologic mechanism (Barsky, 1989). The most common conversion symptoms are those that suggest neurologic disease such as paralysis, aphonia, seizures, coordination disturbance, akinesia, dyskinesia, blindness, tunnel vision, anosmia, anesthesia, and paresthesia.

BODY DYSMORPHIC DISORDER

This disorder, formerly called dysmorphophobia, is characterized by the exaggerated belief that the body is deformed or defective in some specific way. The most common complaints involve imagined or slight flaws of the face or head, such as thinning hair, acne, wrinkles, scars, vascular markings, facial swelling or asymmetry, or excessive facial hair (APA, 1994).

SLEEP DISORDERS

Insomnia

Insomnia is defined as difficulty with initiating or maintaining sleep. It is identified as *primary* when it is not associated with any other physical or mental illness and *secondary* when it is associated with another physical or mental illness.

Hypersomnia

Hypersomnia (sometimes called *somnolence*) is defined as excessive sleepiness or seeking excessive amounts of sleep. Primary hypersomnia refers to the condition when no other cause for the symptom can be found. With this disorder, individuals have difficulty staying awake during what would be considered the waking hours of the sleep-wake cycle.

Narcolepsy

Narcolepsy is a disorder similar to hypersomnia in that both produce excessive sleepiness. The characteristic manifestation of narcolepsy, however, is sleep attacks. When the attack occurs, the individual cannot prevent falling asleep, sometimes in the middle of a task or even in the middle of a sentence. Also associated with the sleep attack in 50% to 70% of the cases is *cataplexy*, a sudden loss of muscle tone, such as jaw drop, head drop, weakness of the knees, or paralysis of all skeletal muscles with collapse (Kaplan, Sadock, and Grebb, 1994).

Nightmare Disorder

Nightmares are frightening dreams that lead to awakenings from sleep (APA, 1994). Nightmare disorder is diagnosed when there is a repeated occurrence of the frightening dreams, which interferes with social or occupational functioning.

Sleep Terror Disorder

The manifestations of sleep terrors include abrupt arousal from sleep with a piercing scream or cry. The individual is difficult to awaken or comfort, and if wakefulness does occur, the individual is usually disoriented and expresses a sense of intense fear, but cannot recall the dream episode. On awakening in the morning, the individual has amnesia for the whole experience.

Sleepwalking

The disorder of sleepwalking is characterized by the performance of motor activity initiated during sleep in which the individual may leave the bed and walk about, dress, go to the bathroom, talk, scream, or even drive (Kaplan, Sadock, and Grebb, 1994). Episodes may last from a few minutes to a half hour. Most often the person returns to bed and has no memory of the event on awakening. Should the individual awaken during the episode, he or she may experience several minutes of confusion and disorientation.

Sleep-Wake Schedule Disturbances

Sleep-wake schedule disturbances can be described as a misalignment between sleep and wake behaviors (Kaplan, Sadock, and Grebb, 1994). *Circadian rhythm sleep disorder* occurs when the normal sleep-wake schedule is disrupted from its usual circadian rhythm. The individual is unable to sleep (or be awake) when he or she wants to sleep (or be awake), but can do so at other times. Sleep-wake schedule disturbances are common among shift workers and airplane travelers (commonly called *jet lag*).

PREDISPOSING FACTORS

1. **Physiologic**
   a. ***Genetic.*** Studies have shown an increased incidence of somatization disorder and hypochondriasis in first-degree relatives, implying a possible inheritable predisposition (McCracken, 1985). Genetic or familial patterns are thought to play a contributing role in primary insomnia, primary hypersomnia, narcolepsy, sleep terror disorder, and sleepwalking.
   b. ***Biochemical.*** Decreased levels of serotonin and endorphins may play a role in the etiology of pain disorder.
   c. ***Medical Conditions.*** A number of medical conditions, including sleep apnea, endocrine or metabolic disorders, infectious or neoplastic disease, and CNS lesions, have been associated with insomnia and/or

hypersomnia. Neurologic abnormalities, particularly in the temporal lobe, may be related to precipitation of night terrors.

2. **Psychosocial**
   a. *Psychodynamic.* This theory emphasizes a disturbance in the early mother-child relationship. McCracken (1985) describes the mother as one who, because of her own conflicts regarding sexuality and dependency, alternately clings to and rejects the child. Out of this conditional nurturing by the mother, the child fails to develop feelings of self-security. He or she defends against this insecurity by learning to gain affection and care through illness.

   Some psychodynamicists view hypochondriasis as an ego defense mechanism. Physical complaints are the expression of low self-esteem and feelings of worthlessness, because it is easier to feel something is wrong with the body than to feel something is wrong with the self (Barsky, 1989).

   The psychodynamic theory of conversion disorder proposes that emotions associated with a traumatic event that the individual cannot express because of moral or ethical unacceptability are "converted" into physical symptoms. The unacceptable emotions are repressed and converted to a somatic hysterical symptom that is symbolic in some way of the original emotional trauma.

   b. *Family Dynamics.* Some families have difficulty expressing emotions openly and resolving conflicts verbally. When this occurs, the child may become ill, and a shift in focus is made from the open conflict to the child's illness, leaving unresolved the underlying issues that the family is unable to confront in an open manner (Stoudemire, 1988). Thus, somatization by the child brings some stability to the family, as harmony replaces discord and the child's welfare becomes the common concern. The child in turn receives positive reinforcement for the illness (Minuchin et al, 1975).

   c. *Sociocultural/Familial Factors.* Somatic complaints are often reinforced when the sick role relieves the individual from the need to deal with a stressful situation, whether it be within society or within the family. When the sick person is allowed to avoid stressful obligations and postpone unwelcome challenges, is excused from troublesome duties, or becomes the prominent focus of attention because of the illness, positive reinforcement virtually guarantees repetition of the response.

d. ***Past Experience with Physical Illness.*** Personal experience, or the experience of close family members, with serious or life-threatening illness can predispose an individual to hypochondriasis. Once an individual has experienced a threat to biologic integrity, he or she may develop a fear of recurrence. The fear of recurring illness generates an exaggerated response to minor physical changes, leading to hypochondriacal behaviors.

SYMPTOMATOLOGY (Subjective and Objective Data)

1. Virtually any physical symptom for which there is no organic basis but for which evidence exists for the implication of psychological factors.
2. Depressed mood is common.
3. Loss or alteration in physical functioning, with no organic basis. Examples include the following:
   a. Blindness or tunnel vision.
   b. Paralysis.
   c. Anosmia (inability to smell).
   d. Aphonia (inability to speak).
   e. Seizures.
   f. Coordination disturbances.
   g. Pseudocyesis (false pregnancy).
   h. Akinesia or dyskinesia.
   i. Anesthesia or paresthesia.
4. "La belle indifference"—a relative lack of concern regarding the severity of the symptoms just described (e.g., a person is suddenly blind, but shows little anxiety over the situation).
5. "Doctor shopping."
6. Excessive use of analgesics.
7. Requests for surgery.
8. Assumption of an invalid role.
9. Impairment in social or occupational functioning because of preoccupation with physical complaints.
10. Psychosexual dysfunction (impotence, dyspareunia [painful coitus experienced by women], sexual indifference).

11. Excessive dysmenorrhea.
12. Excessive preoccupation with physical defect that is out of proportion to the actual condition.
13. Difficulty initiating or maintaining sleep.
14. Excessive sleepiness or seeking excessive amounts of sleep.
15. Sleep attacks.
16. Persistent, frightening nightmares.
17. Sleep terrors (abrupt arousal from sleep with a piercing scream or cry).
18. Physical motor activity initiated during sleep.
19. Inability to sleep (or be awake) when desiring to sleep (or be awake).

COMMON NURSING DIAGNOSES AND INTERVENTIONS

(Interventions are applicable to various health-care settings, such as inpatient and partial hospitalization, community outpatient clinic, home health, and private practice.)

CHRONIC PAIN

Definition: *Sudden or slow onset of any intensity from mild to severe, constant or recurring without anticipated or predictable end, and a duration of greater than 6 months.*

Possible Etiologies ("related to")
[Severe level of anxiety, repressed]
[Low self-esteem]
[Unmet dependency needs]
[Secondary gains from the sick role]

Defining Characteristics ("evidenced by")
[Verbal complaints of pain, in the absence of pathophysiologic evidence]
[Social withdrawal]
Facial mask [of pain]
Guarding behaviors
[Demanding behaviors]
[Refuses to attend therapeutic activities because of pain]
[History of seeking assistance from numerous health-care professionals]

[Excessive use of analgesics, without relief of pain]
Self-focusing

Goals/Objectives
Short-Term Goal
Within 2 weeks, client will verbalize understanding of correlation between pain and psychological problems.

Long-Term Goal
By discharge from treatment, client will verbalize a noticeable, if not complete, relief from pain.

Interventions with *Selected Rationales*
1. Monitor physician's ongoing assessments and laboratory reports *to ascertain that organic pathology is clearly ruled out.*
2. Recognize and accept that the pain is indeed real to the individual, even though no organic etiology can be identified. *Denying the client's feelings is nontherapeutic and hinders the development of a trusting relationship.*
3. Observe and record the duration and intensity of the pain. Note factors that precipitate the onset of pain. *Identification of the precipitating stressor is important for assessment purposes. This information will be used to develop a plan for assisting the client to cope more adaptively.*
4. Provide pain medication as prescribed by physician. *Client comfort and safety are nursing priorities.*
5. Assist with comfort measures, such as back rub, warm bath, and heating pad. Be careful, however, not to respond in a way that reinforces the behavior. *Secondary gains from physical symptoms may prolong maladaptive behaviors.*
6. Offer your attention at times when client is not focusing on pain. *Positive reinforcement encourages repetition of adaptive behaviors.*
7. Identify activities that serve to distract client from focus on self and pain. *These distractors serve in a therapeutic manner as a transition from focus on self or physical manifestations to focus on unresolved psychological issues.*
8. Encourage verbalization of feelings. Explore meaning that pain holds for client. Help client to connect symptoms of pain to times of increased anxiety and to identify specific situations that cause anxiety to rise. *Verbalization of feelings in a nonthreatening environment fa-*

cilitates expression and resolution of disturbing emotional issues.

9. Encourage client to identify alternative methods of coping with stress. *These may avert the physical pain as a maladaptive response to stress.*

10. Explore with client ways to intervene as symptoms begin to intensify, so that pain does not become disabling. (Examples: visual or auditory distractions, guided imagery, breathing exercises, massage, application of heat or cold, relaxation techniques [Carpenito, 1993].)

11. Provide positive reinforcement for adaptive behaviors. *Positive reinforcement enhances self-esteem and encourages repetition of desired behaviors.*

Outcome Criteria
1. Client verbalizes that pain does not interfere with completion of daily activities.
2. Client verbalizes an understanding of the relationship between pain and emotional problems.
3. Client demonstrates ability to intervene as anxiety rises, to prevent the onset or increase in severity of pain.

INEFFECTIVE INDIVIDUAL COPING

Definition: *Impairment of adaptive behaviors and abilities of a person in meeting life's demands and roles.*

Possible Etiologies ("related to")
[Severe level of anxiety, repressed]
[Low self-esteem]
[Unmet dependency needs]
[History of self or loved one having experienced a serious illness or disease]
[Regression to, or fixation in, an earlier level of development]
[Retarded ego development]
[Inadequate coping skills]

Defining Characteristics ("evidenced by")
[Numerous physical complaints verbalized, in the absence of any pathophysiologic evidence]
[Total focus on the self and physical symptoms]
[History of doctor shopping]
[Demanding behaviors]
[Refuses to attend therapeutic activities]

[Does not correlate physical symptoms with psychological
   problems]
Alteration in societal participation
Inability to meet basic needs
Inability to meet role expectations
Inability to problem-solve

Goals/Objectives
Short-Term Goal
Within 2 weeks, client will verbalize understanding of correlation between physical symptoms and psychological problems.

Long-Term Goal
Client will demonstrate ability to cope with stress by means
   other than preoccupation with physical symptoms by discharge from treatment.

Interventions with *Selected Rationales*
1. Monitor physician's ongoing assessments, laboratory reports, and other data to maintain assurance that possibility of organic pathology is clearly ruled out. *Knowledge
   of these data is vital for the provision of adequate and
   appropriate client care.*
2. Recognize and accept that the physical complaint is indeed real to the individual, even though no organic cause
   can be identified. *Denial of the client's feelings is nontherapeutic and interferes with establishment of a
   trusting relationship.*
3. Identify gains that the physical symptom is providing for
   the client: increased dependency, attention, distraction
   from other problems. *These are important assessment
   data to be used in assisting the client with problem
   resolution.*
4. Initially, fulfill client's most urgent dependency needs.
   *Failure to do this may cause client to become ex-
   tremely anxious, with an increase in maladaptive behaviors.*
5. Gradually withdraw attention to physical symptoms. Minimize time given in response to physical complaints. *Lack
   of positive response will discourage repetition of undesirable behaviors.*
6. Explain to client that any new physical complaints will be
   referred to the physician and give no further attention to
   them. Be sure to note physician's assessment of the
   complaint. *The possibility of organic pathology must*

always be taken into consideration. Failure to do so could jeopardize client's safety.

7. Encourage client to verbalize fears and anxieties. Explain that attention will be withdrawn if rumination about physical complaints begins. Follow through. *Without consistency of limit setting, change will not occur.*

8. Help client observe that physical symptoms occur because of, or are exacerbated by, specific stressors. Discuss alternative coping responses to these stressors.

9. Give positive reinforcement for adaptive coping strategies. *Positive reinforcement encourages repetition of desired behaviors.*

10. Help client identify ways to achieve recognition from others without resorting to physical symptoms. *Positive recognition from others enhances self-esteem and minimizes the need for attention through maladaptive behaviors.*

11. Discuss how interpersonal relationships are affected by client's narcissistic behavior. Explain how this behavior alienates others. *Client may not realize how he or she is perceived by others.*

12. Provide instruction in relaxation techniques and assertiveness skills. *These approaches decrease anxiety and increase self-esteem, which facilitate adaptive responses to stressful situations.*

Outcome Criteria

1. Client is able to demonstrate techniques that may be used in response to stress in order to prevent the occurrence or exacerbation of physical symptoms.

2. Client verbalizes an understanding of the relationship between emotional problems and physical symptoms.

BODY IMAGE DISTURBANCE

Definition: Disruption in the way one perceives one's body image.

Possible Etiologies ("related to")
[Severe level of anxiety, repressed]
[Low self-esteem]
[Unmet dependency needs]

Defining Characteristics ("evidenced by")
[Preoccupation with real or imagined change in bodily structure or function]
[Verbalizations about physical appearance that are out of proportion to any actual physical abnormality that may exist]
Fear of rejection or of reaction by others
Negative feelings about body
Change in social involvement

Goals/Objectives
Short-Term Goal
Client will verbalize understanding that changes in bodily structure or function are exaggerated out of proportion to the change that actually exists. (Time frame for this goal must be determined according to individual client's situation.)

Long-Term Goal
Client will verbalize perception of own body that is realistic to actual structure or function by discharge from treatment.

Interventions with *Selected Rationales*
1. Establish trusting relationship with client. *Trust enhances therapeutic interactions between nurse and client.*
2. If there is actual change in structure or function, encourage client to progress through stages of grieving. Assess level of knowledge and provide information regarding normal grieving process and associated feelings. *Knowledge of acceptable feelings facilitates progression through the grieving process.*
3. Identify misperceptions or distortions client has regarding body image. Correct inaccurate perceptions in a matter-of-fact, nonthreatening manner. Withdraw attention when preoccupation with distorted image persists. *Lack of attention may encourage elimination of undesirable behaviors.*
4. Assist client to recognize personal body boundaries. *Use of touch may help him or her recognize acceptance of the individual by others and reduce fear of rejection because of changes in bodily structure or function.*
5. Encourage independent self-care activities, providing assistance as required. *Self-care activities accomplished independently enhance self-esteem and also create the necessity for client to confront reality of his or her bodily condition.*
6. Provide positive reinforcement for client's expressions of realistic bodily perceptions. *Positive reinforcement en-*

hances self-esteem and encourages repetition of desired behaviors.

Outcome Criteria
1. Client verbalizes realistic perception of bodily condition.
2. Client demonstrates acceptance of changes in bodily structure or function, as evidenced by expression of positive feelings about body, ability or willingness to perform self-care activities independently, and a focus on personal achievements rather than preoccupation with distorted body image.

SENSORY-PERCEPTUAL ALTERATION

Definition: *A state in which an individual experiences a change in the amount or patterning of oncoming stimuli [either internally or externally initiated] accompanied by a diminished, exaggerated, distorted, or impaired response to such stimuli.*

Possible Etiologies ("related to")
[Severe level of anxiety, repressed]
[Low self-esteem]
[Unmet dependency needs]
[Regression to, or fixation in, an earlier level of development]
[Retarded ego development]
[Inadequate coping skills]
Psychological stress [narrowed perceptual fields caused by anxiety]

Defining Characteristics ("evidenced by")
[Loss or alteration in physical functioning suggesting a physical disorder (often neurologic in nature), but for which organic pathology is not evident. Common alterations include paralysis, anosmia, aphonia, deafness, blindness.]
[La belle indifference]

Goals/Objectives
Short-Term Goal
Client will verbalize understanding of emotional problems as a contributing factor to alteration in physical functioning within 10 days.

Long-Term Goal
Client will demonstrate recovery of lost function.

Interventions with *Selected Rationales*

1. Monitor physician's ongoing assessments, laboratory reports, and other data to maintain assurance that possibility of organic pathology is clearly ruled out. *Failure to do so may jeopardize client's safety.*
2. Identify gains that the physical symptom is providing for the client: increased dependency, attention, distraction from other problems. *These are important assessment data to be used in assisting the client with problem resolution.*
3. Fulfill client's needs related to activities of daily living (ADL) with which the physical symptom is interfering. *Client comfort and safety are nursing priorities.*
4. Do not focus on the disability and allow client to be as independent as possible. Intervene only when client requires assistance. *Positive reinforcement would encourage continual use of the maladaptive response for secondary gains, such as dependency.*
5. Encourage client to participate in therapeutic activities to the best of his or her ability. Do not allow client to use the disability as a manipulative tool. Withdraw attention if client continues to focus on physical limitation. Reinforce reality as required, but ensure maintenance of a nonthreatening environment.
6. Encourage client to verbalize fears and anxieties. Help client to recognize that the physical symptom appears at a time of extreme stress and is a mechanism used for coping. *Client may be unaware of the relationship between physical symptom and emotional stress.*
7. Help client identify coping mechanisms that he or she could use when faced with stressful situations, rather than retreating from reality with a physical disability.
8. Explain assertiveness techniques and practice use of same through role playing. *Use of assertiveness techniques enhances self-esteem and minimizes anxiety in interpersonal relationships.*
9. Help client identify a satisfactory support system within the community from which he or she may seek assistance as needed to cope with overwhelming stress.

Outcome Criteria

1. Client is no longer experiencing symptoms of altered physical functioning.
2. Client verbalizes an understanding of the relationship between extreme psychological stress and loss of physical functioning.

3. Client is able to verbalize adaptive ways of coping with stress and identify community support systems to which he or she may go for help.

SELF-CARE DEFICIT (Identify Specific Area)

Definition: *A state in which the individual experiences an impaired ability to perform or complete [activities of daily living independently].*

Possible Etiologies ("related to")
[Paralysis of body part]
[Inability to see]
[Inability to hear]
[Inability to speak]
Pain, discomfort

Defining Characteristics ("evidenced by")
Inability to bring food from a receptacle to the mouth
Inability to wash body or body parts; obtain or get to water sources; regulate temperature or flow
Impaired ability to put on or take off necessary items of clothing; obtain or replace articles of clothing; fasten clothing; maintain appearance at a satisfactory level
Inability to get to toilet or commode [impaired mobility]
Inability to manipulate clothing for toileting
Inability to flush toilet or commode
Inability to sit on or rise from toilet or commode
Inability to carry out proper toilet hygiene

Goals/Objectives
Short-Term Goal
Client will perform self-care needs independently, to the extent that physical ability will allow, within 5 days.

Long-Term Goal
By discharge from treatment, client will be able to perform ADL independently and demonstrate a willingness to do so.

Interventions with *Selected Rationales*
1. Assess client's level of disability; note areas of strength and impairment. *This knowledge is required to develop adequate plan of care for client.*

2. Encourage client to perform normal ADL to his or her level of ability. *Successful performance of independent activities enhances self-esteem.*
3. Encourage independence, but intervene when client is unable to perform. *Client comfort and safety are nursing priorities.*
4. Ensure that nonjudgmental attitude is conveyed as nursing assistance with self-care activities is provided. Remember that the physical symptom is real to the client. It is not within the client's conscious control. *A judgmental attitude interferes with the nurse's ability to provide therapeutic care for this client.*
5. Feed client, if necessary, and provide assistance with containers, positioning, and other matters, as required. *Client comfort and safety are nursing priorities.*
6. Bathe client, or assist with bath, depending on his or her level of ability. *Client comfort and safety are nursing priorities.*
7. Assist client with dressing, oral hygiene, combing hair, and applying makeup, as required. *Client comfort and safety are nursing priorities.*
8. Provide bedpan, commode, or assistance to bathroom as determined by client's level of ability. *Client comfort and safety are nursing priorities.*
9. Provide positive reinforcement for ADL performed independently. *Positive reinforcement enhances self-esteem and encourages repetition of desired behaviors.*
10. Take precautions against fostering dependency by intervening when client is capable of performing independently. Allow ample time to complete these activities to the best of his or her ability without assistance.
11. Encourage client to discuss feelings regarding the disability and the need for dependency it creates. Help client to see the purpose this disability is serving for him or her. *Self-disclosure and exploration of feelings with a trusted individual may help client fulfill unmet needs and confront unresolved issues.*

Outcome Criteria
1. Client feeds self without assistance.
2. Client selects appropriate clothing and dresses and grooms self daily.
3. Client maintains optimal level of personal hygiene by bathing daily and carrying out essential toileting procedures without assistance.

KNOWLEDGE DEFICIT (Psychological Causes for Physical Symptoms)

Definition: *Absence or deficiency of cognitive information related to specific topic.*

Possible Etiologies ("related to")
Lack of interest in learning
[Severe level of anxiety]

Defining Characteristics ("evidenced by")
[Denial of emotional problems]
[Statements such as, "I don't know why the doctor put me on the psychiatric unit. I have a physical problem."]
[History of "shopping" for a doctor who will substantiate symptoms as pathophysiologic]
[Noncompliance with psychiatric treatment plan]

Goals/Objectives
Short-Term Goal
Client will verbalize an understanding that no pathophysiologic condition exists to substantiate physical symptoms.

Long-Term Goal
By discharge from treatment, client will be able to verbalize psychological cause(s) for physical symptoms.

Interventions with *Selected Rationales*
1. Assess client's level of knowledge regarding effects of psychological problems on the body. *An adequate database is necessary for the development of an effective teaching plan.*
2. Assess client's level of anxiety and readiness to learn. *Learning does not occur beyond the moderate level of anxiety.*
3. Discuss physical examinations and laboratory tests that have been conducted. Explain purpose and results of each.
4. Explore feelings and fears held by client. Go slowly. These feelings may have been suppressed or repressed for a very long time and their disclosure will undoubtedly be a painful experience. Be supportive.
5. Have client keep a diary of appearance, duration, and intensity of physical symptoms. A separate record of situations that the client finds especially stressful should also be kept. *Comparison of these records may provide ob-*

jective data from which to observe the relationship between physical symptoms and stress.

6. Help client identify needs that are being met through the sick role. Together, formulate a more adaptive means for fulfilling these needs. Practice by role playing.

7. Explain assertiveness techniques to the client. Discuss the importance of recognizing the differences among passive, assertive, and aggressive behaviors, and of respecting the human rights of others while protecting one's own basic human rights. *Use of these techniques enhances self-esteem and facilitates client's interpersonal relationships.*

8. Discuss adaptive methods of stress management: relaxation techniques, physical exercise, meditation, breathing exercises, autogenics. *These techniques may be employed in an attempt to relieve anxiety and discourage the use of physical symptoms as a maladaptive response.*

Outcome Criteria

1. Client verbalizes an understanding of the relationship between psychological stress and physical symptoms.

2. Client demonstrates the ability to use therapeutic techniques in the management of stress.

SLEEP PATTERN DISTURBANCE

Definition: *Disruption of sleep time causing discomfort or interfering with desired lifestyle.*

Possible Etiologies ("related to")
[A specific medical condition]
[Use of, or withdrawal from, substances]
[Anxiety]
[Depression]
[Circadian rhythm disruption]
[Familial patterns]

Defining Characteristics ("evidenced by")
[Insomnia]
[Hypersomnia]
[Nightmares]
[Sleep terrors]
[Sleepwalking]

Goals/Objectives
Short-Term Goal
Client will verbalize causal relationship of sleep disorder.

Long-Term Goal
Client will be able to achieve adequate, uninterrupted sleep.
Client will report feeling rested and demonstrate a sense of well-being.

Interventions with *Selected Rationales*
1. To promote sleep:
   a. Encourage activities that prepare one for sleep: soft music, relaxation exercises, warm bath. *These activities promote relaxation.*
   b. Discourage strenuous exercise within 1 hour of bedtime. *Strenuous exercise can be stimulating and keep one awake.*
   c. Control intake of caffeine-containing substances within 4 hours of bedtime (e.g., coffee, tea, colas, chocolate, and certain analgesic medications). *Caffeine is a CNS stimulant and can interfere with the promotion of sleep.*
   d. Provide a high-carbohydrate snack before bedtime. *Carbohydrates increase the levels of the amino acid tryptophan, a precursor to the neurotransmitter serotonin. Serotonin is thought to play a role in the promotion of sleep.*
   e. Keep the temperature of the room between 68 and 72°F. *This range provides the temperature most conducive to sleep.*
   f. Instruct the client not to use alcoholic beverages to relax. *Although alcohol may initially induce drowsiness and promote falling asleep, a rebound stimulation occurs in the CNS within several hours after drinking alcohol. The individual may fall asleep, only to be wide awake a few hours later.*
   g. Discourage smoking and the use of other tobacco products near sleep time. *These products produce a stimulant effect on the CNS.*
   h. Discourage daytime napping. Increase program of activities to keep the person busy. *Sleeping during the day can interfere with the ability to achieve sleep at night.*
   i. Individuals with chronic insomnia should use sleeping medications judiciously. *Sedatives and hypnotics have serious side effects and are highly addicting.*

Life-threatening symptoms can occur with abrupt withdrawal, and discontinuation should be tapered under a physician's supervision. Long-term use can result in rebound insomnia.

2. To prevent "jet lag" (circadian rhythm disruption):
   a. If time permits, use a preventive strategy of altering mealtimes and sleep times in the appropriate direction *to prepare the body for the oncoming change.*
   b. If preventive measures are impossible, increasing the amount of sleep on arrival sometimes helps *to reduce fatigue and restore the rested feeling.*
   c. Short-term use of sleep medication may be helpful.

Outcome Criteria
1. Client verbalizes a decrease in problems with sleep.
2. Client reports feeling rested and demonstrates a sense of well-being.

RISK FOR INJURY

Definition: *A state in which the individual is at risk of injury as a result of environmental conditions interacting with the individual's adaptive and defensive resources.*

Related/Risk Factors ("related to")
[Excessive sleepiness]
[Sleep terrors]
[Sleepwalking]
[Sleep deprivation]

Goals/Objectives
Short-Term and Long-Term Goal
Client will not experience injury.

Interventions with *Selected Rationales*
1. Ensure that side rails are up on the bed. *An individual who experiences serious nightmares or night terrors can fall from the bed during an episode.*
2. Keep the bed in a low position *to diminish the risk of injury by the person who gets out of bed during a sleepwalking episode.*
3. Equip the bed with a bell (or other noisemaker) that is activated when the bed is exited. *This may alert the caretaker so that supervision to prevent accidental injury can be instituted.*

4. Keep a night light on and arrange the furniture in the bedroom in a manner that promotes safety *to provide a safe environment for the individual who awakens (fully or partially) during the night.*
5. Administer drug therapy as ordered. *Insomnia and parasomnias have been treated effectively with benzodiazepines. The usual treatment for hypersomnia and narcolepsy has been with CNS stimulants such as amphetamines. In some instances, the serotonin-specific reuptake inhibitors (SSRIs) have also been helpful for these problems.*
6. For the child who experiences nightmares, encourage him or her to talk about the dream. Tell the child that all people have dreams. Validate his or her feeling of fearfulness while ensuring safety. Keep a light on in the room or give the child a flashlight. *Talking about the dream helps to promote the unreality of the dream and to differentiate between what is real and what is not real. Light gives the child a feeling of control over the darkness within the room.*

Outcome Criteria
1. Client has not experienced injury from behaviors associated with sleep disorders.
2. Client is following medication regimen and is experiencing no adverse effects.

Chapter 11

DISSOCIATIVE DISORDERS

BACKGROUND ASSESSMENT DATA

The essential feature of the dissociative disorders is a disruption in the usually integrated functions of consciousness, memory, identity, or perception of the environment (APA, 1994). During periods of intolerable stress, the individual blocks off part of his or her life from consciousness. The stressful emotion becomes a separate entity, as the individual "splits" from it and mentally drifts into a fantasy state. The following categories are defined in the *DSM-IV* (APA, 1994):

1. **Dissociative Amnesia.** An inability to recall important personal information, usually of a traumatic or stressful nature. The extent of the disturbance is too great to be explained by ordinary forgetfulness. Types of impairment in recall include the following:
   a. *Localized Amnesia.* Inability to recall all incidents associated with a traumatic event for a specific time period following the event (usually a few hours to a few days).
   b. *Selective Amnesia.* Inability to recall only certain incidents associated with a traumatic event for a specific time period following the event.
   c. *Generalized Amnesia.* Failure of recall encompassing one's entire life.
   d. *Continuous Amnesia.* Inability to recall events subsequent to a specific time up to and including the present. (The memory does not return after a short

period of time, as in localized amnesia. The individual actually is unable to form new memories.)

   e. *Systematized Amnesia.* With this type of amnesia, the individual cannot remember events that relate to a specific category of information, such as one's family, or to one particular person or event.
2. **Dissociative Fugue.** A sudden, unexpected travel away from home or customary work locale with assumption of a new identity and an inability to recall one's previous identity. Following recovery, there is no recollection of events that took place during the fugue. Course is typically brief—hours to days, and rarely, months. Recurrences are rare.
3. **Dissociative Identity Disorder (DID).** The existence within the individual of two or more distinct personalities, each of which is dominant at a particular time. The original personality usually is not aware (at least initially) of the existence of subpersonalities. When there are more than two subpersonalities, however, they are usually aware of each other. Transition from one personality to another is usually sudden and often associated with psychosocial stress. The course tends to be more chronic than in the other dissociative disorders.
4. **Depersonalization Disorder.** Depersonalization disorder is characterized by a temporary change in the quality of self-awareness, which often takes the form of feelings of unreality, changes in body image, feelings of detachment from the environment, or a sense of observing oneself from outside the body (Marciniak, 1985).

PREDISPOSING FACTORS

1. **Physiologic**
   a. *Genetics.* The *DSM-IV* suggests that DID is more common in first-degree relatives of people with the disorder than in the general population. The disorder is often seen in more than one generation of a family.
   b. *Neurobiologic.* Some clinicians have suggested a possible correlation between neurologic alterations and dissociative disorders. Although available information is inadequate, it is possible that dissociative amnesia and dissociative fugue may be related to alterations in the ascending reticular activating system and thalamocortical projections (Nemiah, 1989). Some studies have suggested a possible link between

DID and certain neurologic conditions, such as temporal lobe epilepsy, severe migraine headaches, cerebral cortical damage, and visual alterations. Electroencephalographic abnormalities have been observed in some clients with DID.

2. **Psychosocial**
   a. ***Psychodynamic Theory.*** Freud (1962) believed that dissociative behaviors occurred when individuals repressed distressing mental contents from conscious awareness. He believed that the unconscious was a dynamic entity in which repressed mental contents were stored and unavailable to conscious recall. Current psychodynamic explanations of dissociation are based on Freud's concepts.
   b. ***Psychological Trauma.*** A growing body of evidence points to the etiology of DID as a set of traumatic experiences that overwhelms the individual's capacity to cope by any means other than dissociation. These experiences usually take the form of severe physical, sexual, or psychological abuse by a parent or significant other in the child's life. DID is thought to serve as a survival strategy for the child in this traumatic environment, where he or she creates a new being who is able to experience the overwhelming pain of the cruel reality, while the primary self can then escape awareness of the pain. Kluft (1984) suggests that the number of an individual's alternate personalities is related to the number of different types of abuse he or she suffered as a child.

SYMPTOMATOLOGY (Subjective and Objective Data)

1. Impairment in recall.
   a. Inability to remember specific incidents.
   b. Inability to recall any of one's past life, including one's identity.
2. Sudden travel away from familiar surroundings; assumption of new identity, with inability to recall past.
3. Assumption of additional identities within the personality; behavior involves transition from one identity to another as a method of dealing with stressful situations.
4. Feeling of unreality; detachment from a stressful situation—may be accompanied by dizziness, depression,

obsessive rumination, somatic concerns, anxiety, fear of going insane, and a disturbance in the subjective sense of time.

COMMON NURSING DIAGNOSES AND INTERVENTIONS

(Interventions are applicable to various health-care settings, such as inpatient and partial hospitalization, community outpatient clinic, home health, and private practice.)

INEFFECTIVE INDIVIDUAL COPING

Definition: *Impairment of adaptive behaviors and abilities of a person in meeting life's demands and roles.*

Possible Etiologies ("related to")
[Severe level of anxiety, repressed]
[Childhood trauma]
[Childhood abuse]
[Low self-esteem]
[Unmet dependency needs]
[Regression to, or fixation in, an earlier level of development]
[Retarded ego development]
[Inadequate coping skills]

Defining Characteristics ("evidenced by")
[Dissociating self from painful situation by experiencing:
  Memory loss (partial or complete)
  Sudden travel away from home with inability to recall previous identity
  The presence of more than one personality within the individual
  Detachment from reality]
Inability to problem-solve
Inability to meet role expectations
Alterations in societal participation
Inappropriate use of defense mechanisms

Goals/Objectives
Short-Term Goals
1. Client will verbalize understanding that he or she is employing dissociative behaviors in times of psychosocial stress.

2. Client will verbalize more adaptive ways of coping in stressful situations than resorting to dissociation.

Long-Term Goal
Client will demonstrate ability to cope with stress (employing means other than dissociation).

Interventions with *Selected Rationales*
1. Reassure client of safety and security through your presence. Dissociative behaviors may be frightening to the client. *Presence of a trusted individual provides feeling of security and assurance of freedom from harm.*
2. Identify stressor that precipitated severe anxiety. *This information is necessary to the development of an effective plan of client care and problem resolution.*
3. Explore feelings that client experienced in response to the stressor. Help client to understand that the disequilibrium felt is acceptable—indeed, even expected—in times of severe stress. *Client's self-esteem is preserved by the knowledge that others may experience these behaviors under similar circumstances.*
4. As anxiety level decreases (and memory returns), use exploration and an accepting, nonthreatening environment to encourage client to identify repressed traumatic experiences that contribute to chronic anxiety.
5. Have client identify methods of coping with stress in the past and determine whether the response was adaptive or maladaptive. *In times of extreme anxiety, client is unable to evaluate appropriateness of response. This information is necessary for client to develop a plan of action for the future.*
6. Help client define more adaptive coping strategies. Make suggestions of alternatives that might be tried. Examine benefits and consequences of each alternative. Assist client in the selection of those that are most appropriate for him or her. *Depending on current level of anxiety, client may require assistance with problem solving and decision making.*
7. Provide positive reinforcement for client's attempts to change. *Positive reinforcement enhances self-esteem and encourages repetition of desired behaviors.*
8. Identify community resources to which the individual may go for support if past maladaptive coping patterns return.

Outcome Criteria
1. Client is able to demonstrate techniques that may be used in response to stress in order to prevent dissociation.

2. Client verbalizes an understanding of the relationship between severe anxiety and the dissociative response.

ALTERED THOUGHT PROCESSES

Definition: *A state in which an individual experiences a disruption in cognitive operations and activities.*

Possible Etiologies ("related to")
[Severe level of anxiety, repressed]
[Childhood trauma]
[Childhood abuse]
[Threat to physical integrity]
[Threat to self-concept]

Defining Characteristics ("evidenced by")
[Memory loss—inability to recall selected events related to a
   stressful situation]
[Memory loss—inability to recall events associated with en-
   tire life]
[Memory loss—inability to recall own identity]

Goals/Objectives
Short-Term Goal
Client will verbalize understanding that loss of memory is related to stressful situation and begin discussing stressful
   situation with nurse or therapist.

Long-Term Goal
Client will recover deficits in memory, and develop more
   adaptive coping mechanisms to deal with stressful situations.

Interventions with *Selected Rationales*
1. Obtain as much information as possible about client from
   family and significant others (likes, dislikes, important people, activities, music, pets). *A baseline assessment is important for the development of an effective plan of
   care.*
2. Do not flood client with data regarding his or her past life.
   *Individuals who are exposed to painful information
   from which the amnesia is providing protection may
   decompensate even further into a psychotic state.*
3. Instead, expose client to stimuli that represent pleasant
   experiences from the past, such as smells associated with

enjoyable activities, beloved pets, and music known to have been pleasurable to client.

4. As memory begins to return, engage client in activities that may provide additional stimulation. *Recall may occur during activities that simulate life experiences.*

5. Encourage client to discuss situations that have been especially stressful and to explore the feelings associated with those times. *Verbalization of feelings in a non-threatening environment may help client come to terms with unresolved issues that may be contributing to the dissociative process.*

6. Identify specific conflicts that remain unresolved, and assist client to identify possible solutions. *Unless these underlying conflicts are resolved, any improvement in coping behaviors must be viewed as only temporary.*

7. Provide instruction regarding more adaptive ways to respond to anxiety so that dissociative behaviors are no longer needed.

Outcome Criteria
1. Client is able to recall all events of past life.
2. Client is able to demonstrate adaptive coping strategies that may be used in response to severe anxiety in order to avert amnesic behaviors.

PERSONAL IDENTITY DISTURBANCE

Definition: Inability to distinguish between self and nonself.

Possible Etiologies ("related to")
[Severe level of anxiety, repressed]
[Childhood trauma]
[Childhood abuse]
[Threat to physical integrity]
[Threat to self-concept]
[Underdeveloped ego]

Defining Characteristics ("evidenced by")
[Presence of more than one personality within the individual]

Goals/Objectives
Short-Term Goal
Client will verbalize understanding of the existence of multiple personalities within the self and be able to recognize

stressful situations that precipitate transition from one to another.

Long-Term Goal
Client will verbalize understanding of the need for, enter into, and cooperate with long-term therapy for this disorder, with the ultimate goal being integration into one personality.

Interventions with *Selected Rationales*
1. The nurse must develop a trusting relationship with the original personality and with each of the subpersonalities. *Trust is the basis of a therapeutic relationship. Each of the personalities views itself as a separate entity and must initially be treated as such.*
2. Help the client understand the existence of the subpersonalities. *Client may be unaware of this dissociative response to stressful situations.*
3. Help client identify the need each subpersonality serves in the personal identity of the individual. *Knowledge of these unfulfilled needs is the first step toward integration of the personalities and the client's ability to face unresolved issues without dissociation.*
4. Help the client identify stressful situations that precipitate the transition from one personality to another. Carefully observe and record these transitions. *This knowledge is required to assist the client in responding more adaptively and to eliminate the need for transition to another personality.*
5. Use nursing interventions necessary to deal with maladaptive behaviors associated with individual subpersonalities. For example, if one personality is suicidal, precautions must be taken to guard against client's self-harm. If another personality has a tendency toward physical hostility, precautions must be taken for the protection of others. *Safety of the client and others is a nursing priority.*
6. Help subpersonalities to understand that their "being" will not be destroyed, but integrated into a unified identity within the individual. *Because subpersonalities function as separate entities, the idea of total elimination generates fear and defensiveness.*
7. Provide support during disclosure of painful experiences and reassurance when the client becomes discouraged with lengthy treatment.

Outcome Criteria
1. Client recognizes the existence of more than one personality.

2. Client is able to verbalize the purpose these personalities serve.
3. Client verbalizes the intention of seeking long-term outpatient psychotherapy.

SENSORY/PERCEPTUAL ALTERATION
(Kinesthetic)

Definition: *A state in which an individual experiences a change in the amount or patterning of oncoming stimuli [either internally or externally initiated] accompanied by a diminished, exaggerated, distorted, or impaired response to such stimuli.*

Possible Etiologies ("related to")
[Severe level of anxiety, repressed]
[Childhood trauma]
[Childhood abuse]
[Threat to physical integrity]
[Threat to self-concept]
[Underdeveloped ego]

Defining Characteristics ("evidenced by")
[Alteration in the perception or experience of the self]
[Loss of one's own sense of reality]
[Loss of the sense of reality of the external world]

Goals/Objectives
Short-Term Goal
Client will verbalize adaptive ways of coping with stress.

Long-Term Goal
Client will demonstrate the ability to perceive stimuli correctly and maintain a sense of reality during stressful situations by discharge from treatment.

Interventions with *Selected Rationales*
1. Provide support and encouragement during times of depersonalization. The client manifesting these symptoms may express fear and anxiety at experiencing such behaviors. They do not understand the response and may express a fear of "going insane." *Support and encouragement from a trusted individual provide a feeling of security when fears and anxieties are manifested.*
2. Explain the depersonalization behaviors and the purpose they usually serve for the client. *This knowledge may*

help to minimize fears and anxieties associated with their occurrence.

3. Explain the relationship between severe anxiety and depersonalization behaviors. *The client may be unaware that the occurrence of depersonalization behaviors is related to severe anxiety.*

4. Help client relate these behaviors to times of severe psychological stress that he or she has experienced personally.

5. Explore past experiences and possibly repressed painful situations such as trauma or abuse. *It is thought that traumatic experiences predispose individuals to dissociative disorders.*

6. Discuss these painful experiences with the client and encourage him or her to deal with the feelings associated with these situations. Work to resolve the conflicts these repressed feelings have nurtured. *These interventions serve to decrease the need for the dissociative response to anxiety.*

7. Discuss ways the client may more adaptively respond to stress and role-play with him or her to practice using these new methods.

Outcome Criteria

1. Client perceives stressful situations correctly and is able to maintain a sense of reality.

2. Client demonstrates use of adaptive strategies for coping with stress.

Chapter 12

SEXUAL AND GENDER IDENTITY DISORDERS

BACKGROUND ASSESSMENT DATA

The *DSM-IV* (APA, 1994) identifies two categories of sexual disorders: paraphilias and sexual dysfunctions. Paraphilias are characterized by recurrent, intense sexual urges, fantasies, or behaviors that involve unusual objects, activities, or situations (APA, 1994). Sexual dysfunction disorders can be described as an impairment or disturbance in any of the phases of the sexual response cycle. These include disorders of desire, arousal, orgasm, and disorders that relate to the experience of genital pain during intercourse. Gender identity disorders are characterized by strong and persistent cross-gender identification accompanied by persistent discomfort with one's assigned sex (APA, 1994).

PARAPHILIAS

Abel (1989) identifies the term paraphilia as repetitive or preferred sexual fantasies or behaviors that involve any of the following:

1. The preference for use of a nonhuman object.
2. Repetitive sexual activity with humans involving real or simulated suffering or humiliation.
3. Repetitive sexual activity with nonconsenting partners.

Types of paraphilias include the following:

1. **Exhibitionism.** The major symptoms include recurrent, intense sexual urges, behaviors, or sexually arousing fantasies, of at least 6 months' duration, involving the exposure of one's genitals to an unsuspecting stranger (APA, 1994). Masturbation may occur during the exhibitionism. The condition apparently only occurs in men, and the victims are women in 99% of the cases (Abel, 1989).

2. **Fetishism.** This is identified by recurrent, intense sexual urges or behaviors, or sexually arousing fantasies, of at least 6 months' duration, involving the use of nonliving objects (APA, 1994). Common fetish objects include bras, women's underpants, stockings, shoes, boots, or other wearing apparel. The fetish object is generally used during masturbation or incorporated into sexual activity with another person to produce sexual excitation. When the fetish involves cross-dressing, the disorder is called *transvestic fetishism*.

3. **Frotteurism.** This disorder is defined as the recurrent preoccupation with intense sexual urges or fantasies, of at least 6 months' duration, involving touching or rubbing against a nonconsenting person (APA, 1994). Sexual excitement is derived from the actual touching or rubbing, not from the coercive nature of the act.

4. **Pedophilia.** The *DSM-IV* describes the essential feature of this disorder as recurrent sexual urges, behaviors, or sexually arousing fantasies, of at least 6 months' duration, involving sexual activity with a prepubescent child. The age of the molester is 16 or older, and is at least 5 years older than the child. This category of paraphilia is the most common of sexual assaults (Abel, 1989).

5. **Sexual Masochism.** The identifying feature of this disorder is recurrent, intense sexual urges, behaviors, or sexually arousing fantasies, of at least 6 months' duration, involving the act (real, not simulated) of being humiliated, beaten, bound, or otherwise made to suffer (APA, 1994). These masochistic activities may be fantasized, solitary, or with a partner. Examples include becoming sexually aroused by self-inflicted pain, or by being restrained, raped, or beaten by a sexual partner.

6. **Sexual Sadism.** The essential feature of this disorder is identified as recurrent, intense, sexual urges, behaviors, or sexually arousing fantasies, of at least 6 months' du-

ration, involving acts (real, not simulated) in which the psychological or physical suffering (including humiliation) of the victim is sexually exciting (APA, 1994). The sadistic activities may be fantasized or acted on with a consenting or nonconsenting partner. In all instances, sexual excitation occurs in response to the suffering of the victim. Examples include rape, beating, torture, or even killing.

7. **Voyeurism.** This disorder is identified by recurrent, intense sexual urges, behaviors, or sexually arousing fantasies, of at least 6 months' duration, involving the act of observing an unsuspecting person who is naked, in the process of disrobing, or engaging in sexual activity (APA, 1994). Sexual excitement is achieved through the act of looking, and no contact with the person is attempted. Masturbation usually accompanies the "window peeping" but may occur later as the individual fantasizes about the voyeuristic act.

Predisposing Factors (to Paraphilias)

1. **Physiologic**
   a. *Physical Factors.* Several physical factors have been implicated in the etiology of paraphilias. They include abnormalities in the limbic system of the brain, temporal lobe epilepsy, temporal lobe tumors, and abnormal levels of androgens (Bradford and McLean, 1984). The results of these studies are inconclusive at this time.

2. **Psychosocial**
   a. *Psychoanalytic Theory.* The psychoanalytic approach defines a paraphiliac as one who has failed the normal developmental process toward heterosexual adjustment (Abel, 1989). This occurs when the individual fails to resolve the oedipal crisis, thereby maintaining sexual feelings for the parent of the opposite gender. This creates intense anxiety, which leads the individual to seek sexual gratification in ways that provide a "safe substitution" for the parent (Becker and Kavoussi, 1988).

Symptomatology (Subjective and Objective Data)

1. Exposure of one's genitals to a stranger.
2. Sexual arousal in the presence of nonliving objects.

3. Touching and rubbing one's genitals against an uncon-
   senting person.
4. Sexual attraction to, or activity with, a prepubescent
   child.
5. Sexual arousal from being humiliated, beaten, bound,
   or otherwise made to suffer (through fantasy, self-in-
   fliction, or by a sexual partner).
6. Sexual arousal by inflicting psychological or physical
   suffering on another individual (either consenting or
   nonconsenting).
7. Sexual arousal from dressing in the clothes of the opposite gender.
8. Sexual arousal from observing unsuspecting people either naked or engaged in sexual activity.
9. Masturbation often accompanies the activities described when they are performed solitarily.
10. The individual is markedly distressed by these activities.

SEXUAL DYSFUNCTIONS

Sexual dysfunctions may occur in any phase of the sexual
response cycle. Types of sexual dysfunctions include the
following:

1. **Sexual Desire Disorders**
   a. *Hypoactive Sexual Desire Disorder.* This disorder
      is defined by the *DSM-IV* (APA, 1994) as a persistent
      or recurrent deficiency or absence of sexual fantasies
      and desire for sexual activity. The complaint appears
      to be more common among women than men.
   b. *Sexual Aversion Disorder.* This disorder is charac-
      terized by a persistent or recurrent extreme aversion
      to, and avoidance of, all or almost all genital sexual
      contact with a sexual partner (APA, 1994).
2. **Sexual Arousal Disorders**
   a. *Female Sexual Arousal Disorder.* This disorder is
      identified in the *DSM-IV* (APA, 1994) as a persistent
      or recurrent inability to attain, or to maintain until
      completion of the sexual activity, an adequate lubri-
      cation or swelling response of sexual excitement.
   b. *Male Erectile Disorder.* This disorder is character-
      ized by a persistent or recurrent inability to attain, or
      to maintain until completion of the sexual activity,
      an adequate erection (APA, 1994).

3. **Orgasmic Disorders**
   a. *Female Orgasmic Disorder (Anorgasmia).* This disorder is defined by the *DSM-IV* as a persistent or recurrent delay in, or absence of, orgasm following a normal sexual excitement phase.
   b. *Male Orgasmic Disorder (Retarded Ejaculation).* With this disorder, the man is unable to ejaculate, even though he has a firm erection and has had more than adequate stimulation (Hyde, 1986). The severity of the problem may range from only occasional problems ejaculating to a history of never having experienced an orgasm.
   c. *Premature Ejaculation.* The *DSM-IV* describes this disorder as persistent or recurrent ejaculation with minimal sexual stimulation, or before, on, or shortly after penetration and before the person wishes it.
4. **Sexual Pain Disorders**
   a. *Dyspareunia.* This disorder is defined as recurrent or persistent genital pain associated with sexual intercourse, in either a man or a woman, that is not caused by vaginismus, lack of lubrication, other general medical condition, or the physiologic effects of substance use (APA, 1994).
   b. *Vaginismus.* This disorder is characterized by an involuntary constriction of the outer one-third of the vagina, which prevents penile insertion and intercourse (Sadock, 1989).

Predisposing Factors (to Sexual Dysfunctions)

1. **Physiologic Factors**
   a. *Hypoactive Sexual Desire Disorders.* These have been linked to low levels of serum testosterone in men (Sadock, 1989) and to elevated levels of serum prolactin in both men and women (Segraves, 1988). Various medications, such as antihypertensives, antipsychotics, antidepressants, anxiolytics, and anticonvulsants, as well as chronic use of drugs such as alcohol and cocaine, have also been implicated in sexual desire disorders (Abel, 1985).
   b. *Sexual Arousal Disorders.* These may occur in response to decreased estrogen levels in postmenopausal women. Medications such as antihistamines and cholinergic blockers may produce similar re-

sults. Erectile dysfunctions in men may be attributed to arteriosclerosis, diabetes, temporal lobe epilepsy, multiple sclerosis, some medications (antihypertensives, tranquilizers), spinal cord injury, pelvic surgery, and chronic use of alcohol.

c. ***Orgasmic Disorders.*** In women these may be attributed to some medical conditions (hypothyroidism, diabetes, and hyperprolactinemia), and certain medications (antihypertensives, antidepressants). Medical conditions that may interfere with male orgasm include genitourinary surgery (e.g., prostatectomy), Parkinson's disease, and diabetes. Various medications have also been implicated, including antihypertensives, anticholinergics, and antipsychotics.

d. ***Sexual Pain Disorders.*** In women these can be caused by disorders of the vaginal entrance, irritation or damage to the clitoris, vaginal or pelvic infections, endometriosis, tumors, or cysts. Painful intercourse in men may be attributed to penile infections, phimosis, urinary tract infections, or prostate problems.

2. **Psychosocial Factors**

a. ***Sexual Desire Disorders.*** These may be attributed to a number of early developmental conflicts that have left the individual with unconscious connections between the sexual impulse and overwhelming feelings of shame and guilt (Sadock, 1989). Childhood sexual assault or abuse, as well as repeated painful experiences with coitus, mental depression, aging-related concerns, and relationship difficulties may also be implicated.

b. ***Sexual Arousal Disorders.*** In the female these may be attributed to doubts, fears, guilt, anxiety, shame, conflict, embarrassment, tension, disgust, resentment, grief, anger toward the partner, and puritanical or moralistic upbringing (Tollison and Adams, 1979). A history of sexual abuse may also be an important etiologic factor (Becker, 1989). In men, erectile disorder may be related to an inability to express the sexual impulse because of fear, anxiety, anger, or moral prohibition (Sadock, 1989). Early developmental factors that promote feelings of inadequacy and a sense of being unloving or unlovable may also result in impotence. Difficulties in the relationship may also be a contributing factor.

c. ***Orgasmic Disorders.*** A number of factors have been implicated in the etiology of female orgasm disorders. They include fear of becoming pregnant, hostility toward men, negative cultural conditioning, childhood exposure to rigid religious orthodoxy, and traumatic sexual experiences during childhood or adolescence. Orgasm disorders in men may be related to a rigid, puritanical background where sex was perceived as sinful and the genitals as dirty; or interpersonal difficulties such as ambivalence about commitment, fear of pregnancy, or unexpressed hostility may be implicated.

d. ***Sexual Pain Disorders.*** Vaginismus may occur after having experienced painful intercourse for any organic reason, after which involuntary constriction of the vagina occurs in anticipation and fear of recurring pain. Other psychosocial factors that have been implicated in the etiology of vaginismus include negative childhood conditioning of sex as dirty, sinful, and shameful; early childhood sexual trauma; homosexual orientation; traumatic experience with an early pelvic examination; pregnancy phobia; venereal disease phobia; or cancer phobia (Kolodny et al, 1979).

Symptomatology (Subjective and Objective Data)

1. Absence of sexual fantasies and desire for sexual activity.
2. Discrepancy between partners' levels of desire for sexual activity.
3. Feelings of disgust, anxiety, or panic responses to genital contact.
4. Inability to produce adequate lubrication for sexual activity.
5. Absence of a subjective sense of sexual excitement during sexual activity.
6. Failure to attain or maintain penile erection until completion of sexual activity.
7. Inability to achieve orgasm (in men, to ejaculate) following a period of sexual excitement judged adequate in intensity and duration to produce such a response.
8. Ejaculation occurs with minimal sexual stimulation or before, on, or shortly after penetration and before the individual wishes it.

9. Genital pain occurring before, during, or after sexual intercourse.
10. Constriction of the outer one-third of the vagina prevents penile penetration.

Common Nursing Diagnoses and Interventions
(Interventions are applicable to various health-care settings, such as inpatient and partial hospitalization, community outpatient clinic, home health, and private practice.)

SEXUAL DYSFUNCTION

Definition: *The state in which an individual experiences a change in sexual function that is viewed as unsatisfying, unrewarding, or inadequate.*

Possible Etiologies ("related to")
Ineffectual or absent role models
Physical [or sexual] abuse
Psychosocial abuse
Values conflict
Lack of privacy
Lack of significant other
Altered body structure or function (pregnancy, recent childbirth, drugs, surgery, anomalies, disease process, trauma, radiation)
Misinformation or lack of knowledge
[Depression]
[Pregnancy phobia]
[Venereal disease phobia]
[Cancer phobia]
[Previous painful experience]
[Severe anxiety]
[Relationship difficulties]

Defining Characteristics ("evidenced by")
Verbalization of problem:

- [Absence of desire for sexual activity
- Feelings of disgust, anxiety, or panic responses to genital contact
- Absence of lubrication or subjective sense of sexual excitement during sexual activity

- Failure to attain or maintain penile erection during sexual activity
- Inability to achieve orgasm or ejaculation
- Premature ejaculation
- Genital pain during intercourse
- Constriction of the vagina that prevents penile penetration]

Verbalization of inability to achieve desired sexual satisfaction

Goals/Objectives
Short-Term Goals
1. Client will identify stressors that may contribute to loss of sexual function within 1 week *or*
2. Client will discuss pathophysiology of disease process that contributes to sexual dysfunction within 1 week.

For client with permanent dysfunction due to disease process:
3. Client will verbalize willingness to seek professional assistance from a sex therapist in order to learn alternative ways of achieving sexual satisfaction with partner by (time dimension is individually determined).

Long-Term Goal
Client will resume sexual activity at level satisfactory to self and partner by (time dimension determined by individual situation).

Interventions with *Selected Rationales*
1. Assess client's sexual history and previous level of satisfaction in sexual relationship. *This establishes a database from which to work and provides a foundation for goal setting.*
2. Assess client's perception of the problem. *Client's idea of what constitutes a problem may differ from the nurse's. It is the client's perception on which the goals of care must be established.*
3. Help client determine time dimension associated with the onset of the problem and discuss what was happening in life situation at that time. *Stress in any areas of life can affect sexual functioning. Client may be unaware of correlation between stress and sexual dysfunction.*
4. Assess client's mood and level of energy. *Depression and fatigue decrease desire and enthusiasm for participation in sexual activity.*
5. Review medication regimen; observe for side effects. *Many medications can affect sexual functioning. Eval-*

uation of drug and individual response is important to ascertain whether drug may be contributing to the problem.

6. Encourage client to discuss disease process that may be contributing to sexual dysfunction. Ensure that client is aware that alternative methods of achieving sexual satisfaction exist and can be learned through sex counseling if he or she and partner desire to do so. *Client may be unaware that satisfactory changes can be made in his or her sex life. He or she may also be unaware of the availability of sex counseling.*

7. Encourage client to ask questions regarding sexuality and sexual functioning that may be troubling him or her. *Increasing knowledge and correcting misconceptions can decrease feelings of powerlessness and anxiety and facilitate problem resolution.*

8. Make referral to sex therapist, if necessary. Client may even request that an initial appointment be made for him or her. *Complex problems are likely to require assistance from an individual who is specially trained to treat problems related to sexuality. Client and partner may be somewhat embarrassed to seek this kind of assistance. Support from a trusted nurse can provide the impetus for them to pursue the help that they need.*

Outcome Criteria

1. Client is able to correlate physical or psychosocial factors that interfere with sexual functioning.
2. Client is able to communicate with partner about their sexual relationship without discomfort.
3. Client and partner verbalize willingness and desire to seek assistance from professional sex therapist *or*
4. Client verbalizes resumption of sexual activity at level satisfactory to self and partner.

ALTERED SEXUALITY PATTERNS

Definition: *The state in which an individual expresses concern regarding his or her sexuality.*

Possible Etiologies ("related to")

Lack of significant other
Ineffective or absent role models
[Illness-related alterations in usual sexuality patterns]

Conflicts with sexual orientation or variant preferences
[Unresolved oedipal conflict]
[Delayed sexual adjustment]

Defining Characteristics ("evidenced by")

Reported difficulties, limitations, or changes in sexual behaviors or activities
[Expressed dissatisfaction with sexual behaviors]
[Reports that sexual arousal can only be achieved through variant practices, such as pedophilia, fetishism, masochism, sadism, frotteurism, exhibitionism, voyeurism]
[Desires to experience satisfying sexual relationship with another individual without need for arousal through variant practices]

Goals/Objectives

(Time elements to be determined by individual situation)

Short-Term Goals

1. Client will verbalize aspects about sexuality that he or she would like to change.
2. Client and partner will communicate with each other ways in which each believes their sexual relationship could be improved.

Long-Term Goals

1. Client will express satisfaction with own sexuality pattern.
2. Client and partner will express satisfaction with sexual relationship.

Interventions with *Selected Rationales*

1. Take sexual history, noting client's expression of areas of dissatisfaction with sexual pattern. *Knowledge of what client perceives as the problem is essential for providing the type of assistance he or she may need.*
2. Assess areas of stress in client's life and examine relationship with sexual partner. *Variant sexual behaviors are often associated with added stress in the client's life. Relationship with partner may deteriorate as individual eventually gains sexual satisfaction only from variant practices.*
3. Note cultural, social, ethnic, racial, and religious factors that may contribute to conflicts regarding variant sexual practices. *Client may be unaware of the influence these factors exert in creating feelings of discomfort, shame, and guilt regarding sexual attitudes and behavior.*
4. Be accepting and nonjudgmental. *Sexuality is a very personal and sensitive subject. The client is more likely to*

share this information if he or she does not fear being judged by the nurse.

5. Assist therapist in plan of behavior modification to help client who desires to decrease variant sexual behaviors. *Individuals with paraphilias are treated by specialists who have experience in modifying variant sexual behaviors. Nurses can intervene by providing assistance with implementation of the plan for behavior modification.*

6. If altered sexuality patterns are related to illness or medical treatment, provide information to client and partner regarding the correlation between the illness and the sexual alteration. Explain possible modifications in usual sexual patterns that client and partner may try in an effort to achieve a satisfying sexual experience in spite of the limitation. *Client and partner may be unaware of alternate possibilities for achieving sexual satisfaction, or anxiety associated with the limitation may interfere with rational problem solving.*

7. Explain to client that sexuality is a normal human response and is not synonymous with any one sexual act; that it involves complex interrelationships among one's self-concept, body image, personal history, family and cultural influences; and all interactions with others (VandeVusse and Simandl, 1992). *If client feels "abnormal" or very unlike everyone else, the self-concept is likely to be very low—he or she may even feel worthless. To increase the client's feelings of self-worth and desire to change behavior, help him or her to see that even though the behavior is variant, feelings and motivations are common.*

Outcome Criteria

1. Client is able to verbalize fears about abnormality and inappropriateness of sexual behaviors.
2. Client expresses desire to change variant sexual behavior and cooperates with plan of behavior modification.
3. Client and partner verbalize modifications in sexual activities in response to limitations imposed by illness or medical treatment.
4. Client expresses satisfaction with own sexuality pattern or satisfying sexual relationship with another.

GENDER IDENTITY DISORDERS

Gender identity is the sense of knowing to which sex one belongs—that is, the awareness of one's masculinity or femininity. Gender identity disorders occur when there is an incongruence between anatomic sex and gender identity. An individual with gender identity disorder has an intense desire to be, or insists that he or she is, of the other sex. The *DSM-IV* (APA, 1994) identifies two categories of the disorder:

1. Gender Identity Disorder in Children
2. Gender Identity Disorder in Adolescents and Adults

Kaplan, Sadock, and Grebb (1994) report that intervention with adolescents and adults with gender identity disorder is difficult. Adolescents commonly act out and rarely have the motivation required to alter their cross-gender roles. Adults generally seek therapy to learn how to cope with their altered sexual identity, not to correct it.

Treatment of children with the disorder is aimed at helping them to become more comfortable with their assigned sex and to avoid the possible development of gender dissatisfaction in adulthood.

Predisposing Factors (to Gender Identity Disorder)

1. **Physiologic**
   a. Studies of genetics and physiologic alterations have been conducted in an attempt to determine whether or not a biologic predisposition to gender identity disorder exists. To date, no clear evidence has been demonstrated.
2. **Psychosocial**
   a. ***Family Dynamics.*** Dynamics within a family may have a role in the etiology of gender identity disorder. In Green's (1976, 1985) studies with feminine boys, he found the following:
      (1) Parental indifference to feminine behavior
      (2) Parental encouragement of feminine behavior
      (3) Maternal overprotection of a son and prohibition of "rough, boyish" play
      (4) Excessive maternal attention and physical contact, resulting in lack of separation and individuation of the boy from his mother
      (5) Absence of, or rejection by, the father
      (6) Physical beauty of a boy, influencing adults to treat him in a feminine manner
      (7) Lack of male playmates during early years of socialization

Pauly (1974) found that a disturbed parental relationship was also commonly reported by a substantial majority of adult women with gender identity disorder. The dynamics often included a weak or depressive mother or an aggressive, excessively masculine and often alcoholic father. Encouragement by both parents of masculinity in the daughter was common.

b. ***Psychoanalytic Theory.*** This theory suggests that gender identity problems begin during the struggle of the oedipal conflict. Problems may reflect both real family events and those created in the imagination of the child. These conflicts, whether real or imagined, interfere with the child's loving of the opposite-gender parent and identifying with the same-gender parent, and ultimately with normal gender identity.

Symptomatology (Subjective and Objective Data)

In children or adolescents:

1. Repeatedly stating intense desire to be of the opposite sex.
2. Insistence that one is of the opposite sex.
3. Preference in males for cross-dressing or simulating female attire.
4. Insistence by females on wearing only stereotypical masculine clothing.
5. Fantasies of being of the opposite sex.
6. Intense desire to participate in the stereotypical games and pastimes of the opposite sex.
7. Strong preference for playmates (peers) of the opposite sex.

In adults:

1. A stated desire to be the other sex.
2. Frequently passing as the other sex.
3. Desire to live or be treated as the other sex.
4. Stated conviction that one has the typical feelings and reactions of the other sex.
5. Persistent discomfort with or sense of inappropriateness in the assigned gender role.
6. Request for opposite gender hormones or surgery to alter sexual characteristics.

Common Nursing Diagnoses and Interventions

(Interventions are applicable to various health-care settings, such as inpatient and partial hospitalization, community outpatient clinic, home health, and private practice.)

NOTE: Because adults and adolescents rarely have the desire or motivation to modify their gender identity, nursing interventions in this section are focused on working with gender disordered children.

PERSONAL IDENTITY DISTURBANCE

Definition: *Inability to distinguish between self and nonself.*

Possible Etiologies ("related to")
[Parenting patterns that encourage culturally unacceptable behaviors for assigned gender]
[Unresolved oedipal conflict]

Defining Characteristics ("evidenced by")
[Statements of desire to be other sex]
[Statements that one is the other sex]
[Cross-dressing, or passing as the other sex]
[Strong preference for playmates (peers) of the other sex]
[Stated desire to be treated as the opposite sex]
[Statements of having feelings and reactions of the opposite sex]

Goals/Objectives
Short-Term Goals
Client will verbalize knowledge of behaviors that are appropriate and culturally acceptable for assigned gender.
Client will verbalize desire for congruence between personal feelings and behavior and assigned gender.

Long-Term Goals
Client will demonstrate behaviors that are appropriate and culturally acceptable for assigned gender.
Client will express personal satisfaction and feelings of being comfortable in assigned gender.

Interventions with *Selected Rationales*
1. Spend time with client and show positive regard. *Trust and unconditional acceptance are essential to the establishment of a therapeutic nurse-client relationship.*

2. Be aware of own feelings and attitudes toward this client and his or her behavior. *Attitudes influence behavior. The nurse must not allow negative attitudes to interfere with the effectiveness of interventions.*
3. Allow client to describe his or her perception of the problem. *It is important to know how the client perceives the problem before attempting to correct misperceptions.*
4. Discuss with the client the types of behaviors that are more culturally acceptable. Practice these behaviors through role playing or with play therapy strategies (e.g., male and female dolls). Positive reinforcement or social attention may be given for use of appropriate behaviors. No response is given for opposite-sex-stereotype behaviors. *The goal is to enhance culturally appropriate same-sex behaviors, but not necessarily to extinguish all coexisting opposite-sex behaviors (Rosen et al, 1978).*

Outcome Criteria
1. Client demonstrates behaviors that are culturally appropriate for assigned gender.
2. Client verbalizes and demonstrates self-satisfaction with assigned gender role.
3. Client demonstrates development of a close relationship with the parent of the same gender.

IMPAIRED SOCIAL INTERACTION

Definition: *The state in which an individual participates in an insufficient or excessive quantity or ineffective quality of social exchange.*

Possible Etiologies ("related to")
[Socially and culturally unacceptable behavior]
[Negative role modeling]
[Low self-esteem]

Defining Characteristics ("evidenced by")
Verbalized or observed discomfort in social situations
Verbalized or observed inability to receive or communicate a satisfying sense of belonging, caring, interest, or shared history
Observed use of unsuccessful social interaction behaviors
Dysfunctional interaction with peers, family, or others

Goals/Objectives
Short-Term Goal
Client will verbalize possible reasons for ineffective interactions with others.

Long-Term Goal
Client will interact with others using culturally acceptable behaviors.

Interventions with *Selected Rationales*
1. Once client feels comfortable with the new behaviors in role playing or one-to-one nurse-client interactions, they may be tried in group situations. If possible, remain with the client during initial interactions with others. *Presence of a trusted individual provides security for the client in a new situation. It also provides the potential for feedback to the client about his or her behavior.*
2. Observe client behaviors and the responses he or she elicits from others. Give social attention (e.g., smile, nod) to desired behaviors. Follow up these "practice" sessions with one-to-one processing of the interaction. Give positive reinforcement for efforts. *Positive reinforcement encourages repetition of desirable behaviors. One-to-one processing provides time for discussing the appropriateness of specific behaviors, and why they should or should not be repeated.*
3. Offer support if client is feeling hurt from peer ridicule. Matter-of-factly discuss the behaviors that elicited the ridicule. Offer no personal reaction to the behavior. *Personal reaction from the nurse would be considered judgmental. Validation of client's feelings is important, yet it is important that client understand why his or her behavior was the subject of ridicule, and how to avoid it in the future.*

Outcome Criteria
1. Client interacts appropriately with others demonstrating culturally acceptable behaviors.
2. Client verbalizes and demonstrates comfort in assigned gender role in interactions with others.

SELF-ESTEEM DISTURBANCE

Definition: Negative self-evaluation and feelings about self or self-capabilities, which may be directly or indirectly expressed.

Possible Etiologies ("related to")

[Rejection by peers]
[Lack of positive feedback]
[Repeated negative feedback, resulting in diminished self-worth]
[Dysfunctional family system]
[Lack of personal satisfaction with assigned gender]

Defining Characteristics ("evidenced by")

[Inability to form close, personal relationships]
[Negative view of self]
[Expressions of worthlessness]
[Social isolation]
Hypersensitivity to slight or criticism
Expressions of shame or guilt
Self-negating verbalizations
[Lack of eye contact]

Goals/Objectives
Short-Term Goal
Client will verbalize positive statements about self, including past accomplishments and future prospects.

Long-Term Goal
Client will verbalize and demonstrate behaviors that indicate self-satisfaction with assigned gender, ability to interact with others, and a sense of self as a worthwhile person.

Interventions with *Selected Rationales*

1. *To enhance the child's self-esteem:*
   a. Encourage the child to engage in activities in which he or she is likely to achieve success.
   b. Help the child to focus on aspects of his or her life for which positive feelings exist. Discourage rumination about situations that are perceived as failures or over which the client has no control. Give positive feedback for these behaviors.
2. Help the client identify behaviors or aspects of life he or she would like to change. If realistic, assist the child in problem-solving ways to bring about the change. *Having some control over his or her life may decrease feelings of powerlessness and increase feelings of self-worth.*
3. Offer to be available for support to the child when he or she is feeling rejected by peers. *Having an available support person who does not judge the child's behavior and who provides unconditional acceptance assists*

*the child to progress toward acceptance of self as a
worthwhile person.*

Outcome Criteria

1. Client verbalizes positive perception of self.
2. Client verbalizes self-satisfaction about accomplishments
   and demonstrates behaviors that reflect self-worth.

Chapter 13
EATING DISORDERS

BACKGROUND ASSESSMENT DATA

The *DSM-IV* (APA, 1994) identifies eating disorders as those characterized by severe disturbances in eating behavior. Two such disorders are described in the *DSM-IV*: anorexia nervosa and bulimia nervosa. Obesity is not classified as a psychiatric disorder per se; however, because of the strong emotional factors associated with it, the *DSM-IV* suggests that obesity may be considered within the category of *Psychological Factors Affecting Medical Condition*.

ANOREXIA NERVOSA
Defined
Anorexia nervosa is a clinical syndrome in which the person has a morbid fear of obesity. It is characterized by the individual's gross distortion of body image, preoccupation with food, and refusal to eat. The *DSM-IV* lists the following criteria which must be present to confirm the diagnosis of anorexia nervosa:

1. Refusal to maintain body weight at or above a minimally normal weight for age and height (e.g., weight loss leading to maintenance of body weight less than 85% of that expected; or failure to make expected weight gain during period of growth, leading to body weight less than 85% of that expected).
2. Intense fear of gaining weight or becoming fat, even though underweight.
3. Disturbance in the way one's body weight or shape is

experienced, undue influence of body weight or shape on self-evaluation, or denial of the seriousness of the current low body weight.
4. In postmenarcheal females, amenorrhea, that is, the absence of at least three consecutive menstrual cycles.

The disorder occurs predominantly in females aged 12 to 30 years. Without intervention, death from starvation can occur.

Symptomatology (Subjective and Objective Data)

1. Morbid fear of obesity. Preoccupied with body size. Reports "feeling fat" even when in an emaciated condition.
2. Refusal to eat. Reports "not being hungry," although it is thought that the actual feelings of hunger do not cease until late in the disorder.
3. Preoccupation with food. Thinks and talks about food at great length. Prepares enormous amounts of food for friends and family members, but refuses to eat any of it.
4. Amenorrhea is common, often appearing even before noticeable weight loss has occurred.
5. Delayed psychosexual development.
6. Compulsive behavior, such as excessive hand washing, may be present.
7. Extensive exercising is common.
8. Feelings of depression and anxiety often accompany this disorder.
9. May engage in the binge-and-purge syndrome from time to time (see section on Bulimia Nervosa).

BULIMIA NERVOSA

Defined

Bulimia nervosa is an eating disorder (commonly called "the binge-and-purge syndrome") characterized by extreme overeating, followed by self-induced vomiting and abuse of laxatives and diuretics. Diagnostic criteria for bulimia, as identified by the *DSM-IV*, include the following:

1. Recurrent episodes of binge eating that is characterized by the following:
   a. Eating, within a discrete period of time (e.g., within any 2-hour period), an amount of food that is definitely larger than most people would eat during a

        similar period of time and under similar circumstances.
    b. A sense of lack of control over eating during the episode (e.g., a feeling that one cannot stop eating or control what or how much one is eating).
2. Recurrent, inappropriate compensatory behavior intended to prevent weight gain, such as self-induced vomiting; misuse of laxatives, diuretics, enemas, or other medications; fasting; or excessive exercise.
3. The binge eating and inappropriate compensatory behaviors both occur, on average, at least twice a week for 3 months.
4. Self-evaluation is unduly influenced by body shape and weight.
5. The disturbance does not occur exclusively during episodes of anorexia nervosa.

    The disorder occurs predominantly in females and begins in adolescence or early adult life.

Symptomatology (Subjective and Objective Data)

1. Binges are usually solitary and secret, and the individual may consume thousands of calories in one episode.
2. After the binge has begun, there is often a feeling of loss of control or inability to stop eating.
3. Eating binges may be viewed as pleasurable but are followed by intense self-criticism and depressed mood.
4. Bulimics are usually within normal weight range, some a few pounds underweight, some a few pounds overweight.
5. Obsession with body image and appearance is a predominant feature of this disorder. Individuals with bulimia display undue concern with sexual attractiveness and how they will appear to others.
6. Binges usually alternate with periods of normal eating and fasting.
7. Excessive vomiting may lead to problems with dehydration and electrolyte imbalance. Gastric acid in the vomitus also contributes to the erosion of tooth enamel.

Predisposing Factors to Anorexia Nervosa and Bulimia Nervosa

1. **Physiologic Factors**
    a. *Genetics.* A hereditary predisposition to eating disorders has been hypothesized on the basis of family

histories and an apparent association with other disorders for which the likelihood of genetic influences exist. Anorexia nervosa is more common among sisters and mothers of those with the disorder than among the general population.

b. ***Neuroendocrine Abnormalities.*** Some speculation has occurred regarding a primary hypothalamic dysfunction in anorexia nervosa. Studies consistent with this theory have revealed elevated cerebrospinal-fluid cortisol levels and a possible impairment of dopaminergic regulation in anorexic individuals (Leon and Dinklage, 1989).

2. **Psychosocial Factors**

   a. ***Psychodynamic Theory.*** The psychodynamic theory suggests that behaviors associated with eating disorders reflect a developmental arrest in the very early years of childhood caused by disturbances in mother-infant interactions. The tasks of trust, autonomy, and separation-individuation go unfulfilled, and the individual remains in the dependent position. Ego development is retarded.

   b. ***Family Dynamics.*** This theory proposes that the issue of control becomes the overriding factor in the family of the individual with an eating disorder. These families often consist of a passive father, a domineering mother, and an overly dependent child. A high value is placed on perfectionism in this family, and the child feels he or she must satisfy these standards (Bruch, 1983).

   Parental criticism promotes an increase in obsessive and perfectionistic behavior on the part of the child, who continues to seek love, approval, and recognition. Feelings of helplessness and ambivalence toward the parents eventually develop. In adolescence, these distorted eating patterns may be a rebellion against the parents, viewed by the child as a means of gaining, and remaining in, control. The symptoms are often triggered by a stressor that the adolescent perceives as a loss of control in some aspect of his or her life.

OBESITY

Defined

The following formula is used to determine the degree of obesity in an individual:

$$\text{Body mass index} = \frac{\text{weight (kg)}}{\text{height (m)}^2}$$

The body mass index range for normal weight is 20 to 25 for men and 19 to 24 for women. The individual is considered to be in the obese range once the body mass index range reaches 30. Obesity is known to contribute to a number of health problems, including hyperlipidemia, diabetes mellitus, osteoarthritis, and increased workload on the heart and lungs.

Predisposing Factors to Obesity

1. **Physiologic Factors**
   a. *Genetics.* Genetics have been implicated in the development of obesity in that 80% of children born of two overweight parents will also be overweight. This hypothesis has also been supported by studies of twins reared by normal weight, as well as by overweight, parents.
   b. *Physical Factors.* Overeating and/or obesity has also been associated with lesions in the appetite and satiety centers of the hypothalamus, hypothyroidism, decreased insulin production in diabetes mellitus, and increased cortisone production in Cushing's disease.

2. **Psychosocial Factors**
   a. *Psychoanalytic Theory.* This theory suggests that obesity is the result of unresolved dependency needs, with the individual being fixed in the oral stage of psychosexual development. The symptoms of obesity are viewed as depressive equivalents, attempts to regain "lost" or frustrated nurturance and care.

Common Nursing Diagnoses and Interventions (for Anorexia and Bulimia)

(Interventions are applicable to various health-care settings, such as inpatient and partial hospitalization, community outpatient clinic, home health, and private practice.)

ALTERED NUTRITION: LESS THAN BODY REQUIREMENTS

Definition: *The state in which an individual experiences an intake of nutrients insufficient to meet metabolic needs.*

Possible Etiologies ("related to")
[Refusal to eat]
[Ingestion of large amounts of food, followed by self-induced vomiting]
[Abuse of laxatives, diuretics, and/or diet pills]
[Physical exertion in excess of energy produced through caloric intake]

Defining Characteristics ("evidenced by")
[Loss of 15% of expected body weight (anorexia nervosa)]
Pale conjunctiva and mucous membranes
Poor muscle tone
Excessive loss of hair [or increased growth of hair on body (lanugo)]
[Amenorrhea]
[Poor skin turgor]
[Electrolyte imbalances]
[Hypothermia]
[Bradycardia]
[Hypotension]
[Cardiac irregularities]
[Edema]

Goals/Objectives
Short-Term Goal
Client will gain _____ pounds per week (amount to be established by client, nurse, and dietitian).

Long-Term Goal
By discharge from treatment, client will exhibit no signs or symptoms of malnutrition.

Interventions with *Selected Rationales*
1. If client is unable or unwilling to maintain adequate oral intake, physician may order a liquid diet to be administered via nasogastric tube. Nursing care of the individual receiving tube feedings should be administered according to established hospital procedures. *The client's*

physical safety is a nursing priority, and without adequate nutrition, a life-threatening situation exists. For oral diet:

2. In collaboration with dietitian, determine number of calories required to provide adequate nutrition and realistic (according to body structure and height) weight gain.

3. Explain to client details of behavior modification program as outlined by physician. Explain benefits of compliance with prandial routine and consequences for noncompliance. *Behavior modification bases privileges granted or restricted directly on weight gain and loss. Focus is placed on emotional issues, rather than food and eating specifically.*

4. Sit with client during mealtimes for support and to observe amount ingested. A limit (usually 30 minutes) should be imposed on time allotted for meals. *Without a time limit, meals can become lengthy, drawn-out sessions, providing client with attention based on food and eating.*

5. Client should be observed for at least 1 hour following meals. *Otherwise, this time may be used by client to discard food stashed from tray or to engage in self-induced vomiting.*

6. Client may need to be accompanied to bathroom if self-induced vomiting is suspected.

7. Strict documentation of intake and output. *This information is required to promote client safety and plan nursing care.*

8. Weigh client daily immediately on arising and following first voiding. Always use same scale, if possible. *Client care, privileges, and restrictions will be based on accurate daily weights.*

9. Do not discuss food or eating with client, once protocol has been established. Do, however, offer support and positive reinforcement for obvious improvements in eating behaviors. *Discussing food with client provides positive feedback for maladaptive behaviors.*

10. Client must understand that if, because of poor oral intake, nutritional status does not improve, tube feedings will be initiated *to ensure client's safety.* Staff must be consistent and firm with this action, using a matter-of-fact approach regarding the tube insertion and subsequent feedings.

11. As nutritional status improves and eating habits are established, begin to explore with client the feelings associated with his or her extreme fear of gaining weight.

Emotional issues must be resolved if maladaptive responses are to be eliminated.

Outcome Criteria
1. Client has achieved and maintained at least 85% of expected body weight.
2. Vital signs, blood pressure, and laboratory serum studies are within normal limits.
3. Client verbalizes importance of adequate nutrition.

FLUID VOLUME DEFICIT

Definition: *The state in which an individual experiences vascular, cellular, or intracellular dehydration.*

Possible Etiologies ("related to")
[Decreased fluid intake]
[Abnormal fluid loss caused by self-induced vomiting]
[Excessive use of laxatives or enemas]
[Excessive use of diuretics]
[Electrolyte or acid-base imbalance brought about by malnourished condition or self-induced vomiting]

Defining Characteristics ("evidenced by")
Decreased urine output
Output greater than intake
Concentrated urine
Hemoconcentration
Hypotension
Increased pulse rate
Increased body temperature
Dry skin
Decreased skin turgor
Weakness
Change in mental state
Dry mucous membranes

Goals/Objectives
Short-Term Goal
Client will drink 125 mL of fluid each hour during waking hours.

Long-Term Goal
By discharge from treatment, client will exhibit no signs or symptoms of dehydration (as evidenced by quantity of urinary output sufficient to individual client; normal specific

gravity; vital signs within normal limits; moist, pink mucous membranes; good skin turgor; and immediate capillary refill).

Interventions with *Selected Rationales*
1. Keep strict record of intake and output. Teach client importance of daily fluid intake of 2000 to 3000 mL. *This information is required to promote client safety and plan nursing care.*
2. Weigh client daily immediately on arising and following first voiding. Always use same scale, if possible. *An accurate daily weight is needed to plan nursing care for the client.*
3. Assess and document condition of skin turgor and any changes in skin integrity. *Condition of skin provides valuable data regarding client hydration.*
4. Discourage client from bathing every day if skin is very dry. *Hot water and soap are drying to the skin.*
5. Monitor laboratory serum values, and notify physician of significant alterations. *Laboratory data provide an objective measure for evaluating adequate hydration.*
6. Client should be observed for at least 1 hour following meals and may need to be accompanied to the bathroom if self-induced vomiting is suspected. *Vomiting causes active loss of body fluids and can precipitate fluid volume deficit.*
7. Assess and document moistness and color of oral mucous membranes. *Dry, pale mucous membranes may be indicative of malnutrition or dehydration.*
8. Encourage frequent oral care *to moisten mucous membranes, reducing discomfort from dry mouth, and to decrease bacterial count, minimizing risk of tissue infection.*
9. Help client identify true feelings and fears that contribute to maladaptive eating behaviors. *Emotional issues must be resolved if maladaptive behaviors are to be eliminated.*

Outcome Criteria
1. Client's vital signs, blood pressure, and laboratory serum studies are within normal limits.
2. No abnormalities of skin turgor and dryness of skin and oral mucous membranes are evident.
3. Client verbalizes knowledge regarding consequences of fluid loss due to self-induced vomiting and importance of adequate fluid intake.

INEFFECTIVE INDIVIDUAL COPING

Definition: *The impairment of adaptive behaviors and abilities of a person in meeting life's demands and roles.*

Possible Etiologies ("related to")
[Retarded ego development]
[Unfulfilled tasks of trust and autonomy]
[Dysfunctional family system]
[Unmet dependency needs]
[Feelings of helplessness and lack of control in life situation]
[Possible chemical imbalance caused by malfunction of hypothalamus]
Unrealistic perceptions

Defining Characteristics ("evidenced by")
[Preoccupation with extreme fear of obesity, and distortion of own body image]
[Refusal to eat]
[Obsessed with talking about food]
[Compulsive behavior (e.g., excessive hand washing)]
[Excessive overeating, followed by self-induced vomiting and/or abuse of laxatives and diuretics]
[Poor self-esteem]
[Chronic fatigue]
[Chronic anxiety]
[Chronic depression]
Alteration in societal participation
Inability to problem-solve
Inability to meet role expectations
Destructive behavior toward self

Goals/Objectives
Short-Term Goal
Within 7 days, client will eat regular meals and attend activities without discussing food or physical appearance.

Long-Term Goal
Client will be able to verbalize adaptive coping mechanisms that can be realistically incorporated into his or her lifestyle, thereby eliminating the need for maladaptive eating behaviors.

Interventions with *Selected Rationales*

1. Establish a trusting relationship with client by being honest, accepting, and available and by keeping all promises. *The therapeutic nurse-client relationship is built on trust.*
2. Acknowledge client's anger at feelings of loss of control brought about by established eating regimen (refer to Interventions for Alteration in Nutrition).
3. When nutritional status has improved, begin to explore with client the feelings associated with his or her extreme fear of gaining weight. *Emotional issues must be resolved if maladaptive behaviors are to be eliminated.*
4. Explore family dynamics. Help client to identify his or her role contributions and their appropriateness within the family system. Assist client to identify specific concerns within the family structure and ways to help relieve those concerns. Also, discuss importance of client's separation of self as individual within the family system, and of identifying independent emotions and accepting them as his or her own. *Client must recognize how maladaptive eating behaviors are related to emotional problems—often issues of control within the family structure.*
5. Initially, allow client to maintain dependent role. *To deprive the individual of this role, at this time, could cause his or her anxiety to rise to an unmanageable level.* As trust is developed and physical condition improves, encourage client to be as independent as possible in self-care activities. Offer positive reinforcement for independent behaviors and problem solving and decision making. *Client must learn to function independently. Positive reinforcement increases self-esteem and encourages the client to use behaviors that are more acceptable.*
6. Explore with client ways in which he or she may feel in control within the environment, without resorting to maladaptive eating behaviors.

Outcome Criteria

1. Client is able to assess maladaptive coping behaviors accurately.
2. Client is able to verbalize adaptive coping strategies that can be used in the home environment.

ANXIETY (MODERATE TO SEVERE)

Definition: *A vague uneasy feeling, the source of which is often nonspecific or unknown to the individual.*

Possible Etiologies ("related to")
Situational and maturational crises
[Unmet dependency needs]
[Low self-esteem]
[Dysfunctional family system]
[Feelings of helplessness and lack of control in life situation]
[Unfulfilled tasks of trust and autonomy]

Defining Characteristics ("evidenced by")
Increased tension
Increased helplessness
Overexcited
Apprehensive; fearful
Restlessness
Poor eye contact
[Increased difficulty taking oral nourishment]
[Inability to learn]

Goals/Objectives
Short-Term Goal
Client will demonstrate use of relaxation techniques to maintain anxiety at manageable level within 7 days.

Long-Term Goal
By discharge from treatment, client will be able to recognize events that precipitate anxiety and intervene to prevent disabling behaviors.

Interventions with *Selected Rationales*
1. Be available to stay with client. Remain calm and provide reassurance of safety. *Client safety and security is a nursing priority.*
2. Help client identify the situation that precipitated onset of anxiety symptoms. *Client may be unaware that emotional issues are related to symptoms of anxiety. Recognition may be the first step in elimination of this maladaptive response.*
3. Review client's methods of coping with similar situations in the past. *In seeking to create change, it would be helpful for client to identify past responses and deter-*

mine whether they were successful and if they could be employed again. Client strengths should be identified and used to his or her advantage.

4. Provide quiet environment. Reduce stimuli: low lighting, few people. *Anxiety level may be decreased in calm atmosphere with few stimuli.*

5. Administer antianxiety medications, as ordered by physician. Monitor for effectiveness of medication as well as for adverse side effects. *Antianxiety medications (e.g., diazepam, chlordiazepoxide, alprazolam) provide relief from the immobilizing effects of anxiety, and facilitate client's cooperation with therapy.*

6. Teach client to recognize signs of increasing anxiety and ways to intervene for maintaining the anxiety at a manageable level (e.g., exercise, walking, jogging, relaxation techniques). *Anxiety and tension can be reduced safely and with benefit to the client through physical activities.*

Outcome Criteria

1. Client is able to verbalize events that precipitate anxiety and demonstrate techniques for its reduction.

2. Client is able to verbalize ways in which he or she may gain more control of the environment and thereby reduce feelings of helplessness.

BODY IMAGE/SELF-ESTEEM DISTURBANCE

Definition: *Disruption in the way one perceives one's body image. Negative self-evaluation and feelings about self-capabilities, which may be directly or indirectly expressed.*

Possible Etiologies ("related to")

[Lack of positive feedback]
[Perceived failures]
[Unrealistic expectations (on the part of self and others)]
[Retarded ego development]
[Unmet dependency needs]
[Threat to security caused by dysfunctional family dynamics]
[Morbid fear of obesity]
[Perceived loss of control in some aspect of life]

Defining Characteristics ("evidenced by")

[Distorted body image, views self as fat, even in the presence of normal body weight or severe emaciation]

[Denial that problem with low body weight exists]
[Difficulty accepting] positive reinforcement
Not taking responsibility for self-care (self-neglect)
Nonparticipation in therapy
Self-destructive behavior [self-induced vomiting; abuse of lax-
    atives or diuretics; refusal to eat]
Lack of eye contact
[Depressed mood and self-deprecating thoughts following
    episode of binging and purging]
[Preoccupation with appearance and how others perceive
    them]

Goals/Objectives
Short-Term Goal
Client will verbally acknowledge misperception of body
    image as "fat" within specified time (depending on sever-
    ity and chronicity of condition).

Long-Term Goal
Client will demonstrate an increase in self-esteem as mani-
    fested by verbalizing positive aspects of self and exhibiting
    less preoccupation with own appearance, as a more real-
    istic body image is developed by discharge.

Interventions with *Selected Rationales*
1. Assist client to reexamine negative perceptions of self and
   to recognize positive attributes. *Client's own identification of strengths and positive attributes can increase
   sense of self-worth.*
2. Offer positive reinforcement for independently made decisions influencing client's life. *Positive reinforcement
   enhances self-esteem and may encourage client to
   continue functioning more independently.*
3. Offer positive reinforcement when honest feelings related
   to autonomy and dependence issues remain separated
   from maladaptive eating behaviors.
4. Help client to develop a realistic perception of body image
   and relationship with food. *Client needs to recognize that
   his or her perception of body image is unhealthy and
   that maintaining control through maladaptive eating
   behaviors is dangerous—even life-threatening.*
5. Promote feelings of control within the environment
   through participation and independent decision making.
   Through positive feedback, help client learn to accept self
   as is, including weaknesses as well as strengths. *Client
   must come to understand that he or she is a capable,
   autonomous individual who can perform outside the*

family unit and who is not expected to be perfect. Con-
trol of his or her life must be achieved in other ways
besides dieting and weight loss.
6. Help client realize that perfection is unrealistic, and explore this need with him or her. *As client begins to feel*
   better about self and identifies positive self-attributes,
   as well as develops the ability to accept certain per-
   sonal inadequacies, the need for unrealistic achieve-
   ment should diminish.
7. Help client claim ownership of angry feelings and recognize that expressing them is acceptable if done so in an
   appropriate manner. Be an effective role model. *Unex-*
   pressed anger is often turned inward on the self, re-
   sulting in a depreciation of self-esteem.

Outcome Criteria
1. Client is able to verbalize positive aspects about self.
2. Client expresses interest in welfare of others and less preoccupation with own appearance.
3. Client verbalizes that image of body as "fat" was misperception and demonstrates ability to take control of own
   life without resorting to maladaptive eating behaviors.

Common Nursing Diagnoses and Interventions (for Obesity)
(Interventions are applicable to various health-care set-
tings, such as inpatient and partial hospitalization, com-
munity outpatient clinic, home health, and private prac-
tice.)

ALTERED NUTRITION: MORE THAN BODY REQUIREMENTS

Definition: *The state in which an individual is experiencing*
an intake of nutrients which exceeds metabolic needs.

Possible Etiologies ("related to")
[Compulsive eating]
Excessive intake in relation to metabolic needs
[Sedentary lifestyle]
[Genetics]
[Unmet dependency needs—fixation in oral developmental
  stage]

Defining Characteristics ("evidenced by")
[Weight more than 20% over expected body weight for age and height]
[Body mass index of 30 or more]

Goals/Objectives
Short-Term Goal
Client will verbalize understanding of what must be done to lose weight.

Long-Term Goal
Client will demonstrate change in eating patterns resulting in a steady weight loss.

Interventions with *Selected Rationales*
1. Encourage the client to keep a diary of food intake. *This provides the opportunity for the client to gain a realistic picture of the amount of food ingested and provides a database on which to tailor the dietary program.*
2. Discuss feelings and emotions associated with eating. *This helps to identify when client is eating to satisfy an emotional need rather than a physiologic one.*
3. With input from the client, formulate an eating plan that includes food from the basic food groups with emphasis on low-fat intake. It is helpful to keep the plan as similar to the client's usual eating pattern as possible. *Diet must eliminate calories while maintaining adequate nutrition. Client is more likely to stay on the eating plan if he or she is able to participate in its creation and it deviates as little as possible from usual types of foods.*
4. Identify realistic increment goals for weekly weight loss. *Reasonable weight loss (1–2 lb/wk) results in more lasting effects. Excessive, rapid weight loss may result in fatigue and irritability and may ultimately lead to failure in meeting goals for weight loss. Motivation is more easily sustained by meeting "stair-step" goals.*
5. Plan progressive exercise program tailored to individual goals and choice. *Exercise may enhance weight loss by burning calories and reducing appetite, increasing energy, toning muscles, and enhancing sense of well-being and accomplishment. Walking is an excellent choice for overweight individuals.*
6. Discuss the probability of reaching plateaus when weight remains stable for extended periods. *Client should know that this is likely to happen as changes in metabolism occur. Plateaus cause frustration, and client may need*

additional support during these times to remain on the weight loss program.

7. Administer medications to assist with weight loss if ordered by the physician. *Appetite-suppressant drugs (e.g., phentermine and fenfluramine) may be helpful to someone who is morbidly obese. They should be used for this purpose for only a short period while the individual attempts to adjust to the new pattern of eating.*

Outcome Criteria
1. Client has established a healthy pattern of eating for weight control with weight loss toward a desired goal progressing.
2. Client verbalizes plans for future maintenance of weight control.

BODY IMAGE/SELF-ESTEEM DISTURBANCE

Definition: *Disruption in the way one perceives one's body image. Negative self-evaluation and feelings about self-capabilities, which may be directly or indirectly expressed.*

Possible Etiologies ("related to")
[Dissatisfaction with appearance]
[Unmet dependency needs]
[Lack of adequate nurturing by maternal figure]

Defining Characteristics ("evidenced by")
[Verbalization of negative feelings about the way he or she looks]
[Verbalization of desire to lose weight]
Failure to take responsibility for self-care (self-neglect)
Lack of eye contact
[Expressions of low self-worth]

Goals/Objectives
Short-Term Goal
Client will begin to accept self based on self-attributes rather than on appearance.

Long-Term Goal
Client will pursue loss of weight as desired.

Interventions with *Selected Rationales*
1. Assess client's feelings and attitudes about being obese. *Fat and compulsive eating behaviors may have deep-*

rooted psychological implications, such as compensation for lack of love and nurturing or a defense against intimacy.

2. Ensure that the client has privacy during self-care activities. *The obese individual may be sensitive or self-conscious about his or her body.*

3. Have client recall coping patterns related to food in family of origin and explore how these may affect current situation. *Parents are role models for their children. Maladaptive eating behaviors are learned within the family system and are supported through positive reinforcement. Food may be substituted by the parent for affection and love, and eating is associated with a feeling of satisfaction, becoming the primary defense.*

4. Determine client's motivation for weight loss and set goals. *The individual may harbor repressed feelings of hostility, which may be expressed inward on the self. Because of a poor self-concept, the person often has difficulty with relationships. When the motivation is to lose weight for someone else, successful weight loss is less likely to occur.*

5. Help client identify positive self-attributes. Focus on strengths and past accomplishments unrelated to physical appearance. *It is important that self-esteem not be tied solely to size of the body. Client needs to recognize that obesity need not interfere with positive feelings regarding self-concept and self-worth.*

6. Refer client to support or therapy group. *Support groups can provide companionship, increase motivation, decrease loneliness and social ostracism, and give practical solutions to common problems. Group therapy can be helpful in dealing with underlying psychological concerns.*

Outcome Criteria

1. Client has established a healthy pattern of eating for weight control with weight loss toward a desired goal progressing.

2. Client verbalizes plans for future maintenance of weight control.

Chapter 14

ADJUSTMENT DISORDER

BACKGROUND ASSESSMENT DATA

The essential feature of adjustment disorder is a maladaptive reaction to an identifiable psychosocial stressor that occurs within 3 months after the onset of the stressor and has persisted for no longer than 6 months (APA, 1994). The response is considered maladaptive either because there is impairment in social or occupational functioning or because the behaviors are exaggerated beyond the usual, expected response to such a stressor. The impairment is corrected with the disappearance of, or adaptation to, the stressor. The following categories are defined:

1. **Adjustment Disorder with Depressed Mood.** This category is the most commonly diagnosed adjustment disorder. The major symptoms include depressed mood, tearfulness, and hopelessness. A differential diagnosis with the affective disorders must be considered.
2. **Adjustment Disorder with Anxiety.** The predominant manifestation of this adjustment disorder is anxiety. Major symptoms include nervousness, worry, and jitteriness. A differential diagnosis with the anxiety disorders must be considered.
3. **Adjustment Disorder with Mixed Anxiety and Depressed Mood.** The predominant manifestation of this adjustment disorder is a combination of depression and anxiety. A differential diagnosis must be made considering the affective and anxiety disorders.
4. **Adjustment Disorder with Disturbance of Conduct.** The

major response involves conduct in which there is violation of the rights of others or of major age-appropriate societal norms and rules. A differential diagnosis with conduct disorder or antisocial personality disorder must be considered.

5. **Adjustment Disorder with Mixed Disturbance of Emotions and Conduct.** The predominant manifestations are both emotional symptoms (e.g., depression, anxiety) and disturbances in conduct.

6. **Adjustment Disorder Unspecified.** This diagnosis is used when the maladaptive reaction is not consistent with any of the other categories of adjustment disorder. Manifestations may include physical complaints, social withdrawal, or work or academic inhibition, without significant depressed or anxious mood.

PREDISPOSING FACTORS

1. **Physiologic**
   a. ***Developmental Impairment.*** The presence of chronic disorders, such as organic mental disorder or mental retardation, is thought to limit the general adaptive capacity of an individual (DeWitt, 1984).

2. **Psychosocial Theories**
   a. ***Psychodynamic Theory.*** Erikson (1963) has proposed a systematic development of the personality through the achievement of specific tasks at each stage of the life cycle. Difficulties with adjustment occur when the individual is unable to successfully complete age-appropriate tasks and becomes fixed in a lower developmental level. There is often retarded ego development and the inability to use ego defense mechanisms appropriately. Freud (1964) theorized that traumatic childhood experiences created points of fixation to which the individual, during times of stress, would be likely to regress. This might also apply to other unresolved conflicts or developmental issues.
   b. ***Cognitive Model.*** DeWitt (1984) describes the predisposition to adjustment disorder as an inability to complete the grieving process in response to a painful life change. She describes the presumed cause of this inability to adapt as *psychic overload*, "a level of intrapsychic strain that exceeds the individual's ability to cope and may therefore disrupt normal

functioning and cause psychological or somatic symptoms." Some individuals remain in denial, acting as though the event never occurred. In others, intrusive symptoms may predominate. In all instances, however, it is the persistence of unwanted emotions and images, and the feeling of being powerless to stop them, that precludes the dysfunctional response. Popkin (1989) believes that in adjustment disorder, a specific meaningful stress has found the point of vulnerability in a person of otherwise adequate ego strength.

c. ***Stress-Adaptation Model.*** This model considers the type of stressor the individual experiences, the situational context in which it occurs, and intrapersonal factors in the predisposition to adjustment disorder. Andreasen and Wasek (1980) found that continuous stressors (those to which an individual is exposed over an extended period of time) were more commonly cited than sudden-shock stressors (those that occur without warning) as precipitants to maladaptive functioning.

The situational context in which the stressor occurs may include factors such as personal and general economic conditions; occupational and recreational opportunities; the availability of social supports, such as family, friends, and neighbors; and the availability of cultural or religious support groups.

Intrapersonal factors that have been implicated in the predisposition to adjustment disorder include birth temperament, learned social skills and coping strategies, the presence of psychiatric illness, degree of flexibility, and level of intelligence.

SYMPTOMATOLOGY (Subjective and Objective Data)

1. Depressed mood
2. Tearfulness
3. Hopelessness
4. Nervousness
5. Worry
6. Jitteriness
7. Ambivalence
8. Anger, expressed inappropriately

9. Increased dependency
10. Violation of the rights of others
11. Violation of societal norms and rules, such as truancy, vandalism, reckless driving, fighting
12. Inability to function occupationally or academically
13. Manipulative behavior
14. Social isolation
15. Physical complaints, such as headache, backache, other aches and pains, fatigue

COMMON NURSING DIAGNOSES AND INTERVENTIONS

(Interventions are applicable to various health-care settings, such as inpatient and partial hospitalization, community outpatient clinic, home health, and private practice.)

RISK FOR VIOLENCE: SELF-DIRECTED OR DIRECTED AT OTHERS

Definition: *Behaviors in which an individual demonstrates that he/she can be physically, emotionally, and/or sexually harmful either to self or to others.*

Related/Risk Factors ("related to")
[Fixation in earlier level of development]
[Negative role modeling]
[Dysfunctional family system]
[Low self-esteem]
[Unresolved grief]
[Psychic overload]
[Extended exposure to stressful situation]
[Lack of support systems]
[Biologic factors, such as organic changes in the brain]
Body language—rigid posture, clenching of fists and jaw, hyperactivity, pacing, breathlessness, and threatening stances
[History or threats of violence toward self or others or of destruction to the property of others]
Impulsivity
Suicidal ideation, plan, available means
[Anger; rage]

[Increasing anxiety level]
[Depressed mood]

Goals/Objectives
Short-Term Goals
1. Client will seek out staff member when hostile or suicidal feelings occur.
2. Client will verbalize adaptive coping strategies for use when hostile or suicidal feelings occur.

Long-Term Goals
1. Client will demonstrate adaptive coping strategies for use when hostile or suicidal feelings occur.
2. Client will not harm self or others.

Interventions with *Selected Rationales*
1. Observe client's behavior frequently. Do this through routine activities and interactions; avoid appearing watchful and suspicious. *Close observation is required so that intervention can occur if required to ensure client's (and others') safety.*
2. Observe for suicidal behaviors: verbal statements, such as "I'm going to kill myself" and "Very soon my mother won't have to worry herself about me any longer," and nonverbal behaviors, such as giving away cherished items and mood swings. *Clients who are contemplating suicide often give clues regarding their potential behavior. The clues may be very subtle and require keen assessment skills on the part of the nurse.*
3. Determine suicidal intent and available means. Ask direct questions, such as "Do you plan to kill yourself?" and "How do you plan to do it?" *The risk of suicide is greatly increased if the client has developed a plan and particularly if means exist for the client to execute the plan.*
4. Obtain verbal or written contract from client agreeing not to harm self and to seek out staff in the event that suicidal ideation occurs. *Discussion of suicidal feelings with a trusted individual provides a degree of relief to the client. A contract gets the subject out in the open and places some of the responsibility for his or her safety with the client. An attitude of acceptance of the client as a worthwhile individual is conveyed.*
5. Assist client to recognize when anger occurs and to accept those feelings as his or her own. Have client keep an "anger notebook," in which feelings of anger experienced during a 24-hour period are recorded. Information

regarding source of anger, behavioral response, and client's perception of the situation should also be noted. Discuss entries with client and suggest alternative behavioral responses for those identified as maladaptive.

6. Act as a role model for appropriate expression of angry feelings and give positive reinforcement to client for attempting to conform. *It is vital that the client express angry feelings, because suicide and other self-destructive behaviors are often viewed as the result of anger turned inward on the self.*

7. Remove all dangerous objects from client's environment (e.g., sharp items, belts, ties, straps, breakable items, smoking materials). *Client safety is a nursing priority.*

8. Try to redirect violent behavior with physical outlets for the client's anxiety (e.g., punching bag, jogging). *Physical exercise is a safe and effective way of relieving pent-up tension.*

9. Be available to stay with client as anxiety level and tensions begin to rise. *Presence of a trusted individual provides a feeling of security and may help to prevent rapid escalation of anxiety.*

10. Staff should maintain and convey a calm attitude to client. *Anxiety is contagious and can be transmitted from staff members to client.*

11. Have sufficient staff available to indicate a show of strength to client if necessary. *This conveys to the client evidence of control over the situation and provides some physical security for staff.*

12. Administer tranquilizing medications as ordered by physician or obtain an order if necessary. Monitor client response for effectiveness of the medication and for adverse side effects. *Tranquilizing medications such as anxiolytics or antipsychotics have the capability of inducing a calming effect on the client and may prevent aggressive behaviors.*

13. Use of mechanical restraints or isolation room may be required if less restrictive interventions are unsuccessful. Follow policy and procedure prescribed by the institution in executing this intervention. Most states require that the physician reevaluate the client and issue a new order for restraints every 3 hours, except between the hours of midnight and 8:00 AM. If the client has previously refused medication, administer after restraints have been applied. Most states consider this intervention appropriate in emergency situations or in the event that a client would likely harm self or others.

14. Observe the client in restraints every 15 minutes (or according to institutional policy). Ensure that circulation to extremities is not compromised (check temperature, color, pulses). Assist client with needs related to nutrition, hydration, and elimination. Position client so that comfort is facilitated and aspiration can be prevented. *Client safety is a nursing priority.*

15. As agitation decreases, assess client's readiness for restraint removal or reduction. Remove one restraint at a time, while assessing client's response. *This minimizes risk of injury to the client and staff.*

Outcome Criteria

1. Anxiety is maintained at a level at which client feels no need for aggression.
2. Client denies any ideas of self-destruction.
3. Client demonstrates use of adaptive coping strategies when feelings of hostility or suicide occur.
4. Client verbalizes community support systems from whom assistance may be requested when personal coping strategies are not successful.

ANXIETY (MODERATE TO SEVERE)

Definition: *A vague uneasy feeling, the source of which is often nonspecific or unknown to the individual.*

Possible Etiologies ("related to"):
Situational and maturational crises
[Low self-esteem]
[Dysfunctional family system]
[Feelings of powerlessness and lack of control in life situation]
[Retarded ego development]
[Fixation in earlier level of development]

Defining Characteristics ("evidenced by")
Increased tension
Increased helplessness
Overexcited
Apprehensive; fearful
Restlessness
Poor eye contact
Feelings of inadequacy
Restlessness; insomnia

Focus on the self
Increased cardiac and respiratory rates
[Difficulty learning]

Goals/Objectives
Short-Term Goal
Client will demonstrate use of relaxation techniques to maintain anxiety at manageable level within 7 days.

Long-Term Goal
By discharge from treatment, client will be able to recognize events that precipitate anxiety and intervene to prevent disabling behaviors.

Interventions with *Selected Rationales*
1. Be available to stay with client. Remain calm and provide reassurance of safety. *Client safety and security is a nursing priority.*
2. Help client identify situation that precipitated onset of anxiety symptoms. *Client may be unaware that emotional issues are related to symptoms of anxiety. Recognition may be the first step in elimination of this maladaptive response.*
3. Review client's methods of coping with similar situations in the past. Discuss ways in which client may assume control over these situations. *In seeking to create change, it would be helpful for client to identify past responses and to determine whether they were successful and if they could be employed again. A measure of control reduces feelings of powerlessness in a situation, ultimately decreasing anxiety. Client strengths should be identified and used to his or her advantage.*
4. Provide quiet environment. Reduce stimuli: Low lighting, few people. *Anxiety level may be decreased in calm atmosphere with few stimuli.*
5. Administer antianxiety medications as ordered by physician, or obtain order if necessary. Monitor client's response for effectiveness of the medication as well as for adverse side effects. *Antianxiety medications (e.g., diazepam, chlordiazepoxide, alprazolam) provide relief from the immobilizing effects of anxiety and facilitate client's cooperation with therapy.*
6. Discuss with client signs of increasing anxiety and ways of intervening to maintain the anxiety at a manageable level (e.g., exercise, walking, jogging, relaxation techniques). *Anxiety and tension can be reduced safely and with benefit to the client through physical activities.*

Outcome Criteria
1. Client is able to verbalize events that precipitate anxiety and demonstrate techniques for its reduction.
2. Client is able to verbalize ways in which he or she may gain more control of the environment and thereby reduce feelings of powerlessness.

INEFFECTIVE INDIVIDUAL COPING

Definition: *Impairment of adaptive behaviors and abilities of a person in meeting life's demands and roles.*

Possible Etiologies ("related to")
Situational crises
Maturational crises
[Inadequate support systems]
[Negative role modeling]
[Retarded ego development]
[Fixation in earlier level of development]
[Dysfunctional family system]
[Low self-esteem]
[Unresolved grief]

Defining Characteristics ("evidenced by")
Inability to meet role expectations
Alteration in societal participation
Inability to problem-solve
[Increased dependency]
[Manipulation of others in the environment for purposes of fulfilling own desires]
[Refusal to follow rules]

Goals/Objectives
Short-Term Goal
By the end of 1 week, client will comply with rules of therapy and refrain from manipulating others to fulfill own desires.

Long-Term Goal
By discharge from treatment, client will identify, develop, and use socially acceptable coping skills.

Interventions with *Selected Rationales*
1. Discuss with client the rules of therapy and consequences of noncompliance. Carry out the consequences matter of

factly if rules are broken. *Negative consequences may work to decrease manipulative behaviors.*

2. Do not debate, argue, rationalize, or bargain with the client regarding limit setting on manipulative behaviors. *Ignoring these attempts may work to decrease manipulative behaviors. Consistency among all staff members is vital if this intervention is to be successful.*

3. Encourage discussion of angry feelings. Help client identify the true object of the hostility. Provide physical outlets for healthy release of the hostile feelings (e.g., punching bags, pounding boards). *Verbalization of feelings with a trusted individual may help client work through unresolved issues. Physical exercise provides a safe and effective means of releasing pent-up tension.*

4. Take care not to reinforce dependent behaviors. Encourage client to perform as independently as possible and provide positive feedback. *Independent accomplishment and positive reinforcement enhance self-esteem and encourage repetition of desirable behaviors.*

5. Help client to recognize some aspects of his or her life over which a measure of control is maintained. *Recognition of personal control, however minimal, diminishes the feeling of powerlessness and decreases the need for manipulation of others.*

6. Identify the stressor that precipitated the maladaptive coping. If a major life change has occurred, encourage client to express fears and feelings associated with the change. Assist client through the problem-solving process:
   a. Identify possible alternatives that indicate positive adaptation.
   b. Discuss benefits and consequences of each alternative.
   c. Select the most appropriate alternative.
   d. Implement the alternative.
   e. Evaluate the effectiveness of the alternative.
   f. Recognize areas of limitation and make modifications. Request assistance with this process, if needed.

7. Provide positive reinforcement for application of adaptive coping skills and evidence of successful adjustment. *Positive reinforcement enhances self-esteem and encourages repetition of desirable behaviors.*

Outcome Criteria

1. Client is able to verbalize alternative, socially acceptable, and lifestyle-appropriate coping skills he or she plans to use in response to stress.

2. Client is able to solve problems and fulfill activities of daily living independently.
3. Client does not manipulate others for own gratification.

IMPAIRED ADJUSTMENT*

Definition: *The state in which the individual is unable to modify his or her lifestyle or behavior in a manner consistent with a change in health status.*

Possible Etiologies ("related to")
[Change in health status] requiring modification in life style [e.g.:
  • Normal physiologic changes associated with the aging process
  • Chronic disease such as chronic obstructive pulmonary disease, diabetes, renal failure, coronary heart disease, multiple sclerosis and other progressive neurologic diseases, cancer
  • Disabilities or loss of functioning such as paralysis, limb amputations, hysterectomy, mastectomy, colostomy]
[Lack of adequate support systems or ego strength to respond adaptively to the change]

Defining Characteristics ("evidenced by")
Verbalization of nonacceptance of health status change
[Difficulty with problem solving and decision making]
Lack of movement toward independence or of future-oriented thinking
Extended period of shock, disbelief, or anger regarding health status change [dysfunctional grieving]

Goals/Objectives
Short-Term Goals
1. Client will discuss with primary nurse the kinds of lifestyle changes that will occur because of the change in health status.
2. With the help of primary nurse, client will formulate a plan of action for incorporating those changes into his or her lifestyle.
3. Client will demonstrate movement toward independence, considering change in health status.

---

*According to the North American Nursing Diagnosis Association definition, this diagnosis would only be appropriate for the person with adjustment disorder if the precipitating stressor was a change in health status.

Long-Term Goal

Client will demonstrate competence to function independently to his or her optimal ability, considering change in health status, by discharge from treatment.

Interventions with *Selected Rationales*

1. Encourage client to talk about lifestyle prior to the change in health status. Discuss coping mechanisms that were used at stressful times in the past. *It is important to identify the client's strengths so that they may be used to facilitate adaptation to the change or loss that has occurred.*

2. Encourage client to discuss the change or loss and particularly to express anger associated with it. *Some individuals may not realize that anger is a normal stage in the grieving process. If it is not released in an appropriate manner, it may be turned inward on the self, leading to pathologic depression.*

3. Encourage client to express fears associated with the change or loss, or alteration in lifestyle that the change or loss has created. *Change often creates a feeling of disequilibrium and the individual may respond with fears that are irrational or unfounded. He or she may benefit from feedback that corrects misperceptions about how life will be with the change in health status.*

4. Provide assistance with activities of daily living (ADL) as required, but encourage independence to the limit that client's ability will allow. Give positive feedback for activities accomplished independently. *Independent accomplishments and positive feedback enhance self-esteem and encourage repetition of desired behaviors. Successes also provide hope that adaptive functioning is possible and decrease feelings of powerlessness.*

5. Help client with decision making regarding incorporation of change or loss into lifestyle. Identify problems that the change or loss is likely to create. Discuss alternative solutions, weighing potential benefits and consequences of each alternative. Support client's decision in the selection of an alternative. *The high degree of anxiety that usually accompanies a major lifestyle change often interferes with an individual's ability to solve problems and to make appropriate decisions. Client may need assistance with this process in an effort to progress toward successful adaptation.*

6. Use role playing *to decrease anxiety* as client anticipates stressful situations that might occur in relation to the health status change. *Role playing decreases anxiety*

*and provides a feeling of security by preparing the cli-
ent with a plan of action to respond in an appropriate
manner when a stressful situation occurs.*

7. Ensure that client and family are fully knowledgeable regarding the physiology of the change in health status and
its necessity for optimal wellness. Encourage them to ask
questions, and provide printed material explaining the
change to which they may refer following discharge.

8. Help client identify resources within the community from
which he or she may seek assistance in adapting to the
change in health status. Examples include self-help or support groups and public health nurse, counselor, or social
worker. Encourage client to keep follow-up appointments
with physician, or to call physician's office prior to follow-
up date if problems or concerns arise.

Outcome Criteria
1. Client is able to perform ADL independently.
2. Client is able to make independent decisions regarding
lifestyle considering change in health status.
3. Client is able to express hope for the future with consideration of change in health status.

DYSFUNCTIONAL GRIEVING

Definition: *Extended, unsuccessful use of intellectual and
emotional responses by which individuals (families, communities) attempt to work through the process of modifying
self-concept based upon the perception of [actual or] potential loss.*

Possible Etiologies ("related to")
[Real or perceived loss of any concept of value to the individ-
ual]
[Bereavement overload (cumulative grief from multiple un-
resolved losses)]
[Thwarted grieving response to a loss]
[Absence of anticipatory grieving]
[Feelings of guilt generated by ambivalent relationship with
lost concept]

Defining Characteristics ("evidenced by")
Verbal expression of distress at loss
Idealization of lost [concept]
Denial of loss

[Excessive anger, expressed inappropriately]
Developmental regression
Alterations in concentration or pursuit of tasks
Difficulty in expressing loss
Labile affect
Interference with life functioning
Repetitive use of ineffectual behaviors associated with attempts to reinvest in relationships
Reliving of past experiences with little or no reduction of intensity of the grief
Prolonged interference with life functioning, with onset or exacerbation of somatic or psychosomatic responses

Goals/Objectives
Short-Term Goal
By end of 1 week, client will express anger toward lost concept.

Long-Term Goal
Client will be able to verbalize behaviors associated with the normal stages of grief and identify own position in grief process, while progressing at own pace toward resolution.

Interventions with *Selected Rationales*

1. Determine stage of grief in which client is fixed. Identify behaviors associated with this stage. *Accurate baseline assessment data are necessary to plan effective care for the grieving client.*
2. Develop trusting relationship with client. Show empathy and caring. Be honest and keep all promises. *Trust is the basis for a therapeutic relationship.*
3. Convey an accepting attitude so that the client is not afraid to express feelings openly. *An accepting attitude conveys to the client that you believe he or she is a worthwhile person. Trust is enhanced.*
4. Allow client to express anger. Do not become defensive if initial expression of anger is displaced on nurse or therapist. Assist client to explore angry feelings so that they may be directed toward the intended object or person. *Verbalization of feelings in a nonthreatening environment may help client come to terms with unresolved issues.*
5. Assist client to discharge pent-up anger through participation in large motor activities (e.g., brisk walks, jogging, physical exercises, volleyball, punching bag, exercise bike). *Physical exercise provides a safe and effective method for discharging pent-up tension.*

6. Explain to client the normal stages of grief and the behaviors associated with each stage. Help client to understand that feelings such as guilt and anger toward the lost concept are appropriate and acceptable during the grief process. *Knowledge of the acceptability of the feelings associated with normal grieving may help to relieve some of the guilt that these responses generate.*
7. Encourage client to review relationship with lost concept. With support and sensitivity, point out reality of the situation in areas where misrepresentations are expressed. *Client must give up idealized perception and be able to accept both positive and negative aspects about the lost concept before the grief process is complete.*
8. Communicate to client that crying is acceptable. Use of touch is therapeutic and appropriate with most clients. Knowledge of cultural influences specific to the client is important before employing this technique.
9. Assist client in solving problems as he or she attempts to determine methods for more adaptive coping with the experienced loss. Provide positive feedback for strategies identified and decisions made. *Positive reinforcement enhances self-esteem and encourages repetition of desirable behaviors.*
10. Encourage client to reach out for spiritual support during this time in whatever form is desirable to him or her. Assess spiritual needs of client and assist as necessary in the fulfillment of those needs.

Outcome Criteria
1. Client is able to verbalize normal stages of grief process and behaviors associated with each stage.
2. Client is able to identify own position within the grief process and express honest feelings related to the lost concept.
3. Client is no longer manifesting exaggerated emotions and behaviors related to dysfunctional grieving and is able to carry out ADL independently.

SELF-ESTEEM DISTURBANCE

Definition: *Negative self-evaluation and feelings about self or self-capabilities, which may be directly or indirectly expressed.*

Possible Etiologies ("related to")

[Lack of positive feedback]

[Unmet dependency needs]

[Retarded ego development]

[Repeated negative feedback, resulting in diminished self-worth]

[Personal or situational factors such as dysfunctional family system or absence of social support]

Defining Characteristics ("evidenced by")

[Difficulty accepting positive reinforcement]

[Nonparticipation in therapy]

Self-negating verbalizations

Evaluation of self as unable to deal with events

Hesitant to try new things or situations [because of fear of failure]

Projection of blame or responsibility for problems

Rationalization of personal failures

Hypersensitivity to slight or criticism

Grandiosity

[Lack of eye contact]

[Manipulation of one staff member against another in an attempt to gain special privileges]

[Inability to form close, personal relationships]

[Degradation of others in an attempt to increase own feelings of self-worth]

Goals/Objectives
Short-Term Goal

1. Client will discuss fear of failure with nurse within (realistic time period).
2. Client will verbalize things he or she likes about self within (realistic time period).

Long-Term Goal

1. Client will exhibit increased feelings of self-worth as evidenced by verbal expression of positive aspects about self, past accomplishments, and future prospects.
2. Client will exhibit increased feelings of self-worth by setting realistic goals and trying to reach them, thereby demonstrating a decrease in fear of failure.

Interventions with *Selected Rationales*

1. Ensure that goals are realistic. It is important for client to achieve something, so plan for activities in which success is likely. *Success enhances self-esteem.*
2. Convey unconditional positive regard for the client. Pro-

mote understanding of your acceptance for him or her as a worthwhile human being.

3. Spend time with the client, both on a one-to-one basis and in group activities. *This conveys to client that you feel he or she is worth your time.*

4. Assist client in identifying positive aspects of self and in developing plans for changing the characteristics he or she views as negative. *Individuals with low self-esteem often have difficulty recognizing their positive attributes. They may also lack problem-solving ability and require assistance to formulate a plan for implementing the desired changes.*

5. Encourage and support client in confronting the fear of failure by attending therapy activities and undertaking new tasks. Offer recognition of successful endeavors and positive reinforcement for attempts made. *Recognition and positive reinforcement enhance self-esteem.*

6. Do not allow client to ruminate about past failures. Withdraw attention if he or she persists. *Lack of attention to these behaviors may discourage their repetition. Client must focus on positive attributes if self-esteem is to be enhanced.*

7. Minimize negative feedback to client. Enforce limit setting in matter-of-fact manner, imposing previously established consequences for violations. *Negative feedback can be extremely threatening to a person with low self-esteem, possibly aggravating the problem. Consequences should convey unacceptability of the BEHAVIOR, but not the PERSON.*

8. Encourage independence in the performance of personal responsibilities, as well as in decision making related to own self-care. Offer recognition and praise for accomplishments. *The ability to perform self-care activities independently enhances self-esteem. Positive reinforcement encourages repetition of the desirable behavior.*

9. Help client increase level of self-awareness through critical examination of feelings, attitudes, and behaviors. Help him or her to understand that it is perfectly acceptable for one's attitudes and behaviors to differ from others' as long as they do not become intrusive. *As the client achieves self-awareness and self-acceptance, the need for judging the behavior of others will diminish.*

Outcome Criteria

1. Client verbalizes positive perception of self.
2. Client demonstrates ability to manage own self-care,

make independent decisions, and use problem-solving skills.
3. Client sets goals that are realistic and works to achieve those goals without evidence of fear of failure.

IMPAIRED SOCIAL INTERACTION

Definition: *The state in which an individual participates in an insufficient or excessive quantity or ineffective quality of social exchange.*

Possible Etiologies ("related to")
[Retarded ego development]
[Fixation in an earlier level of development]
[Negative role modeling]
[Low self-esteem]

Defining Characteristics ("evidenced by")
Verbalized or observed discomfort in social situations
Verbalized or observed inability to receive or communicate a satisfying sense of belonging, caring, interest, or shared history
Observed use of unsuccessful social interaction behaviors
Dysfunctional interaction with peers, family, or others
[Exhibiting behaviors unacceptable for age, as defined by dominant cultural group]

Goals/Objectives
Short-Term Goal
Client will develop trusting relationship with staff member within (realistic time period) seeking that staff member out for one-to-one interaction.

Long-Term Goals
1. Client will be able to interact with others on a one-to-one basis with no indication of discomfort.
2. Client will voluntarily spend time with others in group activities demonstrating acceptable, age-appropriate behavior.

Interventions with *Selected Rationales*
1. Develop trusting relationship with client. Be honest; keep all promises; convey acceptance of person, separate from unacceptable behaviors ("It is not *you*, but *your behavior*, that is unacceptable.") *Unconditional acceptance of the client increases his or her feelings of self-worth.*

2. Offer to remain with client during initial interactions with others on the unit. *Presence of a trusted individual provides a feeling of security.*
3. Provide constructive criticism and positive reinforcement for efforts. *Positive reinforcement enhances self-esteem and encourages repetition of desirable behaviors.*
4. Confront client and withdraw attention when interactions with others are manipulative or exploitative. *Attention to the unacceptable behavior may reinforce it.*
5. Act as role model for client through appropriate interactions with him or her, other clients, and staff members.
6. Provide group situations for client. *It is through these group interactions, with positive and negative feedback from his or her peers, that client will learn socially acceptable behavior.*

Outcome Criteria
1. Client seeks out staff member for social as well as therapeutic interaction.
2. Client has formed and satisfactorily maintained one interpersonal relationship with another client.
3. Client willingly and appropriately participates in group activities.
4. Client verbalizes reasons for inability to form close interpersonal relationships with others in the past.

RELOCATION STRESS SYNDROME*

Definition: *A state in which an individual experiences physiologic or psychosocial disturbances as a result of transfer from one environment to another.*

Possible Etiologies ("related to")
Change in environment or location
Past, concurrent, and recent losses
Losses involved with decision to move
Feeling of powerlessness
Lack of adequate support system
Little or no preparation for the impending move

*This diagnosis would be appropriate for the individual with adjustment disorder if the precipitating stressor was relocation to a new environment.

Moderate to high degree of environmental change
History and types of previous transfers
Impaired psychosocial health status
Decreased physical health status

Defining Characteristics ("evidenced by")
Anxiety; restlessness
Apprehension
Depression; sad affect
Loneliness
Verbalization of [opposition] to relocate
Sleep disturbance
Change in eating habits; weight change
Dependency; increased verbalization of needs
Gastrointestinal disturbances
Insecurity in new surroundings; lack of trust
Verbalization of being concerned/upset about [relocation]
Withdrawal; [social isolation]

Goals/Objectives
Short-Term Goal
Client will verbalize at least one positive aspect regarding relocation to new environment within (realistic time period).

Long-Term Goal
Client will demonstrate positive adaptation to new environment, as evidenced by involvement in activities, expression of satisfaction with new acquaintances, and elimination of previously evident physical and psychological symptoms associated with the relocation (time dimension to be determined individually).

Interventions with *Selected Rationales*
1. Encourage individual to discuss feelings (concerns, fears, anger) regarding relocation. *Exploration of feelings with a trusted individual may help the individual perceive the situation more realistically and come to terms with the inevitable change.*
2. Encourage individual to discuss how the change will affect his or her life. Ensure that the individual is involved in decision making and problem solving regarding the move. *Taking responsibility for making choices regarding the relocation will increase feelings of control and decrease feelings of powerlessness.*
3. Assist the individual to identify positive aspects about the move. *Anxiety associated with the opposed relocation may interfere with the individual's ability to recognize*

anything positive about it. Assistance may be required.

4. Assist the individual to identify resources within the new community from whom assistance with various types of services may be obtained. *Because of anxiety and depression, the individual may not be able to identify these resources alone. Assistance with problem solving may be required.*

5. Identify groups within the community that specialize in helping individuals adapt to relocation. Examples include Newcomers' Club, Welcome Wagon Club, senior citizens' groups, school and church organizations. *These groups offer support from individuals who have often encountered similar experiences. Adaptation may be enhanced by the reassurance, encouragement, and support of peers who exhibit positive adaptation to relocation stress.*

6. Refer individual or family for professional counseling if deemed necessary. *An individual who is experiencing dysfunctional grieving over loss of previous residence may require therapy to achieve resolution of the problem. It may be that other unresolved issues are interfering with successful adaptation to the relocation.*

Outcome Criteria

1. The individual no longer exhibits signs of anxiety, depression, or somatic symptoms.
2. The individual verbalizes satisfaction with new environment.
3. The individual willingly participates in social and vocational activities within his or her new environment.

Chapter 15

IMPULSE CONTROL DISORDERS

BACKGROUND ASSESSMENT DATA

Impulse control disorders are characterized by a need or desire that must be satisfied immediately, regardless of the consequences (Booth, 1984). Many of the behaviors have adverse or even destructive consequences for the individuals affected, and seldom do these individuals know why they do what they do or why it is pleasurable.

The *DSM-IV* (APA, 1994) describes the essential features of impulse control disorders as follows:

1. Failure to resist an impulse, drive, or temptation to perform some act that is harmful to the person or others.
2. An increasing sense of tension or arousal before committing the act.
3. An experience of either pleasure, gratification, or relief at the time of committing the act. Following the act, there may or may not be regret, self-reproach, or guilt.

The *DSM-IV* (APA, 1994) describes the following categories of impulse control disorders:

Intermittent Explosive Disorder

This disorder is characterized by discrete episodes of failure to resist aggressive impulses, resulting in serious assaults or destruction of property (APA, 1994). Some clients report changes in sensorium, such as confusion during an episode or amnesia for events that occurred during an episode. Symptoms usually appear suddenly without apparent provocation and terminate abruptly, lasting only minutes to a few hours, followed by feelings of genuine remorse and self-reproach about the behavior.

Kleptomania
Kleptomania is described by the *DSM-IV* as "the recurrent failure to resist impulses to steal items not needed for personal use or for their monetary value" (APA, 1994). Often the stolen items (for which the individual usually has enough money to pay) are given away, discarded, returned, or kept and hidden. The individual with kleptomania steals purely for the sake of stealing and for the sense of relief and gratification that follows an episode.

Pathological Gambling
The *DSM-IV* defines pathological gambling as "persistent and recurrent maladaptive gambling behavior that disrupts personal, family, or vocational pursuits" (APA, 1994). The preoccupation with, and impulse to, gamble intensifies when the individual is under stress. Many pathological gamblers exhibit characteristics associated with narcissism and grandiosity, and often have difficulties with intimacy, empathy, and trust (Booth, 1984).

Pyromania
Pyromania is the inability to resist the impulse to set fires (Booth, 1984). The act itself is preceded by tension or affective arousal, and the individual experiences intense pleasure, gratification, or relief when setting the fires, witnessing their effects, or participating in their aftermath (APA, 1994). Motivation for the behavior is self-gratification, and even though some individuals with pyromania may take precautions to avoid apprehension, many are totally indifferent to the consequences of their behavior.

Trichotillomania
This disorder is defined by the *DSM-IV* as "the recurrent pulling out of one's own hair that results in noticeable hair loss" (APA, 1994). The impulse is preceded by an increasing sense of tension, and the individual experiences a sense of release or gratification from pulling out the hair.

PREDISPOSING FACTORS

1. **Physiologic**
   a. ***Genetics.*** A familial tendency appears to be a factor in some cases of intermittent explosive disorder, pathological gambling, and trichotillomania.
   b. ***Physical Factors.*** Brain trauma or dysfunction and mental retardation have also been implicated in the predisposition to impulse control disorders (Kaplan et al, 1994).

2. **Psychosocial**
   a. ***Family Dynamics.*** Various dysfunctional family patterns have been suggested as contributors in the predisposition to impulse control disorders. These include the following:
      - Child abuse or neglect
      - Parental rejection or abandonment
      - Harsh or inconsistent discipline
      - Emotional deprivation
      - Parental substance abuse
      - Parental unpredictability

SYMPTOMATOLOGY (Subjective and Objective Data)

1. Sudden inability to control violent, aggressive impulses
2. Aggressive behavior accompanied by confusion or amnesia
3. Feelings of remorse following aggressive behavior
4. Inability to resist impulses to steal
5. Increasing tension before committing the theft, followed by pleasure or relief during and following the act
6. Sometimes discards, returns, or hides stolen items
7. Inability to resist impulses to gamble
8. Preoccupation with ways to obtain money with which to gamble
9. Increasing tension that is relieved only by placing a bet
10. The need to gamble or loss of money interferes with social and occupational functioning
11. Inability to resist the impulse to set fires
12. Increasing tension that is relieved only by starting a fire
13. Inability to resist impulses to pull out one's own hair

14. Increasing tension followed by a sense of release or gratification from pulling out the hair
15. Hair pulling may be accompanied by other types of self-mutilation (e.g., head banging, biting, scratching)

COMMON NURSING DIAGNOSES AND INTERVENTIONS

(Interventions are applicable to various health-care settings, such as inpatient and partial hospitalization, community outpatient clinic, home health, and private practice.)

RISK FOR VIOLENCE: DIRECTED TOWARD OTHERS

Definition: *Behaviors in which an individual demonstrates that he/she can be physically, emotionally, and/or sexually harmful to others.*

Related/Risk Factors ("related to")
[Possible familial tendency]
[Central nervous system trauma]
[Dysfunctional family system, resulting in behaviors such as the following:
     Child abuse or neglect
     Parental rejection or abandonment
     Harsh or inconsistent discipline
     Emotional deprivation
     Parental substance abuse
     Parental unpredictability]
Body language—rigid posture, clenching of fists and jaw, hyperactivity, pacing, breathlessness, and threatening stances
[History or threats of violence toward others or of destruction to the property of others]
Impulsivity

Goals/Objectives
Short-Term Goal
Client will recognize signs of increasing tension, anxiety, and agitation, and report to staff (or others) for assistance with intervention (time dimension to be individually determined).

Long-Term Goal
Client will not harm others or the property of others (time dimension to be individually determined).

Interventions with *Selected Rationales*
1. Convey an accepting attitude toward the client. Feelings of rejection are undoubtedly familiar to him or her. Work on the development of trust. Be honest, keep all promises, and convey the message that it is not *him* or *her* but the *behavior* that is unacceptable. *An attitude of acceptance promotes feelings of self-worth. Trust is the basis of a therapeutic relationship.*
2. Maintain low level of stimuli in client's environment (low lighting, few people, simple decor, low noise level). *A stimulating environment may increase agitation and promote aggressive behavior. Make the client's environment as safe as possible* by removing all potentially dangerous objects.
3. Help client identify the true object of his or her hostility. *Because of weak ego development, client may be unable to use ego defense mechanisms correctly. Helping him or her recognize this in a nonthreatening manner may help reveal unresolved issues so that they may be confronted.*
4. Staff should maintain and convey a calm attitude. *Anxiety is contagious and can be transferred from staff to client. A calm attitude provides the client with a feeling of safety and security.*
5. Help the client recognize the signs that tension is increasing and ways in which violence can be averted. *Activities that require physical exertion are helpful in relieving pent-up tension.*
6. Explain to the client that should explosive behavior occur, staff will intervene in whatever way is required (e.g., tranquilizing medication, restraints, isolation) to protect client and others. *This conveys to the client evidence of control over the situation and provides a feeling of safety and security.*

Outcome Criteria
1. Anxiety is maintained at a level at which client feels no need for aggression.
2. The client is able to verbalize the symptoms of increasing tension and adaptive ways for coping with it.
3. The client is able to inhibit the impulse for violence and aggression.

RISK FOR SELF-MUTILATION

Definition: *A state in which an individual is at risk to perform an act on the self to injure, not kill, which produces tissue damage and tension relief.*

Related/Risk Factors ("related to")
[Possible familial tendency]
[Central nervous system trauma]
[Mental retardation]
[Early emotional deprivation]
[Parental rejection or abandonment]
[Child abuse or neglect]
[History of self-mutilative behaviors in response to increasing anxiety: hair pulling, biting, head banging, scratching]

Goals/Objectives
Short-Term Goal
Client will cooperate with plan of behavior modification in an effort to respond more adaptively to stress (time dimension ongoing).

Long-Term Goal
Client will not harm self.

Interventions with *Selected Rationales*
1. Intervene to protect client when self-mutilative behaviors, such as head banging or hair pulling, become evident. *The nurse is responsible to ensure client safety.*
2. A helmet may be used to protect against head banging, hand mitts to prevent hair pulling, and appropriate padding to protect extremities from injury during hysterical movements.
3. Try to determine if self-mutilative behaviors occur in response to increasing anxiety, and if so, to what the anxiety may be attributed. *Self-mutilative behaviors may be averted if the cause can be determined.*
4. Work on one-to-one basis with client *to establish trust.*
5. Assist with plan for behavior modification *in an effort to teach the client more adaptive ways of responding to stress.*
6. Encourage client to discuss feelings, particularly anger, *in an effort to confront unresolved issues and expose internalized rage that may be triggering self-mutilative behaviors.*
7. Offer self to client during times of increasing anxiety, *in*

order to provide feelings of security and decrease need for self-mutilative behaviors.

Outcome Criteria
1. Anxiety is maintained at a level at which client feels no need for self-mutilation.
2. Client demonstrates ability to use adaptive coping strategies in the face of stressful situations.

INEFFECTIVE INDIVIDUAL COPING

Definition: *The impairment of adaptive behaviors and abilities of a person in meeting life's demands and roles.*

Possible Etiologies ("related to")
[Possible hereditary factors]
[Brain trauma or dysfunction]
[Mental retardation]
[Dysfunctional family system, resulting in behaviors such as the following:
    Child abuse or neglect
    Parental rejection or abandonment
    Harsh or inconsistent discipline
    Emotional deprivation
    Parental substance abuse
    Parental unpredictability]

Defining Characteristics ("evidenced by")
[Inability to control impulse of violence or aggression]
[Inability to control impulse to steal]
[Inability to control impulse to gamble]
[Inability to control impulse to set fires]
[Inability to control impulse to pull out own hair]
[Feeling of intense anxiety and tension that precedes, and is relieved by, engaging in these impulsive behaviors]

Goals/Objectives
Short-Term Goal
Client will verbalize adaptive ways to cope with stress by means other than impulsive behaviors (time dimension to be individually determined).

Long-Term Goal
Client will be able to delay gratification and use adaptive coping strategies in response to stress (time dimension to be individually determined).

Interventions with *Selected Rationales*

1. Help client gain insight into his or her own behaviors. Often these individuals rationalize to such an extent that they deny that what they have done is wrong. *Client must come to understand that certain behaviors will not be tolerated within the society and that severe consequences will be imposed on those individuals who refuse to comply. Client must WANT to become a productive member of society before he or she can be helped.*

2. Talk about past behaviors with client. Discuss behaviors that are acceptable by societal norms and those that are not. Help client identify ways in which he or she has exploited others. Encourage client to explore how he or she would feel if the circumstances were reversed. *An attempt may be made to enlighten the client to the sensitivity of others by promoting self-awareness in an effort to assist the client gain insight into his or her own behavior.*

3. Throughout relationship with client, maintain attitude of "It is not *you*, but *your behavior*, that is unacceptable." *An attitude of acceptance promotes feelings of dignity and self-worth.*

4. Work with client to increase the ability to delay gratification. Reward desirable behaviors and provide immediate positive feedback. *Rewards and positive feedback enhance self-esteem and encourage repetition of desirable behaviors.*

5. Help client identify and practice more adaptive strategies for coping with stressful life situations. *The impulse to perform the maladaptive behavior may be so great that the client is unable to see any other alternatives to relieve stress.*

Outcome Criteria

1. Client is able to demonstrate techniques that may be used in response to stress in order to prevent resorting to maladaptive impulsive behaviors.

2. Client verbalizes understanding that behavior is unacceptable and accepts responsibility for own behavior.

Chapter 16

PSYCHOLOGICAL FACTORS AFFECTING MEDICAL CONDITION

BACKGROUND ASSESSMENT DATA

The *DSM-IV* (APA, 1994) identifies *Psychological Factors Affecting Medical Condition* as the presence of one or more specific psychological or behavioral factors that adversely affect a general medical condition. These factors can adversely affect the medical condition in several ways:

1. By influencing the course of the medical condition (i.e., contributing to the development or exacerbation of, or delayed recovery from, the medical condition).
2. By interfering with treatment of the medical condition.
3. By constituting an additional health risk for the individual (e.g., the individual who has peptic ulcers who continues to drink and smoke).

PSYCHOLOGICAL FACTORS AFFECTING MEDICAL CONDITION

Defined

The *DSM-IV* (APA, 1994) designates this diagnosis when there is evidence of a physical symptom(s) or a physical disorder that is adversely affected by psychological factors. Common examples of medical conditions for which this category may be appropriate include, but are not limited to, tension headache, migraine headache, cardiospasm, pylorospasm, rheumatoid arthritis, asthma, ulcers, ulcerative colitis, regional enteritis, hypertension, nausea and vomiting, tachycardia, arrhythmia, acne, angina pectoris, painful menstruation, frequency of micturation, neurodermatitis, and sacroiliac pain. Kaplan (1989) states, "All disease is influenced by psychological factors." Virtually any organic disorder can be considered psychophysiologic.

This category differs from somatoform disorders and conversion disorders in that there is evidence of either demonstrable organic pathology (such as the inflammation associated with rheumatoid arthritis) or a known pathophysiologic process (such as the cerebral vasodilation of migraine headaches).

Several types of psychological factors are implicated by the *DSM-IV* as those that can affect a general medical condition. They include the following:

1. Mental disorders (e.g., major depression)
2. Psychological symptoms (e.g., depressed mood or anxiety)
3. Personality traits or coping style (e.g., denial of the need for medical care)
4. Maladaptive health behaviors (e.g., smoking or overeating)
5. Stress-related physiologic responses (e.g., tension headaches)

Predisposing Factors

1. **Physiologic**
   a. ***Physical Factors.*** Selye (1956) believes that psychophysiologic disorders occur when the body is exposed to prolonged stress, producing a number of physiologic effects under direct control of the pituitary-adrenal axis. He also suggests that genetic predisposition influences which organ system will be affected and determines the type of psychophysiologic disorder the individual will develop.
2. **Psychosocial**
   a. ***Emotional Response Pattern.*** Alexander (1950) proposed that individuals exhibit specific physiologic responses to certain emotions. For example, in response to the emotion of anger, one person may experience peripheral vasoconstriction, resulting in an increase in blood pressure. The same emotion, in an-

other individual, may evoke the response of cerebral vasodilation, manifesting a migraine headache.

b. ***Personality Traits.*** Various studies have suggested that individuals with specific personality traits are predisposed to certain disease processes. Although personality cannot account totally for the development of psychophysiologic disorders, the literature has alluded to the following possible relationships:

Asthma	Dependent personality characteristics
Ulcers, hypertension	Repressed anger
Cancer	Depressive personality
Rheumatoid arthritis, ulcerative colitis	Self-sacrificing and inhibited
Migraine headaches	Compulsive and perfectionistic
Coronary heart disease	Aggressive and competitive

c. ***Learning Theory.*** A third psychosocial theory considers the role of learning in the psychophysiologic response to stress (Pasquali et al, 1989). If a child grows up observing the attention, increased dependency, or other secondary gain an individual receives because of the illness, such behaviors may be viewed as desirable responses and subsequently imitated by the child.

d. ***Theory of Family Dynamics.*** Minuchin and coworkers (1978) have suggested the predisposition of those individuals who are members of dysfunctional family systems that use psychophysiologic problems to cover up interpersonal conflicts. The anxiety in a dysfunctional family situation is shifted from the conflict to the ailing individual. Anxiety decreases, the conflict is avoided, and the person receives positive reinforcement for his or her symptoms. The situation appears more comfortable, but the real problem remains unresolved.

Symptomatology (Subjective and Objective Data)

1. Complaints of physical illness that can be substantiated by objective evidence of physical pathology or known pathophysiologic process.
2. Moderate to severe level of anxiety.
3. Denial of emotional problems; client is unable to see a

relationship between physical problems and response
to stress.
4. Use of physical illness as excuse for noncompliance
   with psychiatric treatment plan.
5. Repressed anger or anger expressed inappropriately.
6. Verbal hostility.
7. Depressed mood.
8. Low self-esteem.
9. Dependent behaviors.
10. Attention-seeking behaviors.
11. Report (or other evidence) of numerous stressors oc-
    curring in person's life.

Common Nursing Diagnoses and Interventions*
*(Interventions are applicable to various health-care set-
tings, such as inpatient and partial hospitalization, community outpatient clinic, home health, and private practice.)*

INEFFECTIVE INDIVIDUAL COPING

Definition: *Impairment of adaptive behaviors and abilities of
a person in meeting life's demands and roles.*

Possible Etiologies ("related to")
[Repressed anxiety]
[Inadequate support systems]
[Inadequate coping methods]
[Low self-esteem]
[Unmet dependency needs]
[Negative role modeling]
[Dysfunctional family system]

Defining Characteristics ("evidenced by")
[Initiation or exacerbation of physical illness (specify)]
[Denial of relationship between physical symptoms and emo-
    tional problems]
[Use of sick role for secondary gains]

---

*A number of nursing diagnoses common to specific physical disorders
or symptoms could be used (e.g., pain, activity intolerance, impaired tissue integrity, diarrhea). For purposes of this chapter, only nursing diagnoses common to the general category are presented.

Inability to meet role expectations
Inability to problem solve

Goals/Objectives
Short-Term Goal
Within 1 week, client will verbalize adaptive ways of coping with stressful situations.

Long-Term Goal
Client will achieve physical wellness and demonstrate the ability to prevent exacerbation of physical symptoms as a coping mechanism in response to stress.

Interventions with *Selected Rationales*
1. Perform thorough physical assessment *in order to determine specific care required for client's physical condition.* Monitor laboratory values, vital signs, intake and output, and other assessments necessary *to maintain an accurate, ongoing appraisal.*
2. Together with the client, identify goals of care and ways in which client believes he or she can best achieve those goals. Client may need assistance with problem solving. *Personal involvement in his or her own care provides a feeling of control and increases chances for positive outcomes.*
3. Encourage client to discuss current life situations that he or she perceives as stressful and the feelings associated with each. *Verbalization of true feelings in a nonthreatening environment may help client come to terms with unresolved issues.*
4. During client's discussion, note times during which a sense of powerlessness or loss of control over life situations emerges. Focus on these times and discuss ways in which the client may maintain a feeling of control. *A sense of self-worth develops and is maintained when an individual feels power over his or her own life situations.*
5. As client becomes able to discuss feelings more openly, assist him or her, in a nonthreatening manner, to relate certain feelings to the appearance of physical symptoms. *Client may be unaware of the relationship between physical symptoms and emotional problems.*
6. Discuss stressful times when physical symptoms did not appear and the adaptive coping strategies that were used during those situations. *Therapy is facilitated by considering areas of strength and using them to the client's benefit.*

7. Provide positive reinforcement for adaptive coping mechanisms identified or used. Suggest alternative coping strategies but allow client to determine which can most appropriately be incorporated into his or her lifestyle. *Positive reinforcement enhances self-esteem and encourages repetition of desirable behaviors. Client may require assistance with problem solving but must be allowed and encouraged to make decisions independently.*

8. Help client to identify a resource within the community (friend, significant other, group) to use as a support system for the expression of feelings *in an effort to prevent maladaptive coping through physical illness.*

Outcome Criteria

1. Client is able to demonstrate techniques that may be used in response to stress in order to prevent the occurrence or exacerbation of physical symptoms.
2. Client verbalizes an understanding of the relationship between emotional problems and physical symptoms.

SELF-ESTEEM DISTURBANCE

Definition: *Negative self-evaluation and feelings about self or self-capabilities, which may be directly or indirectly expressed.*

Possible Etiologies ("related to")
[Lack of positive feedback]
[Unmet dependency needs]
[Retarded ego development]
[Repeated negative feedback, resulting in diminished self-worth]
[Dysfunctional family system]

Defining Characteristics ("evidenced by")
[Difficulty accepting positive reinforcement]
[Nonparticipation in therapy]
Self-negating verbalizations
Evaluation of self as unable to deal with events
Hesitant to try new things or situations [because of fear of failure]
Hypersensitive to slight or criticism
[Lack of eye contact]
[Inability to form close, personal relationships]

[Degradation of others in an attempt to increase own feelings of self-worth]

Goals/Objectives
Short-Term Goals
1. Client will discuss fear of failure with nurse within 3 days.
2. Client will verbalize aspects he or she likes about self within 5 days.

Long-Term Goals
1. Client will exhibit increased feelings of self-worth as evidenced by verbal expression of positive aspects about self, past accomplishments, and future prospects.
2. Client will exhibit increased feelings of self-worth by setting realistic goals and trying to reach them, thereby demonstrating a decrease in fear of failure.

Interventions with *Selected Rationales*
1. Ensure that goals are realistic. It is important for client to achieve something, so plan activities in which success is likely. *Success increases self-esteem.*
2. Minimize amount of attention given to physical symptoms. Client must perceive self as a worthwhile person, separate and apart from the role of client. *Lack of attention may discourage use of undesirable behaviors.*
3. Promote your acceptance of client as a worthwhile person by spending time with him or her. Develop trust through one-to-one interactions, then encourage client to participate in group activities. Support group attendance with your presence until client feels comfortable attending alone. *The feeling of acceptance by others increases self-esteem.*
4. Ask client to make a written list of positive and negative aspects about self. Discuss each item on the list with client. Develop plans of change for the characteristics viewed as negative. Assist client in implementing the plans. Provide positive feedback for successful change. *Individuals with low self-esteem often have difficulty recognizing their positive attributes. They may also lack problem-solving skills and require assistance to formulate a plan for implementing the desired changes. Positive feedback enhances self-esteem and encourages repetition of desired behaviors.*
5. Avoid fostering dependence by "doing for" the client. Allow client to perform as independently as physical condition will permit. Offer recognition and praise for accomplishments. *The ability to perform self-care activities*

independently provides a feeling of self-control and enhances self-esteem. Positive reinforcement encourages repetition of the desirable behavior.

6. Allow client to be an active participant in his or her therapy. Promote feelings of control or power by encouraging input into the decision making regarding treatment, as well as the planning for discharge from treatment. Provide positive feedback for adaptive responses. *Control over own life experiences promotes feelings of self-worth.*

Outcome Criteria

1. Client verbalizes positive perception of self.
2. Client demonstrates ability to manage own self-care, make independent decisions, and use problem-solving skills.
3. Client sets goals that are realistic and works to achieve those goals without evidence of fear of failure.

ALTERED ROLE PERFORMANCE

Definition: *Disruption in the way one perceives one's role performance.*

Possible Etiologies ("related to")

[Physical illness accompanied by real or perceived disabling symptoms]

[Unmet dependency needs]

[Dysfunctional family system]

Defining Characteristics ("evidenced by")

Change in self-perception of role

Change in physical capacity to resume role

[Assumption of dependent role]

Changes in usual patterns of responsibility [because of conflict within dysfunctional family system]

Goals/Objectives
Short-Term Goal

Client will verbalize understanding that physical symptoms interfere with role performance in order to fill an unmet need.

Long-Term Goal

Client will be able to assume role-related responsibilities by discharge from treatment.

Interventions with *Selected Rationales*

1. Determine client's usual role within the family system. Identify roles of other family members. *An accurate database is required in order to formulate appropriate plan of care for the client.*
2. Assess specific disabilities related to role expectations. Assess relationship of disability to physical condition. *It is important to determine the realism of the client's role expectations.*
3. Encourage client to discuss conflicts evident within the family system. Identify how client and other family members have responded to this conflict. *It is necessary to identify specific stressors, as well as adaptive and maladaptive responses within the system, before assistance can be provided in an effort to create change.*
4. Help client identify feelings associated with family conflict, the subsequent exacerbation of physical symptoms, and the accompanying disabilities. *Client may be unaware of the relationship between physical symptoms and emotional problems. An awareness of the correlation is the first step toward creating change.*
5. Help client identify changes he or she would like to occur within the family system.
6. Encourage family participation in the development of plans to effect positive change, and work to resolve the conflict for which the client's sick role provides relief. *Input from the individuals who will be directly involved in the change will increase the likelihood of a positive outcome.*
7. Allow all family members input into the plan for change: knowledge of benefits and consequences for each alternative, selection of appropriate alternatives, methods for implementation of alternatives, alternate plan in the event initial change is unsuccessful. *Family may require assistance with this problem-solving process.*
8. Ensure that client has accurate perception of role expectations within the family system. Use role playing to practice areas associated with his or her role that client perceives as painful. *Repetition through practice may help to desensitize client to the anticipated distress.*
9. As client is able to see the relationship between exacerbation of physical symptoms and existing conflict, discuss more adaptive coping strategies that may be used to prevent interference with role performance during times of stress.

Outcome Criteria
1. Client is able to verbalize realistic perception of role expectations.
2. Client is physically able to assume role-related responsibilities.
3. Client and family are able to verbalize plan for attempt at conflict resolution.

KNOWLEDGE DEFICIT (Psychological Factors Affecting Medical Condition)

Definition: *Absence or deficiency of cognitive information related to specific topic.*

Possible Etiologies ("related to")
Lack of interest in learning
[Severe level of anxiety]
[Low self-esteem]
[Regression to earlier level of development]

Defining Characteristics ("evidenced by")
[Denial of emotional problems]
[Statements such as, "I don't know why the doctor put me on the psychiatric unit. I have a physical problem."]
[History of numerous exacerbations of physical illness]
[Noncompliance with psychiatric treatment]
Inappropriate or exaggerated behaviors, for example, hysterical, hostile, agitated, apathetic

Goals/Objectives
Short-Term Goal
Client will cooperate with plan for teaching provided by primary nurse.

Long-Term Goal
By discharge from treatment, client will be able to verbalize psychological factors affecting his or her medical condition.

Interventions with *Selected Rationales*
1. Assess client's level of knowledge regarding effects of psychological problems on the body. *An adequate database is necessary for the development of an effective teaching plan.*
2. Assess client's level of anxiety and readiness to learn. *Learning does not occur beyond the moderate level of anxiety.*

3. Discuss physical exams and laboratory tests that have been conducted. Explain purpose and results of each. *Fear of the unknown may contribute to elevated level of anxiety. "The client has the right to obtain complete current information concerning his diagnosis, treatment, and prognosis . . ." (AHA, 1975).*

4. Explore client's feelings and fears. Go slowly. These feelings may have been suppressed or repressed for so long that their disclosure may be a very painful experience. Be supportive. *Verbalization of feelings in a nonthreatening environment and with a trusting individual may help the client come to terms with unresolved issues.*

5. Have client keep a diary of appearance, duration, and intensity of physical symptoms. A separate record of situations that the client finds especially stressful should also be kept. *Comparison of these records may provide objective data from which to observe the relationship between physical symptoms and stress.*

6. Help client identify needs that are being met through the sick role. Together, formulate more adaptive means for fulfilling these needs. Practice by role playing. *Repetition through practice serves to reduce discomfort in the actual situation.*

7. Provide instruction in assertiveness techniques, especially the ability to recognize the differences among passive, assertive, and aggressive behaviors and the importance of respecting the human rights of others while protecting one's own basic human rights. *These skills will preserve client's self-esteem while also improving his or her ability to form satisfactory interpersonal relationships.*

8. Discuss adaptive methods of stress management such as relaxation techniques, physical exercise, meditation, breathing exercises, and autogenics. *Use of these adaptive techniques may decrease appearance of physical symptoms in response to stress.*

Outcome Criteria

1. Client verbalizes an understanding of the relationship between psychological stress and exacerbation of physical illness.

2. Client demonstrates the ability to use adaptive coping strategies in the management of stress.

Chapter 17

PERSONALITY DISORDERS

BACKGROUND ASSESSMENT DATA

The *DSM-IV* (APA, 1994) describes personality *traits* as "enduring patterns of perceiving, relating to, and thinking about the environment and oneself that are exhibited in a wide range of social and personal contexts." A personality *disorder* is said to exist only when these traits become inflexible and maladaptive and cause either significant functional impairment or subjective distress.

The *DSM-IV* groups the personality disorders into three clusters. These clusters, and the disorders classified under each, are described as follows:

1. **Cluster A:** Behaviors described as odd or eccentric
   a. Paranoid personality disorder
   b. Schizoid personality disorder
   c. Schizotypal personality disorder
2. **Cluster B:** Behaviors described as dramatic, emotional, or erratic
   a. Antisocial personality disorder
   b. Borderline personality disorder
   c. Histrionic personality disorder
   d. Narcissistic personality disorder
3. **Cluster C:** Behaviors described as anxious or fearful
   a. Avoidant personality disorder
   b. Dependent personality disorder
   c. Obsessive-compulsive personality disorder
   d. Passive-aggressive personality disorder
      Note: Passive-aggressive personality disorder was included in the *DSM-III-R* (APA, 1987) with the cluster

C disorders. In the *DSM-IV*, it is included in the section on *Criteria Provided for Further Study*. For purposes of this text, passive-aggressive personality disorder is described with the cluster C disorders.

Categories of personality disorders described by the *DSM-IV* include the following:

1. **Cluster A**
   a. ***Paranoid Personality Disorder.*** The essential feature is a pervasive and unwarranted suspiciousness and mistrust of people. There is a general expectation of being exploited or harmed by others in some way. Symptoms include guardedness in relationships with others, pathologic jealousy, hypersensitivity, inability to relax, unemotionality, and lack of a sense of humor. These individuals are very critical of others but have much difficulty accepting criticism themselves.
   b. ***Schizoid Personality Disorder.*** This disorder is characterized by an inability to form close, personal relationships. Symptoms include social isolation; absence of warm, tender feelings for others; indifference to praise, criticism, or the feelings of others; flat, dull affect (appears cold and aloof).
   c. ***Schizotypal Personality Disorder.*** This disorder is characterized by peculiarities of ideation, appearance, and behavior, and deficits in interpersonal relatedness that are not severe enough to meet the criteria for schizophrenia. Symptoms include magical thinking; ideas of reference; social isolation; illusions; odd speech patterns; aloof, cold, suspicious behavior; and undue social anxiety.

2. **Cluster B**
   a. ***Antisocial Personality Disorder.*** This disorder is characterized by a pattern of socially irresponsible, exploitative, and guiltless behavior, as evidenced by the tendency to fail to conform to the law, to sustain consistent employment, to exploit and manipulate others for personal gain, to deceive, and to fail to develop stable relationships. The individual must be at least 18 years of age and have a history of conduct disorder before the age of 15. (Symptoms of this disorder are identified later in this chapter, along with predisposing factors and nursing care of the individual with antisocial personality.)

b. ***Borderline Personality Disorder.*** The features of this disorder are described as marked instability in interpersonal relationships, mood, and self-image. The instability is significant to the extent that the individual seems to "hover just across the line from psychosis" (Kaplan and Sadock, 1985). (Symptoms of this disorder are identified later in this chapter, along with predisposing factors and nursing care of the individual with borderline personality.)

c. ***Histrionic Personality Disorder.*** The essential feature of this disorder is described by the *DSM-IV* as a pervasive pattern of excessive emotionality and attention-seeking behavior. Symptoms include exaggerated expression of emotions, incessant drawing of attention to oneself, overreaction to minor events, constantly seeking approval from others, egocentricity, vain and demanding behavior, extreme concern with physical appearance, and inappropriately sexually seductive appearance or behavior.

d. ***Narcissistic Personality Disorder.*** This disorder is characterized by a grandiose sense of self-importance; preoccupation with fantasies of success, power, brilliance, beauty, or ideal love; a constant need for admiration and attention; exploitation of others for fulfillment of own desires; lack of empathy; response to criticism or failure with indifference or humiliation and rage; and preoccupation with feelings of envy.

3. **Cluster C**

a. ***Avoidant Personality Disorder.*** This disorder is characterized by social withdrawal brought about by extreme sensitivity to rejection. Symptoms include unwillingness to enter into relationships unless given unusually strong guarantees of uncritical acceptance; low self-esteem; social withdrawal in spite of a desire for affection and acceptance. Depression and anxiety are common. Social phobia may be a complication of this disorder.

b. ***Dependent Personality Disorder.*** Individuals with this disorder passively allow others to assume responsibility for major areas of life because of their inability to function independently. They lack self-confidence, are unable to make decisions, perceive self as helpless and stupid, possess fear of being alone or abandoned, and seek constant reassurance and approval from others.

c. ***Obsessive-Compulsive Personality Disorder.*** This disorder is characterized by a pervasive pattern of perfectionism and inflexibility. Interpersonal relationships have a formal and serious quality, and others often perceive these individuals as stilted or "stiff." Other symptoms include difficulty expressing tender feelings, insistence that others submit to his or her way of doing things, excessive devotion to work and productivity to the exclusion of pleasure, indecisiveness, perfectionism, preoccupation with details, depressed mood, and being judgmental of self and others.

d. ***Passive-Aggressive Personality Disorder.*** Characteristic of this disorder is a passive resistance to demands for adequate performance in both occupational and social functioning. Symptoms include obstructionism, procrastination, stubbornness, intentional inefficiency, dawdling, "forgetfulness," criticism of persons in authority, dependency, and low self-esteem. Oppositional defiant disorder in childhood or adolescence is a predisposing factor.

Many of the behaviors associated with the various personality disorders may be manifested by clients with virtually every psychiatric diagnosis, as well as by those individuals described as "healthy." It is only when personality traits or styles repetitively "limit the attempts and potential for mastery; disrupt interpersonal relationships; fail to balance dependence and autonomy; or create insufficient moral parameters in human interactions that a diagnosis of personality disorder is assigned" (Burgess, 1990).

Individuals with personality disorders may be encountered in all types of treatment settings. They are not often treated in acute care settings, but because of the instability of the borderline client, hospitalization is necessary from time to time. The individual with antisocial personality disorder also may be hospitalized as an alternative to imprisonment when a legal determination is made that psychiatric intervention may be helpful. Because of these reasons, suggestions for inpatient care of individuals with these disorders are included in this chapter; however, these interventions may be used in other types of treatment settings as well. Undoubtedly, these clients represent the ultimate challenge for the psychiatric nurse.

BORDERLINE PERSONALITY DISORDER

Defined

This personality disorder is characterized by instability of affect, behavior, object relationships, and self-image. The term "borderline" came into being because a group of clients seemed to fall on the border between neurosis and psychosis (Platt-Koch, 1983). Transient psychotic symptoms appear during periods of extreme stress. The disorder is more commonly diagnosed in women than in men.

Predisposing Factors

1. **Theory of Object Relations.** This theory suggests that the basis for borderline personality lies in the ways the child relates to the mother and does *not* separate from her. Mahler and associates (1975) define this process in a series of phases described as follows:
   a. **Phase 1 (Birth to 1 month), Autistic Phase.** Most of the infant's time is spent in a half-waking, half-sleeping state.
   b. **Phase 2 (1 to 5 months), Symbiotic Phase.** A type of psychic fusion of mother and child. Child views self as extension of mother.
   c. **Phase 3 (5 to 10 months), Differentiation Phase.** Child begins to become aware of separateness between self and mother.
   d. **Phase 4 (10 to 16 months), Practicing Phase.** The child displays increased independence in terms of ability to ambulate and explore on his or her own.
   e. **Phase 5 (16 to 24 months), Rapprochement Phase.** Awareness of separateness from mother increases. This is frightening to the child, who wants to regain some lost closeness but not return to symbiosis. The child just wants mother there as needed for "emotional refueling."
   f. **Phase 6 (24 to 36 months), On the Way to Object Constancy Phase.** In this phase the child completes the individuation process and learns to relate to objects in an effective, constant manner.

The theory of object relations suggests that the individual with borderline personality is fixed in the rapprochement phase of development. This fixation occurs when the mother begins to feel threatened by the increasing autonomy of her child and so withdraws her emotional support during those times *or* she may instead reward clinging, dependent behaviors. In this way, the child comes to believe that

"To grow up and be independent = a 'bad' child."
"To stay immature and dependent = a 'good' child."
"Mom withholds nurturing from 'bad' child."

Consequently, the child develops a deep fear of abandonment that persists into adulthood.

Also, because object constancy is never achieved, the child continues to view objects (people) as parts—either good or bad. This is called *splitting*, the primary defense mechanism of borderline personality.

Symptomatology (Subjective and Objective Data)

At least five of the following criteria are required by the *DSM-IV* (APA, 1994) for a diagnosis of borderline personality disorder:

1. Frantic efforts to avoid real or imagined abandonment (does not include suicidal or self-mutilating behavior covered in criterion 5).
2. A pattern of unstable and intense interpersonal relationships characterized by alternating between extremes of idealization and devaluation.
3. Identity disturbance: Markedly and persistently unstable self-image or sense of self.
4. Impulsivity in at least two areas that are potentially self-damaging, such as spending, sex, substance abuse, reckless driving, binge eating (not to include behavior covered in criterion 5).
5. Recurrent suicidal behavior, gestures, or threats, or self-mutilating behavior.
6. Affective instability caused by marked reactivity of mood (e.g., intense episodic dysphoria, irritability, or anxiety, usually lasting a few hours and only rarely more than a few days).
7. Chronic feelings of emptiness.
8. Inappropriate, intense anger or difficulty controlling

anger (e.g., frequent displays of temper, constant anger, recurrent physical fights).

9. Transient, stress-related paranoid ideation or severe dissociative symptoms.

Other symptoms include the following:

10. Alternating clinging and distancing behaviors.
11. Projection—seeing in others those attitudes they fail to see in themselves.
12. Poor reality testing—misinterpretations of the environment and relationships, resulting from poor ego development.

Common Nursing Diagnoses and Interventions
(Interventions are applicable to various health-care settings, such as inpatient and partial hospitalization, community outpatient clinic, home health, and private practice.)

RISK FOR SELF-MUTILATION/RISK FOR VIOLENCE TO SELF OR OTHERS

Definition: *Risk for self-mutilation is a state in which an individual is at risk to perform an act on the self to injure, not kill, which produces tissue damage and tension relief. Risk for violence is defined as: Behaviors in which an individual demonstrates that he/she can be physically, emotionally, and/or sexually harmful either to self or to others.*

Related/Risk Factors ("related to")
[Extreme fears of abandonment]
[Feelings of unreality]
[Depressed mood]
[Use of suicidal gestures for manipulation of others]
[Unmet dependency needs]
[Low self-esteem]
[Unresolved grief]
[Rage reactions]
[Physically self-damaging acts (cutting, burning, drug overdose, etc.)]
Body language—rigid posture, clenching of fists and jaw, hyperactivity, pacing, breathlessness, and threatening stances

[History or threats of violence toward self or others or of destruction to the property of others]
Impulsivity
Suicidal ideation, plan, available means
[History of suicide attempts]

Goals/Objectives
Short-Term Goal
Client will seek out staff member if feelings of harming self or others emerge.

Long-Term Goal
Client will not harm self or others.

Interventions with *Selected Rationales*
1. Observe client's behavior frequently. Do this through routine activities and interactions; avoid appearing watchful and suspicious. *Close observation is required so that intervention can occur if required to ensure client's (and others') safety.*
2. Secure a verbal contract from client that he or she will seek out staff member when urge for self-mutilation is experienced. *Discussing feelings of self-harm with a trusted individual provides a degree of relief to the client. A contract gets the subject out in the open and places some of the responsibility for his or her safety with the client. An attitude of acceptance of the client as a worthwhile individual is conveyed.*
3. If self-mutilation occurs, care for the client's wounds in a matter-of-fact manner. Do not give positive reinforcement to this behavior by offering sympathy or additional attention. *Lack of attention to the maladaptive behavior may decrease repetition of its use.*
4. Encourage client to talk about feelings he or she was having just prior to this behavior. *In order to problem-solve the situation with the client, knowledge of the precipitating factors is important.*
5. Act as a role model for appropriate expression of angry feelings and give positive reinforcement to the client when attempts to conform are made. *It is vital that the client express angry feelings, because suicide and other self-destructive behaviors are often viewed as a result of anger turned inward on the self.*
6. Remove all dangerous objects from the client's environment. *Client safety is a nursing priority.*
7. Try to redirect violent behavior with physical outlets for the client's anxiety (e.g., punching bag, jogging). *Physi-*

cal exercise is a safe and effective way of relieving pent-up tension.

8. Have sufficient staff available to indicate a show of strength to the client if necessary. *This conveys to the client evidence of control over the situation and provides some physical security for staff.*

9. Administer tranquilizing medications as ordered by physician or obtain an order if necessary. Monitor the client for effectiveness of the medication and for the appearance of adverse side effects. *Tranquilizing medications such as anxiolytics or antipsychotics may have a calming effect on the client and may prevent aggressive behaviors.*

10. Use of mechanical restraints or isolation room may be required if less restrictive interventions are unsuccessful. Follow policy and procedure prescribed by the institution in executing this intervention. Most states require that the physician reevaluate and issue a new order for restraints every 3 hours, except between the hours of midnight and 8:00 AM. If the client has previously refused medication, administer after restraints have been applied. Most states consider this intervention appropriate in emergency situations or in the event that a client would likely harm self or others.

11. Observe the client in restraints every 15 minutes (or according to institutional policy). Ensure that circulation to extremities is not compromised (check temperature, color, pulses). Assist the client with needs related to nutrition, hydration, and elimination. Position the client so that comfort is facilitated and aspiration can be prevented. *Client safety is a nursing priority.*

12. May need to assign staff on a one-to-one basis if warranted by acuity of the situation. *Because of their extreme fear of abandonment, leaving clients with borderline personality disorder alone at such a time may cause an acute rise in level of anxiety and agitation.*

Outcome Criteria

1. Client has not harmed self or others.
2. Anxiety is maintained at a level in which client feels no need for aggression.
3. Client denies any ideas of self-harm.
4. Client verbalizes community support systems from which assistance may be requested when personal coping strategies are unsuccessful.

ANXIETY (Severe to Panic)

Definition: *A vague uneasy feeling whose source is often nonspecific or unknown to the individual.*

Possible Etiologies ("related to")
Threat to self-concept
Unmet needs
[Extreme fear of abandonment]
Unconscious conflicts [associated with fixation in earlier level of development]

Defining Characteristics ("evidenced by")
[Transient psychotic symptoms in response to severe stress, manifested by disorganized thinking, confusion, altered communication patterns, disorientation, misinterpretation of the environment]
[Excessive use of projection (attributing own thoughts and feelings to others)]
[Depersonalization (feelings of unreality)]
[Derealization (a feeling that the environment is unreal)]
[Acts of self-mutilation in an effort to find relief from feelings of unreality]

Goals/Objectives
Short-Term Goal
Client will demonstrate use of relaxation techniques to maintain anxiety at manageable level.

Long-Term Goal
Client will be able to recognize events that precipitate anxiety and intervene to prevent disabling behaviors.

Interventions with *Selected Rationales*
1. Symptoms of depersonalization often occur at the panic level of anxiety. Clients with borderline personality disorder often resort to cutting or other self-mutilating acts in an effort to relieve the anxiety. Being able to feel pain or see blood is a reassurance of existence to the person. If injury occurs, care for the wounds in a matter-of-fact manner without providing reinforcement for this behavior. *Lack of reinforcement may discourage repetition of the maladaptive behavior.*

2. During periods of panic anxiety, stay with the client and provide reassurance of safety and security. Orient the client to the reality of the situation. *Client comfort and safety are nursing priorities.*

3. Administer tranquilizing medications as ordered by physician, or obtain order if necessary. Monitor client for effectiveness of the medication as well as for adverse side effects. *Antianxiety medications (e.g., diazepam, chlordiazepoxide, alprazolam) provide relief from the immobilizing effects of anxiety and facilitate client's cooperation with therapy.*

4. Correct misinterpretations of the environment as expressed by client. *Confronting misinterpretations honestly, with a caring and accepting attitude, provides a therapeutic orientation to reality and preserves the client's feelings of dignity and self-worth.*

5. Encourage the client to talk about true feelings. Help him or her recognize ownership of these feelings rather than projecting them onto others in the environment. *Exploration of feelings with a trusted individual may help the client perceive the situation more realistically and come to terms with unresolved issues.*

6. Assist the client to work toward achievement of object constancy. Client may feel totally abandoned when nurse or therapist leaves at shift change or at end of therapy session. There may even be feelings that the therapist ceases to exist. Leaving a signed note or card with the client for reassurance may help. It is extremely important for more than one nurse to develop a therapeutic relationship with the borderline client. It is also necessary that staff maintain open communication and consistency in the provision of care for these individuals. *Individuals with borderline personality disorder have a tendency to cling to one staff member, if allowed, transferring their maladaptive dependency to that individual. This dependency can be avoided if the client is able to establish therapeutic relationships with two or more staff members who encourage independent self-care activities.*

Outcome Criteria

1. Client is able to verbalize events that precipitate anxiety and demonstrate techniques for its reduction.
2. Client manifests no symptoms of depersonalization.
3. Client interprets the environment realistically.

DYSFUNCTIONAL GRIEVING

Definition: Extended, unsuccessful use of intellectual and emotional responses by which individuals (families, communities) attempt to work through the process of modifying self-concept based upon the perception of [actual or] potential loss.

Possible Etiologies ("related to")
[Maternal deprivation during rapprochement phase of development (internalized as a loss, with fixation in the anger stage of the grieving process)]

Defining Characteristics ("evidenced by")
Anger
[Internalized rage]
[Depressed mood]
Labile affect
[Extreme fear of being alone (fear of abandonment)]
[Acting-out behaviors, such as sexual promiscuity, suicidal gestures, temper tantrums, substance abuse]
[Difficulty expressing feelings]
Alterations in eating habits, sleep patterns, dream patterns, activity level, libido
Repetitive use of ineffectual behaviors associated with attempts to reinvest in relationships
Reliving of past experiences with little or no reduction of intensity of the grief
Prolonged interference with life functioning, with onset or exacerbation of somatic or psychosomatic responses

Goals/Objectives
Short-Term Goal
Client will discuss with nurse or therapist maladaptive patterns of expressing anger.

Long-Term Goal
Client will be able to identify the true source of angry feelings, accept ownership of these feelings, and express them in a socially acceptable manner, in an effort to satisfactorily progress through the grieving process.

Interventions with *Selected Rationales*
1. Convey an accepting attitude—one that creates a nonthreatening environment for the client to express feelings. Be honest and keep all promises. *An accepting attitude*

conveys to the client that you believe he or she is a worthwhile person. Trust is enhanced.

2. Identify the function that anger, frustration, and rage serve for the client. Allow the client to express these feelings within reason. *Verbalization of feelings in a nonthreatening environment may help the client come to terms with unresolved issues.*

3. Encourage the client to discharge pent-up anger through participation in large motor activities (e.g., brisk walks, jogging, physical exercises, volleyball, punching bag, exercise bike). *Physical exercise provides a safe and effective method for discharging pent-up tension.*

4. Explore with client the true source of the anger. This is painful therapy that often leads to regression as the client deals with the feelings of early abandonment. It seems that sometimes the client must "get worse before he or she can get better." *Reconciliation of the feelings associated with this stage is necessary before progression through the grieving process can continue.*

5. As anger is displaced onto the nurse or therapist, caution must be taken to guard against the negative effects of countertransference. These are very difficult clients who have the capacity for eliciting a whole array of negative feelings from the therapist. These feelings must be acknowledged but not allowed to interfere with the therapeutic process.

6. Explain the behaviors associated with the normal grieving process. Help the client to recognize his or her position in this process. *Knowledge of the acceptability of the feelings associated with normal grieving may help to relieve some of the guilt that these responses generate.*

7. Help the client to understand appropriate ways to express anger. Give positive reinforcement for behaviors used to express anger appropriately. Act as a role model. *Positive reinforcement enhances self-esteem and encourages repetition of desirable behaviors. It is appropriate to let the client know when he or she has done something that has generated angry feelings in you. Role modeling ways to express anger in an appropriate manner is a powerful learning tool.*

8. Set limits on acting-out behaviors and explain consequences of violation of those limits. Be supportive, yet consistent and firm in caring for this client. *Client lacks sufficient self-control to limit maladaptive behaviors, so assistance is required from staff. Without consistency on the part of all staff members working with*

this client, however, a positive outcome will not be achieved.

Outcome Criteria
1. Client is able to verbalize how anger and acting-out behaviors are associated with maladaptive grieving.
2. Client is able to discuss the original source of the anger and demonstrates socially acceptable ways of expressing the emotion.

IMPAIRED SOCIAL INTERACTION

Definition: *The state in which an individual participates in an insufficient or excessive quantity or ineffective quality of social exchange.*

Possible Etiologies ("related to")
[Fixation in rapprochement phase of development]
[Extreme fears of abandonment and engulfment]
[Lack of personal identity]

Defining Characteristics ("evidenced by")
[Alternating clinging and distancing behaviors]
[Inability to form satisfactory intimate relationship with another person]
Observed use of unsuccessful social interaction behaviors
[Use of primitive dissociation (splitting) in their relationships (viewing others as all good or all bad)]

Goals/Objectives
Short-Term Goal
Client will discuss with nurse or therapist behaviors that impede the development of satisfactory interpersonal relationships.

Long-Term Goals
1. Client will interact with others in the therapy setting in both social and therapeutic activities without difficulty by discharge from treatment.
2. Client will display no evidence of splitting or clinging and distancing behaviors in relationships by discharge from treatment.

Interventions with *Selected Rationales*
1. Encourage client to examine these behaviors (to recognize that they are occurring). *Client may be unaware of split-*

ting or of clinging and distancing pattern of interaction with others.

2. Help client realize that you will be available, without reinforcing dependent behaviors. *Knowledge of your availability may provide needed security for the client.*

3. Give positive reinforcement for independent behaviors. *Positive reinforcement enhances self-esteem and encourages repetition of desirable behaviors.*

4. Rotate staff who work with the client in order to avoid client's developing dependence on particular staff members. *Client must learn to relate to more than one staff member in an effort to decrease use of splitting and to diminish fears of abandonment.*

5. Explore feelings that relate to fears of abandonment and engulfment with the client. Help client understand that clinging and distancing behaviors are engendered by these fears. *Exploration of feelings with a trusted individual may help client come to terms with unresolved issues.*

6. Help client understand how these behaviors interfere with satisfactory relationships. *Client may be unaware of others' perception of him or her and why these behaviors are not acceptable to others.*

7. Assist the client to work toward achievement of object constancy. Be available, without promoting dependency *so that client may resolve fears of abandonment and develop the ability to establish satisfactory intimate relationships.*

Outcome Criteria
1. Client is able to interact with others in both social and therapeutic activities in a socially acceptable manner.
2. Client does not use splitting or clinging and distancing behaviors in relationships and is able to relate the use of these behaviors to failure of past relationships.

PERSONAL IDENTITY DISTURBANCE

Definition: *Inability to distinguish between self and nonself.*

Possible Etiologies ("related to")
[Failure to complete tasks of separation/individuation stage of development]

[Underdeveloped ego]
[Unmet dependency needs]
[Absence of, or rejection by, parental sex-role model]

Defining Characteristics ("evidenced by")

[Excessive use of projection]
[Uncertainties regarding gender identity]
[Uncertainties about long-term goals or career choice]
[Ambiguous value system]
[Vague self-image]
[Unable to tolerate being alone]
[Feelings of depersonalization and derealization]
[Self-mutilation (cutting, burning) to validate existence of self]

Goals/Objectives
Short-Term Goal
Client will describe characteristics that make him or her a unique individual.

Long-Term Goal
Client will be able to distinguish own thoughts, feelings, behaviors, and image from those of others, as the initial step in the development of a healthy personal identity.

Interventions with *Selected Rationales*
1. Help client recognize the reality of his or her separateness. Do not attempt to translate client's thoughts and feelings into words. *Because of the blurred ego boundaries, client may believe you can read his or her mind.* For this reason, caution should be taken in the use of empathetic understanding. For example, avoid statements such as "I know how you must feel about that."
2. Help client to recognize separateness from nurse by clarifying which behaviors and feelings belong to whom. If deemed appropriate, allow client to touch your hand or arm. *Touch and physical presence provide reality for the client and serve to strengthen weak ego boundaries.*
3. Encourage client to discuss thoughts and feelings. Help client recognize ownership of these feelings rather than projecting them onto others in the environment. *Verbalization of feelings in a nonthreatening environment may help client come to terms with unresolved issues.*
4. Confront statements that project client's feelings onto others. Ask client to validate that others possess those

feelings. The expression of *reasonable doubt* as a therapeutic technique may be helpful ("I find that hard to believe").

5. If the problem is with gender identity, ask the client to describe his or her perception of appropriate male and female behaviors. Provide information about role behaviors and sex education, if necessary. Client may require clarification of distorted ideas or misinformation. Convey acceptance of the person regardless of preferred identity. *An attitude of acceptance reinforces client's feelings of self-worth.*

6. Always call client by his or her name. If client experiences feelings of depersonalization or derealization, orientation to the environment and correction of misperceptions may be helpful. *These interventions help to preserve client's feelings of dignity and self-worth.*

7. Help client understand that there are more adaptive ways of validating his or her existence than self-mutilation. Contract with the client to seek out staff member when these feelings occur. *A contract gets the subject out in the open and places some of the responsibility for his or her safety with the client. Client safety is a nursing priority.*

8. Work with client to clarify values. Discuss beliefs, attitudes, and feelings underlying his or her behaviors. Help client to identify those values that have been (or are intended to be) incorporated as his or her own. Care must be taken by the nurse to avoid imposing his or her own value system upon the client. *Because of underdeveloped ego and fixation in early developmental level, client may not have established own value system. In order to accomplish this, ownership of beliefs and attitudes must be identified and clarified.*

9. Use of photographs of the client may help to establish or clarify ego boundaries. *Photographs may help to increase client's awareness of self as separate from others.*

10. Alleviate anxiety by providing assurance to client that he or she will not be left alone. *Early childhood traumas may predispose borderline clients to extreme fears of abandonment.*

11. Use of touch is sometimes therapeutic in identity confirmation. Before this technique is used, however, assess cultural influences and degree of trust. *Touch and physical presence provide reality for the client and serve to strengthen weak ego boundaries.*

Outcome Criteria
1. Client is able to distinguish between own thoughts and feelings and those of others.
2. Client claims ownership of those thoughts and feelings and does not use projection in relationships with others.
3. Client has clarified own feelings regarding sexual identity.

SELF-ESTEEM DISTURBANCE

Definition: Negative self-evaluation and feelings about self or self-capabilities, which may be directly or indirectly expressed.

Possible Etiologies ("related to")
[Lack of positive feedback]
[Unmet dependency needs]
[Retarded ego development]
[Repeated negative feedback, resulting in diminished self-worth]
[Dysfunctional family system]
[Fixation in earlier level of development]

Defining Characteristics ("evidenced by")
[Difficulty accepting positive reinforcement]
[Self-destructive behavior]
[Frequent use of derogatory and critical remarks against the self]
[Lack of eye contact]
[Manipulation of one staff member against another in an attempt to gain special privileges]
[Inability to form close, personal relationships]
[Inability to tolerate being alone]
[Degradation of others in an attempt to increase own feelings of self-worth]
Hesitancy to try new things or situations [because of fear of failure]

Goals/Objectives
Short-Term Goals
1. Client will discuss fear of failure with nurse or therapist.
2. Client will verbalize things he or she likes about self.

Long-Term Goals
1. Client will exhibit increased feelings of self-worth as evidenced by verbal expression of positive aspects about self, past accomplishments, and future prospects.

2. Client will exhibit increased feelings of self-worth by setting realistic goals and trying to reach them, thereby demonstrating a decrease in fear of failure.

Interventions with *Selected Rationales*
1. Ensure that goals are realistic. It is important for client to achieve something, so plan for activities in which success is likely. *Success increases self-esteem.*
2. Convey unconditional positive regard for client. Promote understanding of your acceptance for him or her as a worthwhile human being. *Acceptance by others increases feelings of self-worth.*
3. Set limits on manipulative behavior. Identify the consequences for violation of those limits. Minimize negative feedback to the client. Enforce the limits and impose the consequences for violations in a matter-of-fact manner. Consistency among all staff members is essential. *Negative feedback can be extremely threatening to a person with low self-esteem and possibly aggravate the problem. Consequences should convey unacceptability of the* behavior *but not the* person.
4. Recognize when client is playing one staff member against another. Remember that splitting is the primary defense mechanism of these individuals, and the impressions they have of others as either "good" or "bad" are a manifestation of this defense. Do not listen as client tries to degrade other staff members. Suggest that client discuss the problem directly with staff person involved. *Lack of reinforcement for these maladaptive behaviors may discourage their repetition.*
5. Encourage independence in the performance of personal responsibilities, as well as in decision making related to client's self-care. Offer recognition and praise for accomplishments. *Positive reinforcement enhances self-esteem and encourages repetition of desirable behaviors.*
6. Help client increase level of self-awareness through critical examination of feelings, attitudes, and behaviors. *Self-exploration in the presence of a trusted individual may help the client come to terms with unresolved issues.*
7. Help client identify positive self-attributes, as well as those aspects of the self he or she finds undesirable. Discuss ways to effect change in these areas. *Individuals with low self-esteem often have difficulty recognizing their positive attributes. They may also lack problem-solving ability and require assistance to formulate a plan for implementing the desired changes.*

8. Discuss client's future. Assist client in the establishment of short-term and long-term goals. What are his or her strengths? How can he or she best use those strengths to achieve those goals? Encourage client to perform at a level realistic to his or her ability. Offer positive reinforcement for decisions made.

Outcome Criteria
1. Client verbalizes positive aspects about self.
2. Client demonstrates ability to make independent decisions regarding management of own self-care.
3. Client expresses some optimism and hope for the future.
4. Client sets realistic goals for self and demonstrates willingness to reach them.

ANTISOCIAL PERSONALITY DISORDER

Defined

This personality disorder is characterized by a pattern of antisocial behavior that began before the age of 15. These behaviors violate the rights of others, and individuals with this disorder display no evidence of guilt feelings at having done so. There is often a long history of involvement with law-enforcement agencies. Substance abuse is not uncommon. The disorder is more frequently diagnosed in men than in women. Individuals with antisocial personalities are often labeled *sociopathic* or *psychopathic* in the lay literature.

Predisposing Factors

1. **Physiologic**
   a. ***Genetics.*** Vaillant and Perry (1985) describe findings in which individuals with antisocial personalities, and their parents, display excessive electroencephalographic (EEG) abnormalities, suggesting some genetic involvement. Genetics have also been implicated in a study by Robins (1966). It was found that having a sociopathic or alcoholic father was a powerful predictor of antisocial personality disorder in adult life. Only adequate and strict discipline diminished the risk of antisocial behavior in these children with delinquent parents.

2. **Psychosocial**
   a. ***Psychodynamic Theory.*** Freud (1958) implicated the unmet need for satisfaction and security from sig-

nificant others in the development of antisocial personality. Because of this rejection or indifference, development of the ego is interrupted, and id behavior is maintained. The child also lacks satisfactory role models at the crucial time when he or she would be internalizing standards, values, and morals in the development of a superego. This development is impaired, and the individual becomes an adult who nurtures the need for immediate gratification and lacks feelings of guilt.

  b. ***Theories of Family Dynamics.*** Several sources have implicated family functioning as an important factor in determining whether or not an individual develops antisocial personality (APA, 1987; Birckhead, 1989; Robinson, 1983). They suggest that the following circumstances may predispose to the disorder:
    (1) Absence of parental discipline.
    (2) Extreme poverty.
    (3) Removal from the home.
    (4) Growing up without parental figures of both sexes.
    (5) Erratic and inconsistent methods of discipline.
    (6) Being "rescued" each time they are in trouble (never having to suffer the consequences of their own behavior).
    (7) Maternal deprivation.

Symptomatology (Subjective and Objective Data)

1. Extremely low-self esteem (abuses other people in an attempt to validate his or her own superiority).
2. Inability to sustain satisfactory job performance.
3. Inability to function as a responsible parent.
4. Failure to follow social and legal norms; repeated performance of antisocial acts that are grounds for arrest (whether arrested or not).
5. Inability to develop satisfactory, enduring, intimate relationship with a sexual partner.
6. Aggressive behaviors; repeated physical fights; spouse or child abuse.
7. Extreme impulsivity.
8. Repeated lying for personal benefit.
9. Reckless driving; driving while intoxicated.
10. Inability to learn from punishment.
11. Lack of guilt or remorse felt in response to exploitation of others.

12. Difficulty with interpersonal relationships.
13. Social extroversion; stimulation through interaction with and abuse of others.
14. Repeated failure to honor financial obligations.

Common Nursing Diagnoses and Interventions
(Interventions are applicable to various health-care settings, such as inpatient and partial hospitalization, community outpatient clinic, home health, and private practice.)

RISK FOR VIOLENCE: DIRECTED AT OTHERS

Definition: *Behaviors in which an individual demonstrates that he/she can be physically, emotionally, and/or sexually harmful to others.*

Related/Risk Factors ("related to")
Antisocial character
Rage reactions
[Negative role modeling]
[Temporal lobe involvement (abnormal EEG)]
[Suspiciousness of others]
[Interruption of client's attempt to fulfill own desires]
[Inability to tolerate frustration]
[Learned behavior within client's subculture]
Vulnerable self-esteem
Body language—rigid posture, clenching of fists and jaw, hyperactivity, pacing, breathlessness, and threatening stances
[History or threats of violence toward self or others or of destruction to the property of others]
Impulsivity
Availability and/or possession of weapon(s)
Substance abuse or withdrawal
Provocative behavior: Argumentative, dissatisfied, overreactive, hypersensitive
[History of violent behavior]

Goals/Objectives
Short-Term Goal
Client will discuss angry feelings and situations that precipitate hostility.

Long-Term Goal
Client will not harm others.

Interventions with *Selected Rationales*

1. Convey an accepting attitude toward this client. Feelings of rejection are undoubtedly familiar to him or her. Work on development of trust. Be honest, keep all promises, and convey the message to the client that it is not *him* or *her*, but the *behavior* that is unacceptable. *An attitude of acceptance promotes feelings of self-worth. Trust is the basis of a therapeutic relationship.*

2. Maintain low level of stimuli in client's environment (low lighting, few people, simple decor, low noise level). *A stimulating environment may increase agitation and promote aggressive behavior.*

3. Observe client's behavior frequently. Do this through routine activities and interactions; avoid appearing watchful and suspicious. *Close observation is required so that intervention can occur if needed to ensure client's (and others') safety.*

4. Remove all dangerous objects from client's environment. *Client safety is a nursing priority.*

5. Help client identify the true object of his or her hostility (e.g., "You seem to be upset with . . ."). *Because of weak ego development, client may be misusing the defense mechanism of displacement. Helping him or her recognize this in a nonthreatening manner may help reveal unresolved issues so that they may be confronted.*

6. Encourage client to gradually verbalize hostile feelings. *Verbalization of feelings in a nonthreatening environment may help client come to terms with unresolved issues.*

7. Explore with client alternative ways of handling frustration (e.g., large motor skills that channel hostile energy into socially acceptable behavior). *Physically demanding activities help to relieve pent-up tension.*

8. Staff should maintain and convey a calm attitude toward client. *Anxiety is contagious and can be transferred from staff to client. A calm attitude provides client with a feeling of safety and security.*

9. Have sufficient staff available to present a show of strength to client if necessary. *This conveys to the client evidence of control over the situation and provides some physical security for staff.*

10. Administer tranquilizing medications as ordered by phy-

3. Provide positive feedback or reward for acceptable behaviors. *Positive reinforcement enhances self-esteem and encourages repetition of desirable behaviors.*

4. In an attempt to assist client to delay gratification, begin to increase the length of time requirement for acceptable behavior in order to achieve the reward. For example, 2 hours of acceptable behavior may be exchanged for a phone call; 4 hours of acceptable behavior for 2 hours of television; 1 day of acceptable behavior for a recreational therapy bowling activity; 5 days of acceptable behavior for a weekend pass.

5. A milieu unit provides the appropriate environment for the client with antisocial personality. *The democratic approach, with specific rules and regulations, community meetings, and group therapy sessions emulates the type of societal situation in which the client must learn to live. Feedback from peers is often more effective than confrontation from an authority figure. The client learns to follow the rules of the group as a positive step in the progression toward internalizing the rules of society.*

6. Help client to gain insight into his or her own behaviors. Often these individuals rationalize to such an extent that they deny that what they have done is wrong. (For example, "The owner of this store has so much money, he'll never miss the little bit I take. He has everything, and I have nothing. It's not fair! I deserve to have some of what he has.") *Client must come to understand that certain behaviors will not be tolerated within the society and that severe consequences will be imposed on those individuals who refuse to comply. Client must* want *to become a productive member of society before he or she can be helped.*

7. Talk about past behaviors with client. Discuss which behaviors are acceptable by societal norms and which are not. Help client identify ways in which he or she has exploited others. Encourage client to explore how he or she would feel if the circumstances were reversed. *An attempt may be made to enlighten the client to the sensitivity of others by promoting self-awareness in an effort to assist the client gain insight into his or her own behavior.*

8. Throughout relationship with client, maintain attitude of "It is not *you*, but your *behavior*, that is unacceptable." *An attitude of acceptance promotes feelings of dignity and self-worth.*

Outcome Criteria
1. Client follows rules and regulations of the milieu environment.
2. Client is able to verbalize which of his or her behaviors are not acceptable.
3. Client shows regard for the rights of others by delaying gratification of own desires when appropriate.

DEFENSIVE COPING

Definition: *The state in which an individual repeatedly projects falsely positive self-evaluation based on a self-protective pattern which defends against underlying perceived threats to positive self-regard.*

Possible Etiologies ("related to")
[Low self-esteem]
[Retarded ego development]
[Underdeveloped superego]
[Negative role models]
[Lack of positive feedback]
[Absent, erratic, or inconsistent methods of discipline]
[Dysfunctional family system]

Defining Characteristics ("evidenced by")
Denial of obvious problems or weaknesses
Projection of blame or responsibility
Rationalization of failures
Hypersensitivity to criticism
Grandiosity
Superior attitude toward others
Difficulty establishing or maintaining relationships
Hostile laughter or ridicule of others
Difficulty in reality testing of perceptions
Lack of follow-through or participation in treatment or therapy

Goals/Objectives
Short-Term Goal
Client will verbalize personal responsibility for difficulties experienced in interpersonal relationships within (time period reasonable for client).

Long-Term Goal

Client will demonstrate ability to interact with others without becoming defensive, rationalizing behaviors, or expressing grandiose ideas.

Interventions with *Selected Rationales*

1. Recognize and support basic ego strengths. *Focusing on positive aspects of the personality may help to improve self-concept.*
2. Encourage client to recognize and verbalize feelings of inadequacy and need for acceptance from others, and how these feelings provoke defensive behaviors, such as blaming others for own behaviors. *Recognition of the problem is the first step in the change process toward resolution.*
3. Provide immediate, matter-of-fact, nonthreatening feedback for unacceptable behaviors. *Client may lack knowledge about how he or she is being perceived by others. Providing this information in a nonthreatening manner may help to eliminate these undesirable behaviors.*
4. Help client identify situations that provoke defensiveness and practice through role playing more appropriate responses. *Role playing provides confidence to deal with difficult situations when they actually occur.*
5. Provide immediate positive feedback for acceptable behaviors. *Positive feedback enhances self-esteem and encourages repetition of desirable behaviors.*
6. Help client set realistic, concrete goals and determine appropriate actions to meet those goals. *Success increases self-esteem.*
7. Evaluate with client the effectiveness of the new behaviors and discuss any modifications for improvement. *Because of limited problem-solving ability, assistance may be required to reassess and develop new strategies, in the event that certain of the new coping methods prove ineffective.*

Outcome Criteria

1. Client verbalizes and accepts responsibility for own behavior.
2. Client verbalizes correlation between feelings of inadequacy and the need to defend the ego through rationalization and grandiosity.
3. Client does not ridicule or criticize others.
4. Client interacts with others in group situations without taking a defensive stance.

SELF-ESTEEM DISTURBANCE

Definition: *Negative self-evaluation and feelings about self or self-capabilities, which may be directly or indirectly expressed.*

Possible Etiologies ("related to")
[Lack of positive feedback]
[Unmet dependency needs]
[Retarded ego development]
[Repeated negative feedback, resulting in diminished self-worth]
[Dysfunctional family system]
[Absent, erratic, or inconsistent parental discipline]
[Extreme poverty]

Defining Characteristics ("evidenced by")
Denial of problems obvious to others
Projection of blame or responsibility for problems
Grandiosity
[Aggressive behavior]
[Frequent use of derogatory and critical remarks against others]
[Manipulation of one staff member against another in an attempt to gain special privileges]
[Inability to form close, personal relationships]

Goals/Objectives
Short-Term Goal
Client will verbalize an understanding that derogatory and critical remarks against others reflects feelings of self-contempt.

Long-Term Goal
Client will experience an increase in self-esteem, as evidenced by verbalizations of positive aspects of self and the lack of manipulative behaviors toward others.

Interventions with *Selected Rationales*
1. Ensure that goals are realistic. It is important for client to achieve something, so plan for activities in which success is likely. *Success increases self-esteem.*
2. Identify ways in which client is manipulating others. Set limits on manipulative behavior. *Because client is unable (or unwilling) to limit own maladaptive behaviors, assistance is required from staff.*

3. Explain consequences of manipulative behavior. All staff must be consistent and follow through with consequences in a matter-of-fact manner. *From the onset, client must be aware of the outcomes his or her maladaptive behaviors will effect. Without consistency of follow-through from all staff, a positive outcome cannot be achieved.*

4. Encourage client to talk about his or her behavior, the limits, and consequences for violation of those limits. *Discussion of feelings regarding these circumstances may assist the client in achieving a degree of insight into his or her situation.*

5. Discuss how manipulative behavior interferes with formation of close, personal relationships. *Client may be unaware of others' perception of him or her and of why these behaviors are not acceptable to others.*

6. Help client identify more adaptive interpersonal strategies. Provide positive feedback for nonmanipulative behaviors. *Client may require assistance with solving problems. Positive reinforcement enhances self-esteem and encourages repetition of desirable behaviors.*

7. Encourage client to confront the fear of failure by attending therapy activities and undertaking new tasks. Offer recognition of successful endeavors.

8. Assist client in identifying positive aspects of the self and in developing ways to change the characteristics that are socially unacceptable. *Individuals with low self-esteem often have difficulty recognizing their positive attributes. They may also lack problem-solving ability and require assistance to formulate a plan for implementing the desired changes.*

9. Minimize negative feedback to client. Enforce limit setting in a matter-of-fact manner, imposing previously established consequences for violations. *Negative feedback can be extremely threatening to a person with low self-esteem, possibly aggravating the problem. Consequences should convey unacceptability of the* behavior *but not the* person.

10. Encourage independence in the performance of personal responsibilities and in decision making related to own self-care. Offer recognition and praise for accomplishments. *Positive reinforcement enhances self-esteem and encourages repetition of desirable behaviors.*

11. Help client increase level of self-awareness through critical examination of feelings, attitudes, and behaviors.

Help client to understand that it is perfectly acceptable for attitudes and behaviors to differ from those of others, as long as they do not become intrusive. *As the client becomes more aware and accepting of himself or herself, the need for judging the behavior of others will diminish.*

12. Teach client assertiveness techniques, especially the ability to recognize the differences among passive, assertive, and aggressive behaviors and the importance of respecting the human rights of others while protecting one's own basic human rights. *These techniques increase self-esteem while enhancing the ability to form satisfactory interpersonal relationships.*

Outcome Criteria

1. Client verbalizes positive aspects about self.
2. Client does not manipulate others in an attempt to increase feelings of self-worth.
3. Client considers the rights of others in interpersonal interactions.

IMPAIRED SOCIAL INTERACTION

Definition: *The state in which an individual participates in an insufficient or excessive quantity or ineffective quality of social exchange.*

Possible Etiologies ("related to")

[Low self-esteem]
[Unmet dependency needs]
[Retarded ego development]
[Retarded superego development]
[Negative role modeling]
Knowledge deficit about ways to enhance mutuality

Defining Characteristics ("evidenced by")

Verbalized or observed discomfort in social situations
Verbalized or observed inability to receive or communicate a
    satisfying sense of belonging, caring, interest, or shared
    history
Observed use of unsuccessful social interaction behaviors
Dysfunctional interaction with peers, family, or others
[Exploitation of others for the fulfillment of own desires]

[Inability to develop satisfactory, enduring, intimate relationship with a sexual partner]

[Physical and verbal hostility toward others when fulfillment of own desires is thwarted]

Goals/Objectives
Short-Term Goal
Client will develop satisfactory relationship (no evidence of manipulation or exploitation) with nurse or therapist within 1 week.

Long-Term Goal
Client will interact appropriately with others, demonstrating concern for the needs of others as well as his or her own, by discharge from therapy.

Interventions with *Selected Rationales*
1. Develop therapeutic rapport with client. Establish trust by always being honest; keep all promises; convey acceptance of person, separate from unacceptable behaviors ("It is not *you*, but *your behavior*, that is unacceptable.") *An attitude of acceptance promotes feelings of self-worth. Trust is the basis of a therapeutic relationship.*
2. Offer to remain with client during initial interactions with others on the unit. *Presence of a trusted individual increases feelings of security during uncomfortable situations.*
3. Provide constructive criticism and positive reinforcement for efforts. *Positive feedback enhances self-esteem and encourages repetition of desirable behaviors.*
4. Confront client as soon as possible when interactions with others are manipulative or exploitative. Establish consequences for unacceptable behavior, and always follow through. *Because of the strong id influence on client's behavior, he or she should receive immediate feedback when behavior is unacceptable. Consistency in enforcing the consequences is essential if positive outcomes are to be achieved. Inconsistency creates confusion and encourages testing of limits.*
5. Act as a role model for client through appropriate interactions with him or her and with others. *Role modeling is a powerful and effective form of learning.*
6. Provide group situations for client. *It is through these group interactions with positive and negative feedback from his or her peers, that client will learn socially acceptable behavior.*

Outcome Criteria
1. Client willingly and appropriately participates in group activities.
2. Client has satisfactorily established and maintained one interpersonal relationship with nurse or therapist, without evidence of manipulation or exploitation.
3. Client demonstrates ability to interact appropriately with others, showing respect for self and others.
4. Client is able to verbalize reasons for inability to form close interpersonal relationships with others in the past.

KNOWLEDGE DEFICIT (Self-Care Activities to Achieve and Maintain Optimal Wellness)

Definition: Absence or deficiency of cognitive information related to specific topic.

Possible Etiologies ("related to")
Lack of interest in learning
[Low self-esteem]
[Denial of need for information]
[Denial of risks involved with maladaptive lifestyle]
[Unfamiliarity with sources for acquiring information]

Defining Characteristics ("evidenced by")
[History of substance abuse]
[Statement of lack of knowledge]
[Statement of misconception]
[Request for information]
[Demonstrated lack of knowledge regarding basic health practices]
[Reported or observed inability to take the responsibility for meeting basic health practices in any or all functional pattern areas]
[History of lack of health-seeking behavior]
Inappropriate or exaggerated behaviors (e.g., hysterical, hostile, agitated, apathetic)

Goals/Objectives
Short-Term Goal
Client will verbalize understanding of knowledge required to fulfill basic health needs following implementation of teaching plan.

Long-Term Goal
Client will be able to demonstrate skills learned for fulfillment of basic health needs by discharge from therapy.

Interventions with *Selected Rationales*

1. Assess client's level of knowledge regarding positive self-care practices. *An adequate database is necessary for the development of an effective teaching plan.*
2. Assess client's level of anxiety and readiness to learn. *Learning does not occur beyond the moderate level of anxiety.*
3. Determine method of learning most appropriate for client (e.g., discussion, question and answer, use of audio or visual aids, oral, written). Be sure to consider level of education and development. *Teaching will be ineffective if presented at a level or by a method inappropriate to the client's ability to learn.*
4. Develop teaching plan, including measurable objectives for the learner. Provide information regarding healthful strategies for activities of daily living, as well as harmful effects of substance abuse on the body. Include suggestions for community resources to assist client when adaptability is impaired.
5. Include significant others in the learning activity, if possible. *Input from individuals who are directly involved in the potential change increases the likelihood of a positive outcome.*
6. Implement teaching plan at a time that facilitates, and in a place that is conducive to, optimal learning (e.g., in the evening when family members visit; in an empty, quiet classroom or group therapy room). *Learning is enhanced by an environment with few distractions.*
7. Begin with simple concepts and progress to the more complex. *Retention is increased if introductory material presented is easy to understand.*
8. Provide activities for client and significant others in which to actively participate during the learning exercise. *Active participation increases retention.*
9. Ask client and significant others to demonstrate knowledge gained by verbalizing information regarding positive self-care practices. *Verbalization of knowledge gained is a measurable method of evaluating the teaching experience.*
10. Provide positive feedback for participation, as well as for accurate demonstration of knowledge gained. *Positive*

*feedback enhances self-esteem and encourages rep-
etition of desirable behaviors.*
11. Evaluate the teaching plan. Identify strengths and weaknesses and any changes which may enhance the effectiveness of the plan.

Outcome Criteria
1. Client is able to verbalize information regarding positive
self-care practices.
2. Client is able to verbalize available community resources
for obtaining knowledge regarding, and assistance with,
deficits related to health care.

Chapter 18

PROBLEMS RELATED TO ABUSE OR NEGLECT

BACKGROUND ASSESSMENT DATA

The *DSM-IV* (APA, 1994) lists the following categories for this classification:

1. **Physical Abuse of Child.** Physical injury to a child includes any *nonaccidental* physical injury caused by the parent or caretaker. The most obvious way to detect it is by outward physical signs. However, behavioral indicators may also be evident (Townsend, 1996).
2. **Sexual Abuse of Child.** This category is defined as any sexual act, including but not limited to, indecent exposure, improper touching, and penetration (sexual intercourse), that is carried out with a child for the sexual pleasure of an adult (KCAPC, 1992). Incest has been defined as sexual exploitation of a child under 18 years of age by a relative or a nonrelative who holds a position of trust within the family (Courtois, 1988).
3. **Neglect of Child.** Physical neglect of a child refers to the failure on the part of the parent or caregiver to provide for that child's basic needs, such as food, clothing, shelter, medical and dental care, and supervision (KCAPC, 1992). Emotional neglect refers to a chronic failure by the parent or caretaker to provide the child with the hope, love, and support necessary for the development of a sound, healthy personality (KCAPC, 1992).

4. **Physical Abuse of Adult.** Physical abuse of an adult may be defined as "the infliction of physical pain or injury with the intent to cause harm which may include slaps, punches, biting, and hair pulling, but in frequency or occurrence generally involves more serious assaults including choking, kicking, breaking bones, stabbing, or shooting; or forcible restraint which may include locking in homes or closets, being tied or handcuffed" (Martin, 1988).

5. **Sexual Abuse of Adult.** Sexual abuse of an adult may be defined as the expression of power and dominance by means of sexual violence, most commonly by men over women, although men may also be victims of sexual assault (Hoff, 1985). Sexual assault is identified by the use of force and executed against the person's will.

PREDISPOSING FACTORS (That Contribute to Patterns of Abuse)

1. **Physiologic**
   a. ***Neurophysiologic Influences.*** Alterations in the limbic system of the brain may have an influence on aggressive behavior in some individuals (Goldstein, 1974).
   b. ***Biochemical Influences.*** Goldstein (1974) suggests that various neurotransmitters (e.g., epinephrine, norepinephrine, dopamine, acetylcholine, and serotonin) may play a role in the facilitation and inhibition of aggressive impulses.
   c. ***Genetic Influences.*** Some studies have implicated heredity as a component in the predisposition to aggressive behavior. Both direct genetic links and the genetic karyotype XYY have been investigated as possibilities. Evidence remains inconclusive.
   d. ***Disorders of the Brain.*** Various disorders of the brain including tumors, trauma, and certain diseases (e.g., encephalitis and epilepsy) have been implicated in the predisposition to aggressive behavior (Townsend, 1996).

2. **Psychosocial**
   a. ***Psychoanalytic Theory.*** Various psychoanalytic theorists have hypothesized that aggression and violence are the overt expressions of powerlessness and

low self-esteem, which result when childhood needs for satisfaction and security go unmet (Townsend, 1996).
b. ***Learning Theory.*** This theory postulates that aggressive and violent behaviors are learned from prestigious and influential role models. Individuals who were abused as children or whose parents disciplined with physical punishment are more likely to behave in a violent manner as adults (Owens and Straus, 1975).
c. ***Societal Influences.*** Social scientists believe that aggressive behavior is primarily a product of one's culture and social structure (West, 1979). Societal influences may contribute to violence when individuals come to realize that their needs and desires cannot be met through conventional means, and they resort to delinquent behaviors in an effort to obtain desired ends.

SYMPTOMATOLOGY (Subjective and Objective Data)

1. Signs of physical abuse may include the following:
   a. Bruises over various areas of the body. They may present with different colors of bluish-purple to yellowish-green (indicating various stages of healing).
   b. Bite marks, skin welts, burns.
   c. Fractures, scars, serious internal injuries, even brain damage.
   d. Lacerations, abrasions, or unusual bleeding.
   e. Bald spots indicative of severe hair pulling.
   f. In a child, regressive behaviors (such as thumb sucking and enuresis) are common.
   g. Extreme anxiety and mistrust of others.
2. Signs of neglect of a child may include the following:
   a. Soiled clothing that does not fit and may be inappropriate for the weather.
   b. Poor hygiene.
   c. Always hungry, with possible signs of malnutrition (e.g., emaciated with swollen belly).
   d. Listless and tired much of the time.
   e. Unattended medical problems.
   f. Social isolation; unsatisfactory peer relationships.
   g. Poor school performance and attendance record.

3. Signs of sexual abuse of a child include the following:
   a. Frequent urinary infections.
   b. Difficulty or pain in walking or sitting.
   c. Rashes or itching in the genital area; scratching the area a great deal or fidgeting when seated.
   d. Frequent vomiting.
   e. Seductive behavior; compulsive masturbation; precocious sex play.
   f. Excessive anxiety and mistrust of others.
   g. Sexually abusing another child.
4. Signs of sexual abuse of an adult include (Burgess, 1984) the following:
   a. Contusions and abrasions about various parts of the body.
   b. Headaches, fatigue, sleep-pattern disturbances.
   c. Stomach pains, nausea, and vomiting.
   d. Vaginal discharge and itching, burning on urination, rectal bleeding and pain.
   e. Rage, humiliation, embarrassment, desire for revenge, self-blame.
   f. Fear of physical violence and death.
   g. Overwhelming sense of helplessness and personal violation.

COMMON NURSING DIAGNOSES AND INTERVENTIONS
(Interventions are applicable to various health-care settings, such as inpatient and partial hospitalization, community outpatient clinic, home health, and private practice.)

RAPE-TRAUMA SYNDROME

Definition: *Forced, violent sexual penetration against the victim's will and consent. The trauma syndrome that develops from this attack or attempted attack includes an acute phase of disorganization of the victim's lifestyle and a long-term process of reorganization of lifestyle.*

Possible Etiologies ("related to")
[Having been the victim of sexual violence executed with the use of force and against one's personal will and consent]

[Lacerations over areas of body]
[Fear for personal and children's safety]
[Verbalizations of no way to get out of relationship]

Goals/Objectives
Short-Term Goal
Client will recognize and verbalize choices that are available, thereby perceiving some control over life situation (time dimension to be individually determined).

Long-Term Goal
Client will exhibit control over life situation by making decision about what to do regarding living with cycle of abuse (time dimension to be individually determined).

Interventions with *Selected Rationales*
1. In collaboration with physician, ensure that all physical wounds, fractures, and burns receive immediate attention. It is a good idea to take photographs, if the victim will permit (Smith, 1987b; Burgess, 1990). *Client safety is a nursing priority. Photographs may be called in as evidence if charges are filed.*
2. Take the woman to a private area to do the interview. *If the client is accompanied by the man who did the battering, she is not likely to be truthful about her injuries.*
3. If she has come alone or with her children, assure her of her safety. Encourage her to discuss the battering incident. Ask questions about whether this has happened before; whether the abuser takes drugs; whether the woman has a safe place to go; and whether she is interested in pressing charges. *Some women will attempt to keep secret how their injuries occurred in an effort to protect the partner, or because they are fearful that the partner will kill them if they tell.*
4. Ensure that "rescue" efforts are not attempted by the nurse. Offer support, but remember that the final decision must be made by the client. *Making her own decision gives the client a sense of control over her life situation. Imposing judgments and giving advice are nontherapeutic.*
5. Stress the importance of safety. Smith (1987b) suggests a statement such as, "Yes, it has happened. Now where do you want to go from here?" Burgess (1990) states, "The victim needs to be made aware of the variety of resources that are available to her. These may include crisis hotlines, community groups for women who have been abused, shelters, a variety of counseling opportuni-

ties (i.e., couples, individual, or group), and information regarding the victim's rights in the civil and criminal justice system.'' After a discussion of these available resources, the woman may choose for herself. If her decision is to return to the marriage and home, this choice, too, must be respected. *Knowledge of available choices can serve to decrease the victim's sense of powerlessness, but true empowerment comes only when she chooses to use that knowledge for her own benefit.*

Outcome Criteria

1. The client has received immediate attention to physical injuries.
2. The client verbalizes assurance of her immediate safety.
3. The client discusses life situation with primary nurse.
4. The client is able to verbalize choices available to her from which she may receive assistance.

ALTERED GROWTH AND DEVELOPMENT

Definition: *The state in which an individual demonstrates deviations in norms from his or her age group.*

Possible Etiologies ("related to")

Inadequate caretaking

[The infliction by caretakers of physical pain or injury with the intent to cause harm, usually occurring over an extended period of time]

[Ignoring the child's basic physiologic needs]

[Indifference to the child]

[Ignoring the child's presence]

[Ignoring the child's social, educational, recreational, and developmental needs]

Defining Characteristics ("evidenced by")

Delay or difficulty in performing skills (motor, social, or expressive) typical of age group

Altered physical growth

Inability to perform self-care or self-control activities appropriate for age

Flat affect

Listlessness

Decreased responses

[Evidence of bruises, burns, lacerations, or other types of

physical injury not consistent with performance of every-day activities]

[Expression of fear of parent or caretaker]

[Social isolation]

[Regressive behaviors (e.g., rocking, thumb sucking, enuresis)]

[Wearing clothing inappropriate to weather in order to cover up the injuries]

Goals/Objectives
Short-Term Goal
Client will develop trusting relationship with nurse and report how evident injuries were sustained (time dimension to be individually determined).

Long-Term Goal
Client will demonstrate behaviors consistent with age-appropriate growth and development.

Interventions with *Selected Rationales*
1. Perform complete physical assessment of the child. Take particular note of bruises (in various stages of healing), lacerations, and client complaints of pain in specific areas. Do not overlook or discount the possibility of sexual abuse. Assess for nonverbal signs of abuse: aggressive conduct, excessive fears, extreme hyperactivity, apathy, withdrawal, age-inappropriate behaviors. *An accurate and thorough physical assessment is required in order to provide appropriate care for the client.*
2. Conduct an in-depth interview with the parent or adult who accompanies the child. Consider: If the injury is being reported as an accident, is the explanation reasonable? Is the injury consistent with the explanation? Is the injury consistent with the child's developmental capabilities? *Fear of imprisonment or loss of child custody may place the abusive parent on the defensive. Discrepancies may be evident in the description of the incident, and lying to cover up involvement is a common defense that may be detectable in an in-depth interview.*
3. Use games or play therapy to gain child's trust. Use these techniques to assist in describing his or her side of the story. *Establishing a trusting relationship with an abused child is extremely difficult. They may not even want to be touched. These types of play activities can provide a nonthreatening environment that may enhance the child's attempt to discuss these painful issues (Celano, 1990).*

4. Determine whether nature of the injuries warrant reporting to authorities. Specific state statutes must enter into the decision of whether or not to report suspected child abuse. *A report [is commonly made] if there is reason to suspect that a child has been injured as a result of physical, mental, emotional, or sexual abuse (KCAPC, 1992). "Reason to suspect" exists when there is evidence of a discrepancy or inconsistency in explaining a child's injury. Most states require that the following individuals report cases of suspected child abuse: all health-care workers, all mental health therapists, teachers, child care providers, firefighters, emergency medical personnel, and law enforcement personnel. Reports are made to the Department of Social and Rehabilitative Services (SRS), Department of Human Services (DHS), or a law enforcement agency.*

Outcome Criteria

1. The client has received immediate attention to physical injuries.
2. The client demonstrates trust in primary nurse by discussing abuse through the use of play therapy.
3. The client is demonstrating a decrease in regressive behaviors.

Chapter 19

PREMENSTRUAL DYSPHORIC DISORDER

BACKGROUND ASSESSMENT DATA

DEFINED

Premenstrual dysphoric disorder* is identified by a variety of physical and emotional symptoms that occur during the last week of the luteal phase of the menstrual cycle and that remit within a few days after the onset of the follicular phase. In most women, these symptoms occur in the week before, and remit within a few days after, the onset of menses. The disorder has also been reported in nonmenstruating women who have had a hysterectomy, but retain ovarian function. The diagnosis is given only when the symptoms are sufficiently severe to cause marked impairment in social or occupational functioning, and have occurred during a majority of menstrual cycles in the past year (APA, 1994).

PREDISPOSING FACTORS

1. **Physiologic**
    a. ***Biochemical.*** An imbalance of the hormones estrogen and progesterone have been implicated in the predisposition to premenstrual dysphoric disorder.

---

*Text and criteria are provided in the *DSM-IV* to facilitate systematic clinical research (APA, 1994).

It is postulated that excess estrogen or a high estrogen-to-progesterone ratio during the luteal phase causes water retention and that this hormonal imbalance has other effects as well, resulting in the symptoms associated with premenstrual syndrome (Casey and Dwyer, 1987).

b. ***Nutritional.*** A number of nutritional alterations have been implicated in the etiology of premenstrual dysphoric disorder (Casey and Dwyer, 1987). They include vitamin B_6 deficiency, glucose tolerance fluctuations, abnormal fatty acid metabolism, magnesium deficiency, vitamin E deficiency, and caffeine sensitivity. No definitive evidence exists to support any specific nutritional alteration in the etiology of these symptoms.

2. **Psychosocial**
   a. ***Family Dynamics.*** It is possible that the behaviors associated with premenstrual dysphoric disorder are learned through role modeling during the socialization process (Doenges et al, 1995). Children may observe and identify with this behavior in significant adults and incorporate it into their own responses as they mature. Positive reinforcement in the form of primary or secondary gains for these behaviors may serve to perpetuate the learned patterns of disability.

SYMPTOMATOLOGY (Subjective and Objective Data)

The American Psychiatric Association (1994) has identified the following symptoms as diagnostic for premenstrual (late luteal phase) dysphoric disorder:

1. Markedly depressed mood, feelings of hopelessness, or self-deprecating thoughts
2. Marked anxiety, tension, feelings of being "keyed up," or "on edge"
3. Marked affective lability (e.g., feeling suddenly sad or tearful or increased sensitivity to rejection)
4. Persistent and marked anger or irritability or increased interpersonal conflicts
5. Decreased interest in usual activities (e.g., work, school, friends, hobbies)
6. Subjective sense of difficulty in concentrating
7. Lethargy, easy fatigability, or marked lack of energy

8. Marked change in appetite, overeating, or specific food cravings
9. Hypersomnia or insomnia
10. A subjective sense of being overwhelmed or out of control
11. Other physical symptoms, such as breast tenderness or swelling, headaches, joint or muscle pain, a sensation of "bloating," weight gain

Other subjective symptoms that have been reported include (Doenges et al, 1995):

12. Cramps
13. Alcohol intolerance
14. Acne
15. Cystitis
16. Oliguria
17. Altered sexual drive
18. Forgetfulness
19. Suicidal ideations or attempts

COMMON NURSING DIAGNOSES AND INTERVENTIONS
(Interventions are applicable to various health-care settings, such as inpatient and partial hospitalization, community outpatient clinic, home health, and private practice.)

ACUTE PAIN

Definition: *Sudden or slow onset of any intensity from mild to severe with an anticipated or predictable end and a duration of less than 6 months.*

Possible Etiologies ("related to")
[Imbalance in estrogen and progesterone levels]
[Possible nutritional alterations, including the following:
    Vitamin B_6 deficiency
    Glucose tolerance fluctuations
    Abnormal fatty acid metabolism, which may contribute to alterations in prostaglandin synthesis
    Magnesium deficiency
    Vitamin E deficiency

Caffeine sensitivity
Alcohol intolerance]
[Fluid retention]

Defining Characteristics ("evidenced by")
[Subjective communication of:
Headache
Backache
Joint or muscle pain
A sensation of "bloating"
Abdominal cramping
Breast tenderness and swelling]
Facial mask
Sleep disturbance
Self-focus
Changes in appetite and eating

Goals/Objectives
Short-Term Goal
Client cooperates with efforts to manage symptoms of premenstrual syndrome (PMS) and minimize feelings of discomfort.

Long-Term Goal
Client verbalizes relief from discomfort associated with symptoms of PMS.

Interventions with *Selected Rationales*
1. Assess and record location, duration, and intensity of pain. *Background assessment data is necessary to formulate an accurate plan of care for the client.*
2. Provide nursing comfort measures with a matter-of-fact approach that does not give positive reinforcement to the pain behavior (e.g., backrub, warm bath, heating pad). Give additional attention at times when client is not focusing on physical symptoms. *These measures may serve to provide some temporary relief from pain. Absence of secondary gains in the form of positive reinforcement may discourage client's use of the pain as attention-seeking behavior.*
3. Encourage the client to get adequate rest and sleep and avoid stressful activity during the premenstrual period. *Fatigue exaggerates symptoms associated with PMS. Stress elicits heightened symptoms of anxiety which may contribute to exacerbation of symptoms and altered perception of pain.*

4. Assist client with activities that distract from focus on self and pain. Demonstrate techniques such as visual or auditory distractions, guided imagery, breathing exercises, massage, application of heat or cold, and relaxation techniques that may provide symptomatic relief. *These techniques may help to maintain anxiety at manageable level and prevent the discomfort from becoming disabling.*

5. *In an effort to correct the possible nutritional alterations that may be contributing to PMS,* the following guidelines may be suggested (Doenges et al, 1995):
   a. Reduce intake of fats in the diet, particularly saturated fats.
   b. Limit intake of dairy products to two servings a day (excessive dairy products block the absorption of magnesium).
   c. Increase intake of complex carbohydrates (vegetables, legumes, cereals, and whole grains) and cis-linoleic acid-containing foods (e.g., safflower oil).
   d. Decrease refined and simple sugars. (Excess sugar is thought to cause nervous tension, palpitations, headache, dizziness, drowsiness, and excretion of magnesium in the urine, thus preventing the body from breaking down sugar for energy.)
   e. Decrease salt intake to 3 g per day but not less than 0.5 g per day. (Salt restriction prevents edema; too little salt stimulates norepinephrine and causes sleep disturbances.)
   f. Limit intake of caffeine (coffee, tea, colas, and chocolate) and alcohol (one to two drinks a week). Caffeine increases breast tenderness and pain. Alcohol can cause reactive hypoglycemia and fluid retention.
   g. Because some women crave junk food during the premenstrual period, it is important to take a multiple vitamin or mineral tablet daily to ensure that adequate nutrients are consumed.

6. Administer medications as prescribed. Monitor client response for effectiveness of the medication, as well as for appearance of adverse side effects. *When other measures are insufficient to bring about relief,* physician may prescribe symptomatic drug therapy. Provide client with information about the medication to be administered. *Client has the right to know about the treatment she is receiving.* Some medications commonly used for symptomatic treatment of PMS are presented in Table 19–1.

TABLE 19–1. **Medications for Symptomatic Relief of PMS**

Medication	Indication
Hydrochlorothiazide (Esidrix, HydroDiuril), furosemide (Lasix)	Diuretics may provide relief from edema when diet and sodium restriction are not sufficient.
Ibuprofen (Advil, Motrin, Nuprin), naproxen (Naprosyn)	Nonsteroidal anti-inflammatory agents may provide relief from joint, muscle, and lower abdominal pain related to increased prostaglandins.
Propranolol (Inderal), verapamil (Isoptin)	β-Blockers and calcium channel blockers are often given for prophylactic treatment of migraine headaches.
Sumatriptan (Imitrex)	This cerebral vasoconstrictor is highly effective in the treatment of acute migraine attack.
Carisoprodol (Soma), chlorzoxazone (Parafon Forte)	Muscle relaxants may provide relief of muscular tension.
Bromocriptine (Parlodel)	This drug may be prescribed to relieve breast pain and other symptoms of PMS that may be caused by elevated prolactin.

Outcome Criteria
1. Client demonstrates ability to manage premenstrual symptoms with minimal discomfort.
2. Client verbalizes relief of painful symptoms.

INEFFECTIVE INDIVIDUAL COPING

Definition: *Impairment of adaptive behaviors and abilities of a person in meeting life's demands and roles.*

Possible Etiologies ("related to")

[Imbalance in estrogen and progesterone levels]

[Possible nutritional alterations, including the following:

Vitamin B_6 deficiency

Glucose tolerance fluctuations

Abnormal fatty acid metabolism, which may contribute to alterations in prostaglandin systhesis

Magnesium deficiency

Vitamin E deficiency

Caffeine sensitivity

Alcohol intolerance]

[Learned coping patterns through early role modeling]

Defining Characteristics ("evidenced by")

[Affective liability (sad one minute, angry the next)]

[Marked anger or irritability]

[Feelings of elevated anxiety, tension, being "keyed up" or "on edge"]

[Depressed mood, feelings of hopelessness, or self-deprecating thoughts]

[Decreased interest in usual activities]

[Easy fatigability or marked lack of energy]

[Difficulty concentrating; forgetfulness]

[Changes in appetite]

[Hypersomnia or insomnia]

[Altered sexual drive]

[Suicidal ideations or attempts]

Inability to problem-solve

Inability to meet role expectations

Goals/Objectives
Short-Term Goals

1. Client will seek out support person when having thoughts of suicide.
2. Client will verbalize ways to express anger in an appropriate manner and maintain anxiety at a manageable level.

Long-Term Goals

1. Client will not harm self while experiencing symptoms associated with PMS.
2. Client will demonstrate adaptive coping strategies to use in an effort to minimize disabling behaviors during the premenstrual and perimenstrual period.

Interventions with *Selected Rationales*

1. Assess client's potential for suicide. Has she expressed feelings of not wanting to live? Does she have a plan? A

means? *Depression is the most prevalent disorder that precedes suicide. The risk of suicide is greatly increased if the client has developed a plan and particularly if means exist for the client to execute the plan.*

2. Formulate a short-term verbal contract with the client that she will not harm herself during specific time period. When that contract expires, make another, and so forth. *Discussion of suicidal feelings with a trusted individual provides a degree of relief to the client. A contract gets the subject out in the open and places some of the responsibility for the client's safety with the client. An attitude of acceptance of the client as a worthwhile individual is conveyed.*

3. Secure a promise from client that she will seek out a staff member if thoughts of suicide emerge. *Suicidal clients are often very ambivalent about their feelings. Discussion of feelings with a trusted individual may provide assistance before the client experiences a crisis situation.*

4. Encourage client to express angry feelings within appropriate limits. Provide safe method of hostility release. Help client to identify source of anger, if possible. Work on adaptive coping skills for use outside the health care system. *Depression and suicidal behaviors are sometimes viewed as anger turned inward on the self. If this anger can be verbalized in a nonthreatening environment, the client may be able to resolve these feelings, regardless of the discomfort involved.*

5. Encourage client to discharge pent-up anger through participation in large motor activities (e.g., brisk walks, jogging, physical exercises, volleyball, punching bag, exercise bike). *Physical exercise provides a safe and effective method for discharging pent-up tension.*

6. Assist client to identify stressors that precipitate anxiety and irritability and to learn new methods of coping with these situations (e.g., stress reduction techniques, relaxation, and visualization skills). *Knowing stress factors and ways of handling them reduces anxiety and allows client to feel a greater measure of control over the situation.*

7. Identify extent of feelings and situations when loss of control occurs. Assist with problem solving to identify behaviors for protection of self and others (e.g., call support person, remove self from situation). *Recognition of potential for harm to self or others and development*

of a plan enables client to take effective actions to meet safety needs.

8. Encourage client to reduce or shift workload and social activities during the premenstrual period as part of a total stress management program. *By coping realistically with life stresses, the decreased responsibility should relieve stress and therefore help relieve symptoms.*

9. At each visit, evaluate symptoms, and discuss those that may be most troublesome and continue to persist well after initiation of therapy. *If traditional measures are inadequate, pharmacologic intervention may be required to enhance coping abilities. For example, antidepressants may be administered for depression that remains unresolved after other symptoms have been relieved.*

10. Encourage participation in support group, psychotherapy, marital counseling, or other type of therapy as deemed necessary. *Professional assistance may be required to help the client and family members learn effective coping strategies and support lifestyle changes that may be needed.*

Outcome Criteria

1. Client participates willingly in treatment regimen, and initiates necessary lifestyle changes.
2. Client demonstrates adaptive coping strategies to deal with episodes of depression and anxiety.
3. Client verbalizes that she has no suicidal thoughts or intentions.

Chapter 20

PSYCHO-
PHARMACOLOGY

INTRODUCTION

Psychotropic medications give many individuals a chance, without which they would be unable to function. Psychotropic medications have also provided researchers and clinicians with information to study the origins and etiologies of mental illness. Knowledge gained from learning how these drugs work has promoted advancement in understanding how behavioral disorders develop.

Psychotropic medications are not intended to "cure" mental illness. Most physicians who prescribe these medications for their clients use them as an adjunct to individual or group psychotherapy. Although their contribution to psychiatric care cannot be minimized, it must be emphasized that psychotropic medications relieve physical and behavioral symptoms. They do not resolve emotional problems.

Nurses must have knowledge about these medications in order to safely administer them to their clients. Advanced practice nurses now have prescriptive authority in many states. It is essential for these nurses to have in-depth knowledge about how these drugs work, the potential effects, and dosing considerations if they are to meet the exacting standards set forth by the profession.

ANTIANXIETY AND SEDATIVE-HYPNOTIC AGENTS

INDICATIONS
Antianxiety agents are also called *anxiolytics* and *minor tranquilizers*. (Table 20–1). They are used in the treatment of anxiety disorders, anxiety symptoms, acute alcohol withdrawal, skeletal muscle spasms, convulsive disorders, status epilepticus, and preoperative sedation. Sedative-hypnotics are used in the short-term management of various anxiety states and to treat insomnia. Selected agents are used as anticonvulsants and to reduce the anxiety associated with drug withdrawal.

MECHANISM OF ACTION
These drugs work by depressing the central nervous system (CNS).

Exception: Buspirone (BuSpar) does not depress the CNS. Its action is unknown, but the drug is believed to produce the desired effects through interactions with serotonin, dopamine, and other neurotransmitter receptors.

CONTRAINDICATIONS
These drugs are contraindicated in clients with known hypersensitivity. They should not be taken in combination with other CNS depressants and are contraindicated in narrow-angle glaucoma, pregnancy and lactation, shock, and coma. Caution should be taken in administering these drugs to individuals with a history of drug abuse or addiction and with those who are depressed or suicidal.

POSSIBLE NURSING DIAGNOSES
1. Risk for injury related to seizures, panic anxiety, acute agitation from alcohol withdrawal (indications); abrupt withdrawal from the medication after long-term use; effects of medication intoxication or overdose.
2. Anxiety (specify) related to threat to physical integrity or self-concept.
3. Risk for activity intolerance related to medication side effects of sedation, confusion, lethargy.

TABLE 20–1. **Commonly Used Groups of Antianxiety and Sedative-Hypnotic Agents**

Chemical Class	Generic (Trade) Name	CC*	Daily Dosage
Antihistamines	Diphenhydramine (Benadryl)		25–200 mg
	Hydroxyzine (Vistaril, Atarax)		100–400 mg 100–400 mg
Barbiturates	Amobarbital (Amytal)	CII	30–200 mg
	Aprobarbital (Alurate)	CIII	40–160 mg
	Butabarbital (Butisol)	CIII	45–120 mg
	Pentobarbital (Nembutal)	CII	40–200 mg
	Phenobarbital (Luminal)	CIV	30–320 mg
	Secobarbital (Seconal)	CII	90–200 mg
Benzodiazepines	Alprazolam (Xanax)	CIV	0.75–4 mg
	Chlordiazepoxide (Librium)	CIV	15–100 mg
	Clorazepate (Tranxene)	CIV	15–60 mg
	Estazolam (ProSom)	CIV	1–2 mg
	Flurazepam (Dalmane)	CIV	15–30 mg
	Diazepam (Valium)	CIV	4–40 mg
	Halazepam (Paxipam)	CIV	60–160 mg
	Lorazepam (Ativan)	CIV	2–6 mg
	Oxazepam (Serax)	CIV	30–120 mg
	Prazepam (Centrax)	CIV	10–60 mg
	Quazepam (Doral)	CIV	7.5–15 mg
	Temazepam (Restoril)	CIV	15–30 mg
	Triazolam (Halcion)	CIV	0.25–0.5 mg
Metathiazanones	Chlormezanone (Trancopal)		100–800 mg
Propanediols	Meprobamate (Equanil, Miltown)	CIV CIV	400–2400 mg 400–2400 mg
Miscellaneous	Buspirone (BuSpar)		15–60 mg
	Chloral hydrate (Noctec)	CIV	500–1000 mg
	Ethchlorvynol (Placidyl)	CIV	500–1000 mg
	Ethinamate (Valmid)	CIV	500–1000 mg
	Glutethimide (Doriden)	CII	250–500 mg
	Methyprylon (Noludar)	CIII	200–400 mg
	Zolpidem (Ambien)	CIV	5–10 mg

*Controlled categories.
Adapted from Townsend, 1996, p. 273.

4. Sleep pattern disturbance related to situational crises, physical condition, severe level of anxiety.
5. Knowledge deficit related to medication regimen.

SIDE EFFECTS AND NURSING IMPLICATIONS

1. **Drowsiness, Confusion, Lethargy** (most common side effects)
   - Instruct client not to drive or operate dangerous machinery while taking the medication.
2. **Tolerance, Physical and Psychological Dependence** (does not apply to buspirone)
   - Instruct client receiving long-term therapy not to quit taking the drug abruptly. Abrupt withdrawal can be life-threatening. Symptoms include depression, insomnia, increased anxiety, abdominal and muscle cramps, tremors, vomiting, sweating, convulsions, and delirium.
3. **Potentiates the Effects of Other CNS Depressants.**
   - Instruct client not to drink alcohol or take other medications that depress the CNS while taking this medication.
4. **May Aggravate Symptoms in Depressed Persons.**
   - Assess mood daily.
   - Take necessary precautions for potential suicide.
5. **Orthostatic Hypotension**
   - Monitor lying and standing blood pressure and pulse every shift.
   - Instruct client to arise slowly from a lying or sitting position.
6. **Paradoxical Excitement**
   - Withhold drug and notify the physician.
7. **Dry Mouth**
   - Have client take frequent sips of water, ice chips, suck on hard candy, or chew sugarless gum.
8. **Nausea and Vomiting.**
   - Have client take drug with food or milk.
9. **Blood Dyscrasias**
   - Symptoms of sore throat, fever, malaise, easy bruising, or unusual bleeding should be reported to the physician immediately.

10. **Delayed Onset** (Buspirone [BuSpar] Only)
    - Ensure that client understands there is a lag time of 10 days to 2 weeks between onset of therapy and subsiding of anxiety symptoms. Client should continue to take the medication during this time. (*Note:* This medication is not recommended for prn administration because of this delayed therapeutic onset. There is no evidence that buspirone creates tolerance or physical dependence as do the CNS depressant anxiolytics.)

CLIENT/FAMILY EDUCATION

The client should:

- Not drive or operate dangerous machinery. Drowsiness and dizziness can occur.
- Not stop taking the drug abruptly. Can produce serious withdrawal symptoms, such as depression, insomnia, anxiety, abdominal and muscle cramps, tremors, vomiting, sweating, convulsions, delirium.
- (With buspirone only): Be aware of lag time between start of therapy and subsiding of symptoms. Relief is usually evident within 10 to 14 days. The client must take the medication regularly, as ordered, so that it has sufficient time to take effect.
- Not consume other CNS depressants (including alcohol).
- Not take nonprescription medication without approval from physician.
- Rise slowly from the sitting or lying position to prevent a sudden drop in blood pressure.
- Report to physician immediately, symptoms of sore throat, fever, malaise, easy bruising, unusual bleeding, or motor restlessness.
- Be aware of risks of taking these drugs during pregnancy. (Congenital malformations have been associated with use during the first trimester). If pregnancy is suspected or planned, the client should notify the physician of the desirability to discontinue the drug.
- Be aware of possible side effects. The client should refer to written materials furnished by health-care providers regarding the correct method of self-administration.
- Carry card or piece of paper at all times stating names of medications being taken.

ANTIDEPRESSANTS

INDICATIONS

Antidepressant medications are used in the treatment of dysthymic disorder; major depression with melancholia or psychotic symptoms; depression associated with organic disease, alcoholism, schizophrenia, or mental retardation; depressive phase of bipolar disorder; and depression accompanied by anxiety (Table 20–2). These drugs elevate mood and alleviate other symptoms associated with moderate to severe depression. Symptomatic relief is usually achieved in 1 to 4 weeks.

TABLE 20–2. **Commonly Used Groups of Antidepressants**

Chemical Class	Generic (Trade) Name	Daily Dosage
Tricyclics	Amitriptyline (Elavil)	75–300 mg
	Clomipramine (Anafranil)	75–300 mg
	Desipramine (Norpramin)	75–300 mg
	Doxepin (Sinequan, Adapin)	75–300 mg
	Imipramine (Tofranil)	75–300 mg
	Nortryptyline (Aventyl, Pamelor)	75–150 mg
	Protriptyline (Triptil, Vivactil)	15–60 mg
	Trimipramine (Surmontil)	75–300 mg
Heterocyclics	Amoxapine (Asendin)	100–600 mg
	Bupropion (Wellbutrin)	200–450 mg
	Maprotiline (Ludiomil)	75–225 mg
	Trazodone (Desyrel)	150–600 mg
Selective serotonin reuptake inhibitors	Fluoxetine (Prozac)	20–80 mg
	Sertraline (Zoloft)	50–200 mg
	Paroxetine (Paxil)	20–50 mg
Nonselective reuptake inhibitors	Venlafaxine (Effexor)	75–375 mg
	Nefazodone (Serzone)	200–600 mg
Monoamine oxidase inhibitors	Phenelzine (Nardil)	45–90 mg
	Isocarboxazid (Marplan)	10–30 mg
	Tranylcypromine (Parnate)	30–60 mg

Adapted from Townsend, 1996, p. 275.

MECHANISM OF ACTION

These drugs ultimately work to increase the concentration of norepinephrine, serotonin, and/or dopamine in the body. This is accomplished in the brain by blocking the reuptake of these neurotransmitters by the neurons (tricyclics, tetracyclics, selective serotonin reuptake inhibitors, and others). It also occurs when an enzyme, monoamine oxidase (MAO), that is known to inactivate norepinephrine, serotonin, and dopamine is inhibited at various sites in the nervous system (MAO inhibitors [MAOIs]).

CONTRAINDICATIONS

Contraindications include hypersensitivity, acute recovery phase following myocardial infarction, angle-closure glaucoma, and concomitant use of more than one antidepressant.

   Caution: As these drugs take effect, and mood begins to lift, the individual may have increased energy with which to implement a suicide plan. Suicide potential often increases as level of depression decreases. The nurse should be particularly alert for *sudden* lifts in mood.

POSSIBLE NURSING DIAGNOSES

1. Risk for self-directed violence related to depressed mood.
2. Risk for injury related to medication side effects (blurred vision, sedation, hypertensive crisis, priapism).
3. Social isolation related to depressed mood.
4. Risk for activity intolerance related to medication side effects.
5. Knowledge deficit related to medication regimen.

SIDE EFFECTS AND NURSING IMPLICATIONS

1. **Anticholinergic Effects**
   a. *Dry Mouth*
      • Offer sugarless candy, ice, frequent sips of water.
      • Ensure that client practices strict oral hygiene.
   b. *Blurred Vision*
      • Offer reassurance that symptom should subside after a few weeks.

- Instruct the client not to drive until vision is clear.
- Clear small items from routine pathway to prevent falls.

c. *Constipation*
  - Order foods high in fiber; increase fluid intake if not contraindicated; and encourage the client to increase physical exercise, if possible.

d. *Urinary Retention*
  - Instruct the client to report hesitancy or inability to urinate.
  - Monitor intake and output.

2. **Sedation**
   - Request an order from the physician for the drug to be given at bedtime.
   - Request that the physician decrease the dosage or consider ordering a less sedating drug.
   - Instruct the client not to drive or use dangerous equipment while experiencing sedation.

3. **Orthostatic Hypotension**
   - Instruct the client to rise slowly from a lying or sitting position.
   - Monitor blood pressure (lying and standing) frequently, and document and report significant changes.
   - Avoid long hot showers or tub baths.

4. **Reduction of Seizure Threshold**
   - Clients with history of seizures should be observed closely.
   - Institute seizure precautions as specified in hospital procedure manual.
   - Bupropion (Wellbutrin) should be administered in doses of no more than 150 mg and should be given at least 4 hours apart. Bupropion has been associated with a relatively high incidence of seizure activity in anorexic and cachectic clients.

5. **Tachycardia, Arrhythmias**
   - Carefully monitor blood pressure and pulse rate and rhythm, and report any significant change to the physician.

6. **Photosensitivity** (with Tricyclics)
   - Ensure that the client wears protective sunscreens, clothing, and sunglasses outdoors.

7. **Hypertensive Crisis** (with MAOIs)
   - This occurs if the individual consumes foods containing tyramine while receiving MAOI therapy.

- Products containing tyramine include aged cheeses; other aged, overripe, and fermented foods; broad beans; pickled herring; beef and chicken liver; preserved sausages; beer; wine (especially chianti); yeast extract (found in some packaged soups); chocolate; caffeinated drinks; sour cream; yogurt; soy sauce; over-the-counter cold medications; and diet pills.
- Symptoms of hypertensive crisis include severe occipital headache, palpitations, nausea and vomiting, nuchal rigidity, fever, sweating, marked increase in blood pressure, chest pain, and coma.
- *Treatment of hypertensive crisis:* Discontinue drug immediately; monitor vital signs; administer short-acting antihypertensive medication, as ordered by physician; use external cooling measures to control hyperpyrexia.

8. **Priapism** (with trazodone)
   - This is a rare side effect, but it has occurred in some men taking trazodone (Desyrel).
   - If the client complains of prolonged or inappropriate penile erection, withhold medication dosage and notify the physician immediately.
   - This can become very problematic, requiring surgical intervention, and, if not treated successfully, can result in impotence.

9. **Weight Loss** (with SSRIs)
   - Weight loss has been noted as a side effect of selective serotonin reuptake inhibitors (SSRIs). This is especially significant in underweight, depressed clients.
   - Caution should be used in prescribing this drug for anorectic clients.
   - Client should be weighed daily or every other day, at same time and on the same scale if possible.

CLIENT/FAMILY EDUCATION

The client should:

- Continue to take the medication even though the symptoms have not subsided. The therapeutic effect may not be seen for as long as 4 weeks. If after this length of time no improvement is noted, the physician may prescribe a different medication.
- Use caution when driving or operating dangerous machinery. Drowsiness and dizziness can occur. If these side effects become persistent or interfere with activities

of daily living, the client should report them to the physician. Dosage adjustment may be necessary.

- Not stop taking the drug abruptly. To do so might produce withdrawal symptoms, such as nausea, vertigo, insomnia, headache, malaise, and nightmares.
- (If taking a tricyclic), use sun screens and wear protective clothing when spending time outdoors. The skin may be sensitive to sunburn.
- Report occurrence of any of the following symptoms to physician immediately: sore throat, fever, malaise, unusual bleeding, easy bruising, persistent nausea and vomiting, severe headache, rapid heart rate, difficulty urinating, anorexia and weight loss, seizure activity, stiff or sore neck, or chest pain.
- Rise slowly from a sitting or lying position to prevent a sudden drop in blood pressure.
- Take frequent sips of water, chew sugarless gum, or suck on hard candy if dry mouth is a problem. Good oral care (frequent brushing, flossing) is very important.
- Not consume the following foods or medications while taking MAOIs: aged cheese, wine (especially chianti), beer, chocolate, colas, coffee, tea, beef or chicken livers, soy sauce, overripe and fermented foods, pickled herring, preserved sausages, yeast extract, broad beans, over-the-counter cold remedies or diet pills. To do so could cause a life-threatening hypertensive crisis.
- Avoid smoking while on tricyclic therapy. Smoking increases the metabolism of tricyclics, requiring an adjustment in dosage to achieve a therapeutic effect.
- Not drink alcohol while on antidepressant therapy. These drugs potentiate the effects of each other.
- Not consume other medications (including over-the-counter medications) without the physician's approval while on antidepressant therapy. Many medications contain substances that, in combination with antidepressant medication, could precipitate a life-threatening hypertensive crisis.
- Notify the physician immediately if inappropriate or prolonged penile erections occur while taking trazodone (Desyrel). If the erection persists longer than 1 hour, seek emergency room treatment. This condition is rare, but has occurred in some men who have taken trazodone. If measures are not instituted immediately, impotence can result.
- Not "double up" on medication if a dose of bupropion (Wellbutrin) is missed, unless advised to do so by the

physician. Taking bupropion in divided doses will decrease the risk of seizures and other adverse effects.
- Be aware of possible risks of taking antidepressants during pregnancy. Safe use during pregnancy and lactation has not been fully established. These drugs are thought to readily cross the placental barrier; if so, the fetus could experience adverse effects of the drug. Inform the physician immediately if pregnancy occurs, is suspected, or is planned.
- Be aware of the side effects of antidepressants. Refer to written materials furnished by health-care providers for safe self-administration.
- Carry a card or other identification at all times describing the medications being taken.

ANTIMANIC AGENTS

The drug of choice for the treatment and management of bipolar disorder, mania, is lithium carbonate. However, in recent years, a number of investigators and clinicians in practice have achieved satisfactory results with several other medications, either alone or in combination with lithium. These include clonazepam, carbamazepine, valproic acid, and verapamil (Table 20–3).

INDICATIONS
Lithium carbonate is used in the prevention and treatment of manic episodes associated with bipolar disorder. It is also used to treat depression associated with bipolar disorder.

Following initiation of lithium therapy, there is a lag period of 1 to 3 weeks before the symptoms of mania are alleviated. During this time, antipsychotics such as chlorpromazine (Thorazine) or haloperidol (Haldol) are often administered to decrease the level of hyperactivity.

Treatment of bipolar affective disorder is an unlabeled use for clonazepam, carbamazepine, valproic acid, and verapamil.

MECHANISM OF ACTION
The exact mechanism of action of lithium carbonate is unknown; however, it is thought to enhance the reuptake of

TABLE 20–3. **Commonly Used Groups of Antimanic Agents**

Classification	Generic (Trade) Name	Daily Dosage
Antimanic	Lithium carbonate (Eskalith, Lithane)	Acute mania: 1800–2400 mg Maintenance: 300–1200 mg
Anti- convulsants	Clonazepam (Klonopin)	2–20 mg
	Carbamazepine (Tegretol)	400–1200 mg
	Valproic acid (Depakene, Depakote)	500–1500 mg
Calcium channel blocker	Verapamil (Calan, Isoptin)	240–320 mg

Adapted from Townsend, 1996, p. 280.

the biogenic amines (norepinephrine and serotonin) in the brain, thus lowering their levels in the body. Another theory relates the effectiveness of lithium to an alteration in sodium metabolism within nerve and muscle cells.

The action of clonazepam, carbamazepine, valproic acid, and verapamil in the treatment of bipolar disorder is unclear.

CONTRAINDICATIONS

Lithium carbonate is contraindicated in severe cardiovascular or renal disease, severe dehydration, concomitant use with diuretics, pregnancy and lactation, and children under 12 years of age.

Anticonvulsants (clonazepam, carbamazepine, valproic acid) are contraindicated in clients with hypersensitivity to the medication and those with hepatic insufficiency.

Verapamil is contraindicated in clients with hypersensitivity, second-degree or third-degree AV block, severe hypotension, cardiogenic shock, and congestive heart failure.

POSSIBLE NURSING DIAGNOSES

1. Risk for injury related to extreme hyperactivity or toxicity due to elevated serum levels of the medication.
2. Risk for violence to self or others related to biochemical alterations or excessive hyperactivity.
3. Risk for alteration in nutrition, more than body requires, related to lithium-induced changes in glucose metabolism; excessive intake of high-calorie beverages in response to lithium's side effect of polydipsia.
4. Risk for activity intolerance related to medication side effects of lethargy, drowsiness, dizziness, muscular weakness, ataxia.
5. Knowledge deficit related to medication regimen.

SIDE EFFECTS AND NURSING IMPLICATIONS
(for Lithium Carbonate)

1. **Drowsiness, Dizziness, Headache**
   - Ensure that until response has stabilized, client does not participate in activities that require alertness.
2. **Dry Mouth, Thirst**
   - Offer sugarless candy, ice, frequent sips of water.
   - Ensure that client practices strict oral hygiene.
3. **GI Upset, Nausea/Vomiting**
   - Schedule medication dosages with meals to minimize GI upset.
4. **Fine Hand Tremors**
   - Physician may decrease dose of medication.
   - Some physicians prescribe small doses of the beta blocker propranolol (Inderal) to counteract this side effect.
5. **Hypotension, Pulse Irregularities, Arrhythmias**
   - Monitor vital signs on a regular basis (bid or tid).
   - Physician may decrease dose of medication.
6. **Polyuria, Dehydration**
   - May subside after initial week or two.
   - Monitor daily I&O and weight.
   - Monitor skin turgor daily.
   - Report changes (e.g., altered ratio of I&O, sudden weight gain or loss) to physician immediately.
7. **Weight Gain**
   - Instruct client regarding reduced calorie diet.
   - Emphasize importance of maintaining adequate intake of sodium.

TOXICITY

There is a narrow margin between the therapeutic and toxic levels of lithium carbonate. The usual ranges of therapeutic serum concentrations are as follows:

- **For acute mania:**   1.0 to 1.5 mEq/L
- **For maintenance:**   0.6 to 1.2 mEq/L

Serum lithium levels should be monitored once or twice a week after initial treatment until dosage and serum levels are stable, then monthly during maintenance therapy. Blood samples should be drawn 12 hours after the last dose.

Symptoms of lithium toxicity begin to appear at blood levels greater than 1.5 mEq/L and are dosage determinate. Symptoms include the following:

- **At serum levels of 1.5 to 2.0 mEq/L:** Blurred vision, ataxia, tinnitis, persistent nausea and vomiting, and severe diarrhea.
- **At serum levels of 2.0 to 3.5 mEq/L:** Excessive output of dilute urine, increasing tremors, muscular irritability, psychomotor retardation, mental confusion, and giddiness.
- **At serum levels above 3.5 mEq/L:** Impaired consciousness, nystagmus, seizures, coma, oliguria or anuria, arrhythmias, myocardial infarction, and cardiovascular collapse.

Lithium levels should be monitored before medication administration, and dosage should be withheld and the physician notified if the level reaches 1.5 mEq/L, or at the earliest observation or report by the client of even the mildest symptom. If left untreated, lithium toxicity is a life-threatening situation for the client.

Lithium is similar in chemical structure to sodium, behaving in the body in much the same manner and competing at various sites in the body with sodium. If sodium intake is reduced, or the body is depleted of its normal sodium (e.g., because of excessive sweating, fever, diuresis), lithium is reabsorbed by the kidneys, increasing the possibility of toxicity. It is therefore extremely important that the client consumes a diet adequate in sodium, as well as 2500 to 3000 mL of fluid per day. Accurate records of intake, output, and client's weight should be kept on a daily basis.

CLIENT/FAMILY EDUCATION (for Lithium Carbonate)

The client should:

- Take medication on a regular basis, even when feeling well. Discontinuation can result in return of symptoms.
- Not drive or operate dangerous machinery until lithium levels are stabilized. Drowsiness and dizziness can occur.
- Not skimp on dietary sodium intake. Choose nutritious food and avoid "junk" foods. Drink six to eight large glasses of water each day. Avoid excessive use of beverages containing caffeine (coffee, tea, colas), which promote increased urine output.
- Notify physician if vomiting or diarrhea occurs. These symptoms can result in sodium loss and an increased risk of toxicity.
- Carry card or other identification noting client is taking lithium.
- Be aware of appropriate diet should weight gain become a problem. Include adequate intake of sodium and other nutrients while decreasing number of calories.
- Be aware of risks of becoming pregnant while on lithium therapy. Use information furnished by health-care providers regarding methods of contraception. If pregnancy is suspected or planned, notify physician as soon as possible.
- Be aware of side effects and symptoms associated with toxicity. Notify physician if any of the following symptoms occur: persistent nausea and vomiting, severe diarrhea, ataxia, blurred vision, tinnitus, excessive output of urine, increasing tremors, mental confusion.
- Refer to written materials furnished by health-care providers while receiving self-administered maintenance therapy. Keep appointments for outpatient follow-up; have serum lithium level checked every 1 or 2 months, or as advised by physician.

SIDE EFFECTS AND NURSING IMPLICATIONS (for Anticonvulsants)

1. **Drowsiness, Dizziness**
   - Ensure that client does not operate dangerous machinery or participate in activities that require alertness.
2. **Nausea and Vomiting**
   - May give with food or milk to minimize GI upset.

3. **Leukopenia**
   - Ensure that client understands the importance of regular blood tests while receiving anticonvulsant therapy.
4. **Prolonged Bleeding Time** (valproic acid)
   - Ensure that platelet counts and bleeding time are determined before initiation of therapy with valproic acid. Monitor for spontaneous bleeding or bruising.

CLIENT/FAMILY EDUCATION
(for Anticonvulsants)
The client should:

- Not stop taking drug abruptly. Physician will administer orders for tapering the drug when therapy is to be discontinued.
- Report any of the following symptoms to physician immediately: unusual bleeding, spontaneous bruising, sore throat, fever, malaise, dark urine, yellow skin or eyes.
- Not drive or operate dangerous machinery until reaction to medication has been established.
- Avoid alcohol and nonprescription medication without approval from physician.
- Carry card at all times identifying name of medications being taken.

SIDE EFFECTS AND NURSING IMPLICATIONS
(for Verapamil)

1. **Drowsiness, Dizziness**
   - Ensure that client does not operate dangerous machinery or participate in activities that require alertness.
2. **Hypotension, Bradycardia**
   - Take vital signs just before initiation of therapy and before daily administration of the drug. Physician will provide acceptable parameters for administration. Report pronounced changes immediately.
3. **Nausea**
   - May be given with food to minimize GI upset.
4. **Constipation**
   - Encourage increased fluid (if not contraindicated) and fiber in diet.

CLIENT/FAMILY EDUCATION (for Verapamil)
The client should:

- Take medication with meals to minimize GI upset.
- Use caution when driving or when operating dangerous machinery. Dizziness, drowsiness, and blurred vision can occur.
- Not discontinue taking the drug abruptly. To do so may precipitate cardiovascular problems.
- Report occurrence of any of the following symptoms to physician immediately: irregular heartbeat, shortness of breath, swelling of the hands and feet, pronounced dizziness, chest pain, profound mood swings, severe and persistent headache.
- Take radial pulse as instructed before each dose. Report to physician any significant increase or decrease from baseline normal.
- Rise slowly from a sitting or lying position to prevent a sudden drop in blood pressure.
- Not consume other medications (including over-the-counter medications) without physician's approval.
- Carry card at all times describing medications being taken.

ANTIPSYCHOTIC AGENTS

INDICATIONS
Also called *major tranquilizers* and *neuroleptics*, these medications are used in the treatment of acute and chronic psychoses, particularly when accompanied by increased psychomotor activity (Table 20–4). Selected agents are used as antiemetics (chlorpromazine, perphenazine, prochlorperazine), in the treatment of intractable hiccoughs (chlorpromazine, perphenazine), and for the control of tics and vocal utterances in Tourette's disorder (haloperidol, pimozide).

MECHANISM OF ACTION
The exact mechanism of action is not known. These drugs are thought to work by blocking postsynaptic dopamine receptors in the basal ganglia, hypothalamus, limbic system, brain stem, and medulla. Antipsychotic effects may also be related to the inhibition of dopamine-mediated transmission of neural impulses at the synapses.

TABLE 20–4. **Commonly Used
Groups of Antipsychotic Agents**

Chemical Class	Generic (Trade) Name	Daily Dosage
Phenothiazines	Acetophenazine (Tindal)	60–120 mg
	Chlorpromazine (Thorazine)	40–800 mg
	Fluphenazine (Prolixin)	1–40 mg
	Mesoridazine (Serentil)	30–400 mg
	Perphenazine (Trilafon)	12–64 mg
	Prochlorperazine (Compazine)	15–150 mg
	Promazine (Sparine)	40–1200 mg
	Thioridazine (Mellaril)	150–800 mg
	Trifluoperazine (Stelazine)	4–40 mg
	Triflupromazine (Vesprin)	60–150 mg
Thioxanthenes	Chlorprothixene (Taractan)	75–600 mg
	Thiothixene (Navane)	8–30 mg
Benzisoxazole	Resperidone (Risperdal)	4–6 mg
Butyrophenone	Haloperidol (Haldol)	1–100 mg
Dibenzoxazepine	Loxapine (Loxitane)	20–250 mg
Dihydroindolones	Molindone (Moban)	15–225 mg
Dibenzodiazepine	Clozapine (Clozaril)	300–900 mg
Diphenyl-butylpiperidine	Pimozide (Orap)	2–10 mg

Adapted from Townsend, 1996, p. 284.

CONTRAINDICATIONS
These drugs are contraindicated in clients with known hypersensitivity, in comatose or severely CNS-depressed clients, when blood dyscrasias exist, in client's with Parkinson's disease, or those with liver, renal, or cardiac insufficiency.

POSSIBLE NURSING DIAGNOSES
1. Risk for violence to others related to mistrust and panic anxiety.
2. Risk for injury related to medication side effects of sedation, dizziness, ataxia, weakness, lowered seizure threshold; abrupt withdrawal after prolonged use; overdose.
3. Sensory-perceptual alteration related to panic anxiety evidenced by hallucinations.

4. Altered thought processes related to inability to trust and panic anxiety evidenced by suspiciousness and delusional thinking.
5. Social isolation related to inability to trust others.
6. Risk for activity intolerance related to medication side effects of drowsiness, dizziness, ataxia, and weakness.
7. Noncompliance with medication regimen related to suspiciousness and mistrust of others.
8. Knowledge deficit related to medication regimen.

SIDE EFFECTS AND NURSING IMPLICATIONS

1. **Anticholinergic Effects**
   a. *Dry Mouth*
      - Offer sugarless candy or gum, ice, frequent sips of water.
      - Ensure that client practices strict oral hygiene.
   b. *Blurred Vision*
      - Explain that symptom will most likely subside after a few weeks.
      - Offer to assist with tasks requiring visual acuity.
   c. *Constipation*
      - Order foods high in fiber; encourage increase in physical activity and fluid intake if not contraindicated.
   d. *Urinary Retention*
      - Instruct client to report any difficulty urinating; monitor intake and output.
2. **Nausea, GI Upset**
   - Tablets or capsules may be administered with food to minimize GI upset.
   - Concentrates may be diluted and administered with fruit juice or other liquid; they should be mixed immediately before administration.
3. **Skin Rash**
   - Report appearance of any rash on skin to physician.
   - Avoid spilling any of the liquid concentrate on skin; contact dermatitis can occur.
4. **Sedation**
   - Discuss with physician possibility of administering drug at bedtime.
   - Discuss with physician possible decrease in dosage or order for less sedating drug.
   - Instruct client not to drive or operate dangerous equipment while experiencing sedation.

5. **Orthostatic Hypotension**
   - Instruct client to rise slowly from a lying or sitting position; monitor blood pressure (lying and standing) each shift; document and report significant changes.

6. **Photosensitivity**
   - Ensure that client wears protective sunscreens, clothing, sunglasses while spending time outdoors.

7. **Hormonal Effects**
   a. *Decreased Libido, Retrograde Ejaculation, Gynecomastia (males)*
      - Provide explanation of the effects and reassurance of reversibility; may discuss with physician possibility of ordering alternate medication.

   b. *Amenorrhea (females)*
      - Offer reassurance of reversibility; instruct client to continue use of contraception, because amenorrhea does not indicate cessation of ovulation.

   c. *Weight Gain*
      - Weigh client every other day; order calorie-controlled diet; provide opportunity for physical exercise; provide diet and exercise instruction.

8. **Reduction of Seizure Threshold**
   - Closely observe clients with history of seizures.

9. **Agranulocytosis**
   - Potentially very serious side effect, but relatively rare with most of the antipsychotic drugs. Usually occurs within the first 3 months of treatment. Observe for symptoms of sore throat, fever, malaise; a complete blood count (CBC) should be monitored if these symptoms appear.
   - *Exception:* With clozapine (Clozaril), agranulocytosis occurs in 1% to 2% of all clients taking the drug (Pokalo, 1991). This is a potentially fatal blood disorder in which the client's white blood cell (WBC) count can drop to extremely low levels. Individuals receiving clozapine therapy are required to have blood levels drawn weekly to continue therapy. They are administered a 1-week supply of medication at a time. If the WBC count falls below 3000 mm^3 or the granulocyte count falls below 1500 mm^3, clozapine therapy is discontinued. The disorder is reversible if discovered in the early stages.

10. **Extrapyramidal Symptoms (EPS)**
    - Observe for symptoms and report; administer antiparkinsonian drugs, as ordered; notify physician if antiparkinsonian agent has not been ordered.
    a. *Pseudoparkinsonism (tremor, shuffling gait, drooling, rigidity)*
       - Symptoms may appear 1 to 5 days following initiation of antipsychotic medication; occurs most often in women, the elderly, and dehydrated clients.
    b. *Akinesia (muscular weakness)*
       - Same as above.
    c. *Akathisia (continuous restlessness and fidgeting)*
       - Occurs most frequently in women; symptoms may occur 50 to 60 days after initiation of therapy.
    d. *Dystonia (involuntary muscular movements [spasms] of face, arms, legs, and neck)*
       - Occurs most often in men and clients under 25 years of age.
    e. *Oculogyric crisis (uncontrolled rolling back of the eyes)*
       - May appear as part of syndrome described as dystonia; may be mistaken for seizure activity; dystonia and oculogyric crisis should be treated as emergency situations; contact physician; IV benztropine (Cogentin) is commonly administered; stay with the client and offer reassurance and support during this frightening time.

11. **Tardive Dyskinesia (bizarre facial and tongue movements, stiff neck, and difficulty swallowing)**
    - All clients receiving long-term (months or years) antipsychotic therapy are at risk.
    - Symptoms are potentially irreversible.
    - Drug should be withdrawn at first sign, which is usually vermiform movements of the tongue; prompt action may prevent irreversibility.

12. **Neuroleptic Malignant Syndrome (NMS)**
    - A rare, but potentially fatal, complication of treatment with neuroleptic drugs.
    - Onset can occur within hours or even years after drug initiation, and progression is rapid over the following 24 to 72 hours.
    - Symptoms include severe parkinsonian muscle rigidity, hyperpyrexia up to 107°F, tachycardia, tachy-

pnea, fluctuations in blood pressure, diaphoresis, and rapid deterioration of mental status to stupor and coma.
- Discontinue neuroleptic medication immediately.
- Monitor vital signs, degree of muscle rigidity, intake and output, level of consciousness.
- Physician may order bromocriptine (Parlodel) or dantrolene (Dantrium) to counteract the effects of NMS.

CLIENT/FAMILY EDUCATION
The client should:
- Use caution when driving or operating dangerous machinery. Drowsiness and dizziness can occur.
- Not stop taking the drug abruptly after long-term use. To do so might produce withdrawal symptoms, such as nausea, vomiting, gastritis, headache, tachycardia, insomnia, tremulousness.
- Use sunscreens and wear protective clothing when spending time outdoors. Skin is more susceptible to sunburn. Can happen in as little as 30 minutes.
- Report occurrence of any of the following symptoms to the physician immediately: sore throat, fever, malaise, unusual bleeding, easy bruising, persistent nausea and vomiting, severe headache, rapid heart rate, difficulty urinating, muscle twitching, tremors, darkly colored urine, pale stools, yellow skin or eyes, muscular incoordination, or skin rash.
- Be aware that the drug may turn urine pink to reddish-brown. This is neither significant nor harmful.
- Rise slowly from a sitting or lying position to prevent a sudden drop in blood pressure.
- Take frequent sips of water, chew sugarless gum, or suck on hard candy, if experiencing a problem with dry mouth. Good oral care (frequent brushing, flossing) is very important.
- Wash liquid concentrate off immediately if some is spilled on skin; otherwise, a rash may appear.
- Consult physician regarding smoking while on neuroleptic therapy. Smoking increases the metabolism of neuroleptics, possibly requiring adjustment in dosage to achieve therapeutic effect.
- Dress warmly in cold weather and avoid extended exposure to very high or low temperatures. Body temperature is harder to maintain with this medication.

- Not drink alcohol while on neuroleptic therapy. These drugs potentiate each other's effects.
- Not consume other medications (including over-the-counter products) without physician's approval. Many medications contain substances that interact with neuroleptics in a way that may be harmful.
- Be aware of possible risks of taking neuroleptics during pregnancy. Safe use during pregnancy and lactation has not been established. It is thought that neuroleptics readily cross the placental barrier, so a fetus could experience adverse effects of the drug. Inform physician immediately if pregnancy occurs, is suspected, or is planned.
- Be aware of side effects of neuroleptic drug. Refer to written materials furnished by health-care providers for safe self-administration.
- Continue to take medication, even if feeling well and as though it is not needed. Symptoms may return if medication is discontinued.
- Carry card or other identification at all times describing medications being taken.

ANTIPARKINSONIAN AGENTS

INDICATIONS
Antiparkinsonian agents are indicated for the treatment of all forms of parkinsonism and for the relief of drug-induced extrapyramidal reactions (Table 20–5).

TABLE 20–5. **Commonly Used
Groups of Antiparkinsonian Agents**

Chemical Class	Generic (Trade) Name	Daily Dosage
Anticholinergics	Benztropine (Cogentin)	0.5–6 mg
	Biperiden (Akineton)	2–8 mg
	Ethopropazine (Parsidol)	50–600 mg
	Procyclidine (Kemadrin)	5–20 mg
	Trihexyphenidyl (Artane)	1–15 mg
Antihistamine	Diphenhydramine (Benadryl)	10–400 mg
Dopaminergic agonists	Amantadine (Symmetrel)	100–300 mg
	Bromocriptine (Parlodel)	2.5–100 mg

Adapted from Townsend, 1996, p. 287.

MECHANISM OF ACTION
The action of these drugs is aimed at restoring the natural balance of two major neurotransmitters in the CNS: acetylcholine and dopamine. The imbalance is a deficiency in dopamine that results in excessive cholinergic activity. Drugs used are either *anticholinergics* (which block the acetylcholine receptor to diminish excess cholinergic effect) or *dopaminergic agonists* (which increase the content of dopamine in the brain directly by stimulation of dopamine receptors or indirectly by blocking neuronal reuptake of dopamine).

CONTRAINDICATIONS
These drugs are contraindicated in clients with known hypersensitivity, angle-closure glaucoma, peptic ulcers, prostatic hypertrophy, and myasthenia gravis. Extreme caution must be used in administering to clients with tachycardia, cardiac arrhythmias, hypertension, hypotension, tendency toward urinary retention, and clients exposed to high environmental temperatures.

POSSIBLE NURSING DIAGNOSES

1. Risk for injury related to symptoms of Parkinson's disease or drug-induced EPS.
2. Hyperthermia related to anticholinergic effect of decreased sweating.
3. Activity intolerance related to side effects of drowsiness, dizziness, ataxia, weakness, confusion.
4. Knowledge deficit related to medication regimen.

SIDE EFFECTS AND NURSING IMPLICATIONS

1. **Anticholinergic Effects.** These side effects are identical to those produced by antipsychotic drugs. Taking both medications compounds these effects. For this reason, the physician may elect to prescribe an antiparkinsonian agent only at the onset of EPS, rather than as routine adjunctive therapy.
   a. *Dry Mouth*
      - Offer sugarless candy or gum, ice, frequent sips of water.
      - Ensure that client practices strict oral hygiene.

   b. *Blurred Vision*
- Explain that symptom will most likely subside after a few weeks.
- Offer to assist with tasks requiring visual acuity.

   c. *Constipation*
- Order foods high in fiber; encourage increase in physical activity and fluid intake, if not contraindicated.

   d. *Paralytic Ileus*
- A rare, but potentially very serious side effect of anticholinergic drugs. Monitor for abdominal distension, absent bowel sounds, nausea, vomiting, epigastric pain.
- Report any of these symptoms to physician immediately.

   e. *Urinary Retention*
- Instruct client to report any difficulty urinating; monitor intake and output.

   f. *Tachycardia, Decreased Sweating, Elevated Temperature*
- Assess vital signs each shift; document and report significant changes to physician.
- Ensure that client remains in cool environment, because the body is unable to cool itself naturally with this medication.

2. **Nausea, GI Upset**
- May administer tablets or capsules with food to minimize GI upset.

3. **Sedation, Drowsiness, Dizziness**
- Discuss with physician possibility of administering drug at bedtime.
- Discuss with physician possible decrease in dosage or order for less sedating drug.
- Instruct client not to drive or use dangerous equipment while experiencing sedation or dizziness.

4. **Exacerbation of Psychoses**
- Assess for signs of loss of contact with reality.
- Intervene during a hallucination; talk about real people and real events; reorient client to reality.
- Stay with client during period of agitation and delirium; remain calm and reassure client of his or her safety.
- Discuss with physician possible decrease in dosage or change in medication.

5. **Orthostatic Hypotension**
   - Instruct client to rise slowly from a lying or sitting position; monitor blood pressure (lying and standing) each shift; document and report significant changes.

CLIENT/FAMILY EDUCATION
The client should:

- Take the medication with food if GI upset occurs.
- Use caution when driving or operating dangerous machinery. Drowsiness and dizziness can occur.
- Not stop taking the drug abruptly. To do so might produce unpleasant withdrawal symptoms.
- Report occurrence of any of the following symptoms to the physician immediately: pain or tenderness in area in front of ear; extreme dryness of mouth; difficulty urinating; abdominal pain; constipation; fast, pounding heart beat; rash; visual disturbances; mental changes.
- Rise slowly from a sitting or lying position to prevent a sudden drop in blood pressure.
- Stay inside in air-conditioned room when weather is very hot. Perspiration is decreased with antiparkinsonian agents, and the body cannot cool itself as well. There is greater susceptibility to heat stroke. Inform physician if air-conditioned housing is not available.
- Take frequent sips of water, chew sugarless gum, or suck on hard candy, if dry mouth is a problem. Good oral care (frequent brushing, flossing) is very important.
- Not drink alcohol while on antiparkinsonian therapy.
- Not consume other medications (including over-the-counter products) without physician's approval. Many medications contain substances that interact with antiparkinsonian agents in a way that may be harmful.
- Be aware of possible risks of taking antiparkinsonian agents during pregnancy. Safe use during pregnancy and lactation has not been fully established. It is thought that antiparkinsonian agents readily cross the placental barrier; if so, fetus could experience adverse effects of the drug. Inform physician immediately if pregnancy occurs, is suspected, or is planned.
- Be aware of side effects of antiparkinsonian agents. Refer to written materials furnished by health-care providers for safe self-administration.

- Continue to take medication, even if feeling well and as though it is not needed. Symptoms may return if medication is discontinued.
- Carry card or other identification at all times describing medications being taken.

CENTRAL NERVOUS SYSTEM STIMULANTS

INDICATIONS

CNS stimulants are used in the management of narcolepsy and in attention deficit disorder with hyperactivity in children, and as adjunctive therapy to caloric restriction in the treatment of exogenous obesity (Table 20–6).

MECHANISM OF ACTION

CNS stimulants increase levels of neurotransmitters (probably norepinephrine, dopamine, and serotonin) in the CNS. They produce CNS and respiratory stimulation, dilated pu-

TABLE 20–6.   **Commonly Used Groups of CNS Stimulants**

Chemical Class	Generic (Trade) Name	CC*	Daily Dosage
Amphetamines	Amphetamine sulfate	CII	5–60 mg
	Dextroamphetamine sulfate (Dexedrine)	CII	6–40 mg
	Methamphetamine (Desoxyn)	CII	5–25 mg
Anorexigenics	Benzphetamine (Didrex)	CIII	25–150 mg
	Diethylpropion (Tenuate)	CIV	75–100 mg
	Fenfluramine (Pondimin)	CIV	60–120 mg
	Mazindol (Mazanor)	CIV	1–3 mg
	Phendimetrazine (Anorex)	CIII	35–210 mg
	Phenmetrazine (Preludin)	CII	75 mg
	Phentermine (Fastin)	CIV	15–37.5 mg
Miscellaneous	Methylphenidate (Ritalin)	CII	10–60 mg
	Pemoline (Cylert)	CIV	37.5–112.5 mg

*Controlled categories.
Adapted from Townsend, 1996, p. 291.

pils, increased motor activity and mental alertness, diminished sense of fatigue, and brighter spirits.

CONTRAINDICATIONS
CNS stimulants are contraindicated in individuals with hypersensitivity to sympathomimetic amines. They should not be used in advanced arteriosclerosis, symptomatic cardiovascular disease, hypertension, hyperthyroidism, glaucoma, agitated or hyperexcitability states, in clients with a history of drug abuse, during or within 14 days of receiving therapy with MAOIs, in children under 3 years of age, and in pregnancy.

POSSIBLE NURSING DIAGNOSES
1. Risk for injury related to overstimulation and hyperactivity.
2. Risk for self-directed violence related to abrupt withdrawal after extended use.
3. Alteration in nutrition, less than body requirements, related to side effects of anorexia and weight loss.
4. Alteration in nutrition, more than body requirements, related to excess intake in relation to metabolic needs.
5. Sleep pattern disturbance related to overstimulation resulting from use of the medication.

SIDE EFFECTS AND NURSING IMPLICATIONS

1. **Overstimulation, Restlessness, Insomnia**
   - Assess mental status for changes in mood, level of activity, degree of stimulation, and aggressiveness.
   - Ensure that the client is protected from injury.
   - Keep stimuli low and environment as quiet as possible to discourage overstimulation.
   - To prevent insomnia, administer the last dose at least 6 hours before bedtime. Administer sustained-release forms in the morning.
2. **Palpitations, Tachycardia**
   - Monitor and record vital signs at regular intervals (2 or 3 times a day) throughout therapy. Report significant changes to the physician immediately.

3. **Anorexia, Weight Loss**
   - If this drug is being taken by children with behavior disorders (and not as an anorexigenic): To reduce anorexia, the medication may be administered immediately after meals. The client should be weighed regularly (at least weekly) during hospitalization and at home while receiving therapy with CNS stimulants because of the potential for anorexia or weight loss and temporary interruption of growth and development.

4. **Tolerance, Physical, and Psychological Dependence**
   - Tolerance develops rapidly. If anorexigenic effects begin to diminish, the client should notify the physician immediately. The client should be on a reduced-calorie diet and program of regular exercise in addition to the medication.
   - In children with behavior disorders, a drug "holiday" should be attempted periodically under direction of the physician to determine the effectiveness of the medication and the need for continuation.
   - The drug should not be withdrawn abruptly. To do so could initiate the following syndrome of symptoms: nausea, vomiting, abdominal cramping, headache, fatigue, weakness, mental depression, suicidal ideation, increased dreaming, and psychotic behavior.

CLIENT/FAMILY EDUCATION

The client should:

- Use caution in driving or operating dangerous machinery. Dizziness and blurred vision can occur.
- Not stop taking the drug abruptly. To do so could produce serious withdrawal symptoms.
- Avoid taking medication late in the day to prevent insomnia. Take no later than 6 hours before bedtime.
- Not take other medications (including over-the-counter drugs) without physician's approval. Many medications contain substances that, in combination with CNS stimulants, can be harmful.
- Diabetic clients should monitor blood sugar 2 or 3 times a day or as instructed by the physician. Be aware of need for possible alteration in insulin requirements owing to changes in food intake, weight, and activity.
- Avoid consumption of large amounts of caffeinated products (coffee, tea, colas, chocolate), because they may enhance the stimulant effect of these medications.

- Follow a reduced-calorie diet provided by the dietitian, as well as a program of regular exercise. Do not exceed the recommended dose if the appetite suppressant effect diminishes. Contact the physician.
- Notify physician if restlessness, insomnia, anorexia, or dry mouth becomes severe or if rapid, pounding heartbeat becomes evident.
- Be aware of possible risks of taking CNS stimulants during pregnancy. Safe use during pregnancy and lactation has not been established. Inform the physician immediately if pregnancy is suspected or planned.
- Be aware of potential side effects of CNS stimulants. Refer to written materials furnished by health care providers for safe self-administration.
- Carry a card or other identification at all times describing medications being taken.

BIBLIOGRAPHY

Abel, GG: Paraphilias. In Kaplan, HI, and Sadock, BJ (eds): Comprehensive Textbook of Psychiatry, Vol 1, ed 5. Williams & Wilkins, Baltimore, 1989.

Abrams, R: Electroconvulsive Therapy. Oxford University Press, New York, 1988.

Ackerman, S: The management of obesity. Hosp Pract 18(3):117–135, 1983.

Aguilera, DC, and Messick, JM: Crisis Intervention: Theory and Methodology, ed 4. CV Mosby, St. Louis, 1982.

Alexander, F: Psychosomatic Medicine. WW Norton, New York, 1950.

American Hospital Association: A Patient's Bill of Rights. American Hospital Association, Chicago, 1975.

American Nurses' Association: Nursing: A Social Policy Statement. American Nurses' Association, Kansas City, MO, 1980.

American Nurses' Association: Standards of Clinical Nursing Practice. American Nurses' Association, Kansas City, MO, 1991.

American Psychiatric Association: Diagnostic and Statistical Manual of Mental Disorders, ed 3—revised. American Psychiatric Association, Washington, DC, 1987.

American Psychiatric Association: Diagnostic and Statistical Manual of Mental Disorders, ed 4. American Psychiatric Association, Washington, DC, 1994.

Andreasen, NC, and Wasek, P: Adjustment disorders in adolescents and adults. Arch Gen Psychiatry 37:1166–1170, 1980.

Barsky, AJ: Somatoform disorders. In Kaplan, HI, and Sadock, BJ (eds): Comprehensive Textbook of Psychiatry, Vol 1, ed 5. Williams & Wilkins, Baltimore, 1989.

Beck, A, et al: Cognitive Theory of Depression. Guilford Press, New York, 1979.

Beck, CK, Rawlins, RP, and Williams, SR: Mental Health—Psychiatric Nursing: A Holistic Life—Cycle Approach, ed 2. CV Mosby, St. Louis, 1988.

Becker, JV: Impact of sexual abuse on sexual functioning. In Leiblum, SR, and Rosen, RC (eds): Principles and Practice of Sex Therapy: Update for The 1990s, ed 2. Guilford Press, New York, 1989.

Becker, JV, and Kavoussi, RJ: Sexual disorders. In Talbot, JA, Hales, RE, and Yudofsky, SC (eds): Textbook of Psychiatry. The American Psychiatric Press, Washington, DC, 1988.

Bennett, G, and Woolf, DS: Substance Abuse: Pharmacologic, Developmental, and Clinical Perspectives, ed 2. John Wiley & Sons, New York, 1991.

Birchwood, MJ, et al.: Schizophrenia: An Integrated Approach to Research and Treatment. New York University Press, New York, 1989.

Birckhead, LM: Psychiatric/Mental Health Nursing. JB Lippincott, Philadelphia, 1989.

Booth, GK: Disorders of impulse control. In Goldman, HH (ed): Review of General Psychiatry. Lange Medical Publications, Los Altos, CA, 1984.

Bowen, M: Family Therapy in Clinical Practice. Jason Aronson, New York, 1978.

Bowlby, J: Attachment and Loss: Separation, Anxiety, and Anger. Basic Books, New York, 1973.

Bradford, JM, and McLean, D: Sexual offenders, violence, and testosterone: A clinical study. Can J Psychiatry 29:335–343, 1984.

Bruch, H: Eating disorders in adolescence. Proc Am Psychopathol Assoc 59:181–202, 1970.

Bruch, H: Psychotherapy in anorexia nervosa and developmental obesity. In Goodstein, RK (ed): Eating and Weight Disorders. Springer, New York, 1983.

Burgess, AW: Intra-familial sexual abuse. In Campbell, J, and Humphreys, J (eds): Nursing Care of Victims of Family Violence. Reston Publishing, Reston, VA, 1984.

Burgess, AW: Psychiatric Nursing in the Hospital and the Community, ed 5. Appleton & Lange, Norwalk, CT, 1990.

Caplan, G: Principles of Preventive Psychiatry. Basic Books, New York, 1964.

Carpenito, LJ: Nursing Diagnosis: Application to Clinical Practice, ed 5. JB Lippincott, Philadelphia, 1993.

Carroll-Johnson, RM: Classification of Nursing Diagnoses: Proceedings of the Eighth National Conference. JB Lippincott, Philadelphia, 1989.

Casey, V, and Dwyer, JT: Premenstrual syndrome: Theories and evidence. Nutrition Today (Nov/Dec):4–12, 1987.

Celano, MP: Activities and games for group psychotherapy with sexually abused children. Int J Group Psychother 40(4):419–428, 1990.

Chess, S, Thomas, A, and Birch, H: The origins of personality. Sci Am 223:102, 1970.

Clunn, P: Child Psychiatric Nursing. Mosby–Year Book, St. Louis, MO, 1991.

Courtois, C: Healing the Incest Wound. WW Norton, New York, 1988.

Deglin, JH, and Vallerand, AH: Davis's Drug Guide for Nurses, ed 4. FA Davis, Philadelphia, 1996.

DeWitt, KN: Adjustment disorder. In Goldman, HH (ed): Review of General Psychiatry. Lange Medical Publications, Los Altos, CA, 1984.

Doenges, M, and Moorhouse, M: Nurse's Pocket Guide: Nursing Diagnoses with Interventions, ed 5. FA Davis, Philadelphia, 1996.

Doenges, M, Townsend, M, and Moorhouse, M: Psychiatric Care Plans: Guidelines for Client Care, ed 2. FA Davis, Philadelphia, 1995.

Drug Enforcement Administration: Drug Abuse, Drug Enforcement. US Department of Justice, Washington, DC, 1979.

Duespohl, TA: Nursing Diagnosis Manual for the Well and Ill Client. WB Saunders, Philadelphia, 1986.

Dunbar, HF: Emotions and Bodily Changes. Columbia University Press, New York, 1954.

Egeland, JA, et al: Amish study: Lithium-sodium countertransport and catechol O-methyltransferase in pedigrees of bipolar probands. Am J Psychiatry 141:1049, 1984.

Engel, G: Grief and grieving. Am J Nurs 64:93, 1964.

Erikson, EH: Childhood and Society. WW Norton, New York, 1963.

Estes, NJ, and Heinemann, ME: Alcoholism: Development, Consequences, and Interventions, ed 2. CV Mosby, St. Louis, MO, 1982.

Estes, NJ, Smith-DiJulio, K, and Heinemann, ME: Nursing Diagnosis of the Alcoholic Person. CV Mosby, St. Louis, MO, 1980.

Freeman, CP, et al: ECT: Patients who complain. Br J Psychiatry 137:17–25, 1980.

Freud, S: The neuro-psychoses of defense (1894). In Strachey, J (ed): Standard Edition of the Complete Psychological Works of Sigmund Freud, Vol 3. Hogarth Press (original work published 1894), London, 1962.

Freud, S: Collected Papers of Sigmund Freud. (Ernest Jones, ed). Basic Books, New York, 1959.

Freud, S: New introductory lectures on psychoanalysis and other works. In Strachey (ed): The Standard Edition of the Complete Psychological Works of Sigmund Freud, Vol 22. Hogarth Press, London, 1964.

Gibbons, JL: Total body sodium and potassium in depressive illness. Clin Sci 19:133, 1960.

Goldstein, M: Brain research and violent behavior. Arch Neurol 30(1):1–35, 1974.

Gordon, M: Nursing Diagnosis: Process and Application, ed 2. McGraw-Hill, New York, 1987.

Gottesman, II: Schizophrenia and genetics: Where are we? Are you sure? In Wynne, LC, Cromwell, RD, and Mathesses, S (eds): The Nature of Schizophrenia. John Wiley & Sons, New York, 1978.

Govoni, LE, and Hayes, JE: Drugs and Nursing Implications, ed 7. Appleton & Lange, Norwalk, CT, 1992.

Grace, HK, and Camilleri, D: Mental Health Nursing: A Sociopsychological Approach, ed 2. WC Brown, Dubuque, IA, 1981.

Green, R: One hundred and ten feminine and masculine boys: Behavioral contrasts and demographic similarities. Arch Sex Behav 5:425–446, 1976.

Green, R: Gender identity in childhood and later sexual orientation: Follow up of 78 males. Am J Psychiatry 142:339–341, 1985.

Haber, J, Leach, AM, Schudy, SM, and Sideleau, BF: Comprehensive Psychiatric Nursing, ed 3. McGraw-Hill, New York, 1987.

Haber, J, McMahon, AL, Price-Hoskins, P, and Sideleau, BF: Comprehensive Psychiatric Nursing, ed 4. CV Mosby, St. Louis, MO, 1992.

Hartmann, H: Contributions to the metapsychology of schizophrenia. In Hartmann, H (ed): Essays on Ego Psychology. International Universities Press, New York, 1964.

Hays, JS, and Larson, KH: Interacting with Patients. Macmillan, New York, 1963.

Heston, LL: Genetic factors. Hosp Pract June, 1977.

Hoff, LA: Rape and sexual assault: Evaluation and treatment. Surgeon General's Workshop on Violence and Public Health (DHHS Publication No. HRS-D-MC86-1). U.S. Government Printing Office, Washington, DC, 1985.

Hollandsworth, JG: The Physiology of Psychological Disorders. Plenum Press, New York, 1990.

Horney, K: New Ways in Psychoanalysis. WW Norton, New York, 1939.

Hyde, JS: Understanding Human Sexuality, ed 3. McGraw-Hill, New York, 1986.

Janosik, EH, and Davies, JL: Psychiatric Mental Health Nursing, ed 2. Jones and Bartlett, Boston, 1989.

Janowsky, DS, et al: Neurochemistry of depression and mania. In Georgotas, A, and Cancro, R (eds): Depression and Mania. Elsevier Science Publishing, New York, 1988.

Johnson, BS: Psychiatric-Mental Health Nursing: Adaptation and Growth, ed 3. JB Lippincott, Philadelphia, 1993.

Kanner, L: To what extent is early infantile autism determined by constitutional inadequacies? Childhood Psychosis: Initial Studies and New Insights. VH Winston, Washington, DC, 1973.

Kansas Child Abuse Prevention Council (KCAPC): A Guide About Child Abuse and Neglect. National Committee for Prevention of Child Abuse and Parents Anonymous, Inc, Wichita, KS, 1992.

Kaplan, HI: History of psychosomatic medicine. In Kaplan, HI, and Sadock, BJ (eds): Comprehensive Textbook of Psychiatry. Williams & Wilkins, Baltimore, 1989.

Kaplan, HI, and Sadock, BJ: Modern Synopsis of Comprehensive Textbook of Psychiatry, ed 5. Williams & Wilkins, Baltimore, 1989.

Kaplan, HI, Sadock, BJ, and Grebb, JA: Kaplan and Sadock's Synopsis of Psychiatry, ed 7. Williams & Wilkins, Baltimore, 1994.

Kicey, C: Catecholamines and depression: A physiological theory of depression. Am J Nursing 74:2018, 1974.

Kim, MJ, McFarland, GK, and McLane, AM: Classification of Nursing Diagnoses: Proceedings of the Fifth National Conference. CV Mosby, St. Louis, MO, 1984.

Klein, M: A contribution to the psychogenesis of manic-depressive states. In Kline, M (ed): Contributions to Psychoanalysis. Hogarth Press, London, 1934.

Kluft, RP: Multiple personality in childhood. Psychiatric Clin N Am 7:121–134, 1984.

Kohlberg, L: Moral development. International Encyclopedia of Social Science. Macmillan, New York, 1968.

Kolata, G: Manic-depressive gene tied to chromosome 11. Science 235:1139, 1987.

Kolb, LC: Modern Clinical Psychiatry, ed 9. WB Saunders, Philadelphia, 1977.

Kolodny, RC, Masters, WH, and Johnson, VE: Textbook of Sexual Medicine. Little, Brown, Boston, 1979.

Kübler-Ross, E: On Death and Dying. Macmillan, New York, 1969.

Leahy, RL, and Beck, AT: Cognitive therapy of depression and mania. In Georgotas, A, and Cancro, R (eds): Depression and Mania. Elsevier Science Publishing, New York, 1988.

Leigh, G: Psychosocial factors in the etiology of substance abuse. In Bratter, TE, and Forrest, GG (eds): Alcoholism and Substance Abuse: Strategies for Clinical Intervention. The Free Press, New York, 1985.

Leon, GR, and Dinklage, D: Obesity and anorexia nervosa. In Ollendick, TH, and Hersen, M (eds): Handbook of Child Psychopathology, ed 2. Plenum Press, New York, 1989.

Mahler, M, et al: Psychological Birth of the Human Infant: Symbiosis and Individuation. Basic Books, New York, 1975.

Marciniak, RD: Other psychiatric disorders. In Walker, JI (ed): Essentials of Clinical Psychiatry. JB Lippincott, Philadelphia, 1985.

Mark, B: Hospital treatment of borderline patients: Toward a better understanding of problematic issues. J Psychosocial Nursing Mental Health Services 18(8):25–31, 1980.

Martin, M: Battered women. In Hutchings, N (ed): The Violent Family: Victimization of Women, Children, and Elders. Human Sciences Press, New York, 1988.

Masters, JC, and Spitler, R: Neuroleptic malignant syndrome. J Psychosocial Nursing 24(9):11–16, 1986.

Mathewson, MK: Pharmacotherapeutics: A Nursing Process Approach, ed 2. FA Davis, Philadelphia, 1991.

Matthysse, S, and Kety, SS: Catecholamines and Schizophrenia. Pergamon Press, Elmsford, NY, 1975.

McCracken, JT: Somatoform disorders. In Walker, JI (ed): Essentials of Clinical Psychiatry. JB Lippincott, Philadelphia, 1985.

McFarland, G, Wasli, E, and Gerety, EK: Nursing Diagnoses and Process in Psychiatric Mental Health Nursing, ed 2. JB Lippincott, Philadelphia, 1992.

Minuchin, S, et al: Family organization and family therapy. Arch Gen Psychiatry 32:1031–1038, 1975.

Minuchin, S, Rosman, B, and Baker, L: Psychosomatic Families. Harvard University Press, Cambridge, MA, 1978.

Mulaik, JS: Nurses' questions about electroconvulsive therapy. J Psychosocial Nursing Mental Health Services 17:15–19, 1979.

Murray, RB, and Huelskoetter, MMW: Psychiatric/Mental Health Nursing, Giving Emotional Care, ed 3. Appleton & Lange, Norwalk, CT, 1991.

National Council of State Boards of Nursing: The National Council Licensure Examination for Registered Nurses, ed 3. The Council, Chicago, 1985.

Nemiah, JC: Dissociative disorders (hysterical neuroses, dissociative type). In Kaplan, HI, and Sadock, BJ (eds): Comprehensive Textbook of Psychiatry, Vol 1, ed 5. Williams & Wilkins, Baltimore, 1989.

North American Nursing Diagnosis Association: Nursing Diagnoses: Definitions and Classification, 1995–1996. NANDA, Philadelphia, 1994.

Owens, DJ, and Straus, MA: The social structure of violence in childhood and approval of violence as an adult. Aggressive Behav 1:193–211, 1975.

Pasquali, EA, Arnold, HM, DeBasio, N, and Alesi, EG: Mental Health Nursing: A Holistic Approach, ed 3. CV Mosby, St. Louis, 1989.

Pauls, DL, and Leckman, JF: The inheritance of Gilles de la Tourette's syndrome and associated behaviors. N Engl J Med 315:993–997, 1986.

Pauly, IB: Female transsexualism. Arch Sex Behav 3:487–526, 1974.

Peplau, HE: Interpersonal techniques: The crux of psychiatric nursing. Am J Nurs 62(6):50–54, 1962.

Peplau, HE: Interpersonal Relations in Nursing. Springer, New York, 1991.

Peschel, E, and Peschel, R: Neurobiological disorders. J California Alliance for the Mentally Ill 2(4):4, 1991.

Piaget, J and Inhelder, B: The Psychology of the Child. Basic Books, New York, 1969.

Platt-Koch, LM: Borderline personality disorder: A therapeutic approach. Am J Nursing 83(12):1666–1671, 1983.

Pokalo, CL: Clozapine: Benefits and controversies. J Psychosocial Nursing 29(2):33–36, 1991.

Popkin, MK: Adjustment disorder and impulse control disorder. In Kaplan, HI, and Sadock, BJ (eds): Comprehensive Textbook of Psychiatry, Vol 2, ed 5. Williams & Wilkins, Baltimore, 1989.

Popper, CW, and Steingard, RJ: Disorders usually first diagnosed in infancy, childhood, or adolescence. In Hales, RE, Yudofsky, SC, and Talbott, JA (eds): The American Psychiatric Press Textbook of Psychiatry, ed 2. The American Psychiatric Press, Washington, DC, 1994.

Robins, LN: Deviant Children Grown Up: A Sociological and Psychiatric Study of Sociopathic Personality. Williams & Wilkins, Baltimore, 1966.

Robinson, L: Psychiatric Nursing as a Human Experience, ed 3. WB Saunders, Philadelphia, 1983.

Rosen, AC, Rekers, GA, and Bentler, PM: Ethical issues in the treatment of children. J Soc Issues 32:84, 1978.

Rosner, TA, and Pollice, SA: Tourette's syndrome. J Psychosocial Nursing 29(1):4–9, 1991.

Sadock, VA: Normal human sexuality and sexual disorders. In Kaplan, HI, and Sadock, BJ (eds): Comprehensive textbook of psychiatry, Vol 1, ed 5. Williams & Wilkins, Baltimore, 1989.

Scanlon, VC, and Sanders, T: Essentials of Anatomy and Physiology, ed 2. FA Davis, Philadelphia, 1995.

Scheibel, A: Schizophrenia: cells in disarray. Journal of the California Alliance for the Mentally Ill, 2(4):9–10, 1991.

Schultz, JM, and Dark, SL: Manual of Psychiatric Nursing Care Plans, ed 3. Scott, Foresman and Company, Glenview, IL, 1990.

Segraves, RT: Hormones and libido. In Leiblum, SR, and Rosen, RC (eds): Sexual Desire Disorders. The Guilford Press, New York, 1988.

Seligman, M: Depression and learned helplessness. In Friedman, R, and Katz, M (eds): The Psychology of Depression: Contemporary Theory and Research. VH Winston & Sons, Washington, DC, 1974.

Selye, H: The Stress of Life. McGraw-Hill, New York, 1956.

Shives, LR: Basic Concepts of Psychiatric-Mental Health Nursing, ed 2. JB Lippincott, Philadelphia, 1990.

Smith, LS: Sexual Assault: The Nurse's Role. AD Nurse 2(2):24–28, 1987a.

Smith, LS: Battered women: The nurse's role. AD Nurse 2(5):21–24, 1987b.

Smith, SF, Karasik, DA, and Meyer, BJ: Psychiatric and Psychosocial Nursing: A Review for NCLEX in the Nursing Process. National Nursing Review, Los Altos, CA, 1984.

Stoudemire, GA: Somatoform disorders, factitious disorders, and malingering. In Talbott, JA, Hales, RE, and Yudofsky, SC (eds): Textbook of Psychiatry. American Psychiatric Press, Washington, DC, 1988.

Stuart, GW, and Sundeen, SJ: Principles and Practice of Psychiatric Nursing, ed 5. CV Mosby, St. Louis, 1995.

Sullivan, HS: The Interpersonal Theory of Psychiatry. WW Norton, New York, 1953.

Sullivan, HS: Clinical Studies in Psychiatry. WW Norton, New York, 1956.

Sullivan, HS: Schizophrenia as a Human Process. WW Norton, New York, 1962.

Sundel, M, and Sundel, SS: Behavior Modification in the Human Services: A Systematic Introduction to Concepts and Applications, ed 2. Prentice-Hall, Englewood Cliffs, NJ, 1982.

Swearingen, PL: Manual of Nursing Therapeutics. Addison-Wesley, Menlo Park, CA, 1986.

Taylor, CM: Mereness' Essentials of Psychiatric Nursing, ed 13. CV Mosby, St. Louis, 1990.

Thompson, JM, McFarland, GK, Hirsch, JE, Tucker, SM, and Bowers, AC: Clinical Nursing. CV Mosby, St. Louis, 1986.

Tollison, CD, and Adams, HE: Sexual Disorders: Treatment, Theory. Gardner Press, New York, 1979.

Townsend, MC: Psychiatric Mental Health Nursing: Concepts of Care. FA Davis, Philadelphia, 1993.

Townsend, MC: Psychiatric Mental Health Nursing: Concepts of Care, ed 2. FA Davis, Philadelphia, 1996.

Townsend, MC: Drug Guide for Psychiatric Nursing, ed 2. FA Davis, Philadelphia, 1995.

Vaillant, GE, and Perry, JC: Personality disorders. In Kaplan, HI, and Sadock, BJ (eds): Comprehensive Textbook of Psychiatry, ed 4. Williams & Wilkins, Baltimore, 1985.

VandeVusse, L and Simandl, G: Sexuality patterns, altered. In Gettrust, KV and Brabec, PD (eds): Nursing Diagnosis in Clinical Practice: Guides for Care Planning. Delmar, Albany, New York, 1992.

West, DJ: The response to violence. J Med Ethics, 5:128–131, 1979.

Wilson, HS, and Kneisl, CR: Psychiatric Nursing, ed 4. Addison-Wesley, Menlo Park, CA, 1992.

Wise, MG, and Gray, KF: Delirium, dementia, and amnestic disorders. In Hales, RE, Yudofsky, SC, and Talbott, JA (eds): The American Psychiatric Press Textbook of Psychiatry, ed 2. American Psychiatric Press, Washington, DC, 1994.

Wolpe, J: The Practice of Behavior Therapy, ed 2. Pergamon Press, New York, 1973.

Yalom, IE: The Theory and Practice of Group Psychotherapy, ed 3. Basic Books, New York, 1985.

Appendix A

COMPARISON OF DEVELOPMENTAL THEORIES

Age	Stage	Major Developmental Tasks
S. FREUD'S STAGES OF PSYCHOSEXUAL DEVELOPMENT		
Birth–18 months	Oral	Relief from anxiety through oral gratification of needs
18 months–3 years	Anal	Learning independence and control, with focus on the excretory function
3–6 years	Phallic	Identification with parent of same sex; development of sexual identity; focus is on genital organs
6–12 years	Latency	Sexuality is repressed; focus is on relationships with same-sex peers
13–20 years	Genital	Libido is reawakened as genital organs mature; focus is on relationships with members of the opposite sex

(continued)

		STAGES OF DEVELOPMENT IN H.S. SULLIVAN'S INTERPERSONAL THEORY
Birth–18 months	Infancy	Relief from anxiety through oral gratification of needs
18 months–6 years	Childhood	Learning to experience a delay in personal gratification without undo anxiety
6–9 years	Juvenile	Learning to form satisfactory peer relationships
9–12 years	Preadolescence	Learning to form satisfactory relationships with persons of the same sex; the initiation of feelings of affection for another person
12–14 years	Early adolescence	Learning to form satisfactory relationships with persons of the opposite sex; developing a sense of identity
14–21 years	Late adolescence	Establishing self-identity; experiencing satisfying relationships; working to develop a lasting, intimate opposite-sex relationship

		STAGES OF DEVELOPMENT IN ERIC ERIKSON'S PSYCHOSOCIAL THEORY
Infancy (Birth–18 months)	Trust vs. mistrust	To develop a basic trust in the mothering figure and be able to generalize it to others
Early childhood (18 months–3 years)	Autonomy vs. shame and doubt	To gain some self-control and independence within the environment

Late childhood (3–6 years)	Initiative vs. guilt	To develop a sense of purpose and the ability to initiate and direct own activities
School age (6–12 years)	Industry vs. inferiority	To achieve a sense of self-confidence by learning, competing, performing successfully, and receiving recognition from significant others, peers, and acquaintances
Adolescence (12–20 years)	Identity vs. role confusion	To integrate the tasks mastered in the previous stages into a secure sense of self
Young adulthood (20–30 years)	Intimacy vs. isolation	To form an intense, lasting relationship or a commitment to another person, a cause, an institution, or a creative effort
Adulthood (30–65 years)	Generativity vs. stagnation	To achieve the life goals established for oneself, while also considering the welfare of future generations
Old age (65 years–death)	Ego integrity vs. despair	To review one's life and derive meaning from both positive and negative events, while achieving a positive sense of self-worth

STAGES OF DEVELOPMENT IN M. MAHLER'S THEORY OF OBJECT RELATIONS

Birth–1 month	I. Normal autism	Fulfillment of basic needs for survival and comfort
1–5 months	II. Symbiosis	Developing awareness of external source of need fulfillment
	III. Separation-individuation	

(continued)

5–10 months	a. Differentiation	Commencement of a primary recognition of separateness from the mothering figure
10–16 months	b. Practicing	Increased independence through locomotor functioning; increased sense of separateness of self
16–24 months	c. Rapprochement	Acute awareness of separateness of self; learning to seek "emotional refueling" from mothering figure to maintain feeling of security
24–36 months	d. Consolidation	Sense of separateness established; on the way to object constancy: able to internalize a sustained image of loved object/person when it is out of sight; resolution of separation anxiety

J. PIAGET'S STAGES OF COGNITIVE DEVELOPMENT

| Birth–2 years | Sensorimotor | With increased mobility and awareness, develops a sense of self as separate from the external environment; the concept of object permanence emerges as the ability to form mental images evolves |
| 2–6 years | Preoperational | Learning to express self with language; develops understanding of symbolic gestures; achievement of object permanence |

6–12 years	Concrete operations	Learning to apply logic to thinking; develops understanding of reversibility and spatiality; learning to differentiate and classify; increased socialization and application of rules
12–15+ years	Formal operations	Learning to think and reason in abstract terms; makes and tests hypotheses; logical thinking and reasoning ability expand and are refined; cognitive maturity achieved

L. KOHLBERG'S STAGES OF MORAL DEVELOPMENT

Preconventional (common from ages 4–10 years)	1. Punishment and obedience orientation	Behavior is motivated by fear of punishment
	2. Instrumental relativist orientation	Behavior is motivated by egocentrism and concern for self
Conventional (common from ages 10–13 years and into adulthood)	3. Interpersonal concordance orientation	Behavior is motivated by the expectations of others; strong desire for approval and acceptance
	4. Law and order orientation	Behavior is motivated by respect for authority

(continued)

| Postconventional (can occur from adolescence on) | 5. Social contract legalistic orientation | Behavior is motivated by respect for universal laws and moral principles and guided by an internal set of values |
| | 6. Universal ethical principle orientation | Behavior is motivated by internalized principles of honor, justice, and respect for human dignity and guided by the conscience |

STAGES OF DEVELOPMENT IN H. PEPLAU'S INTERPERSONAL THEORY

Infancy	Learning to count on others	Learning to communicate in various ways to the primary caregiver in order to have comfort needs fulfilled
Toddlerhood	Learning to delay gratification	Learning the satisfaction of pleasing others by delaying self-gratification in small ways
Early childhood	Identifying oneself	Learning appropriate roles and behaviors by acquiring the ability to perceive the expectations of others
Late childhood	Developing skills in participation	Learning the skills of compromise, competition, and cooperation with others. Establishment of a more realistic view of the world and a feeling of one's place in it.

Adapted from Townsend, 1993, pp 40, 42, 43, 46–48.

Appendix B

EGO DEFENSE MECHANISMS

Defense Mechanisms	Example	Defense Mechanisms	Example
Compensation: Covering up a real or perceived weakness by emphasizing a trait one considers more desirable.	A physically handicapped boy who is unable to participate in football compensates by becoming a great scholar.	**Projection:** Attributing feelings or impulses unacceptable to one's self to another person.	Sue felt a strong sexual attraction to her track coach. She tells her friend, "He's coming on to me!"
Denial: Refusing to acknowledge the existence of a real situation or the feelings associated with it.	A woman who drinks alcohol every day and cannot stop fails to acknowledge that she has a problem.	**Rationalization:** Attempting to make excuses or formulate logical reasons to justify unacceptable feelings or behaviors.	John tells the rehab nurse, "I drink because it's the only way I can deal with my bad marriage and my worse job."

(continued)

Displacement:
The transfer of feelings from one target to another that is considered less threatening or neutral.

A client is angry at his physician, does not express it, but becomes verbally abusive with the nurse.

Identification:
An attempt to increase self-worth by acquiring certain attributes and characteristics of an individual one admires.

A teenager who required lengthy rehabilitation after an accident decides to become a physical therapist as a result of his experiences.

Intellectualization:
An attempt to avoid expressing actual emotions associated with a stressful situation by using the

S's husband is being transferred with his job to a city far away from her parents. She hides her anxiety by explain-

Reaction formation:
Preventing unacceptable or undesirable thoughts or behaviors from being expressed by exaggerating opposite thoughts or types of behaviors.

Jane hates nursing. She attended nursing school to please her parents. During career day, she speaks to prospective students about the excellence of nursing as a career.

Regression:
Retreating in response to stress to an earlier level of development and the comfort measures associated with that level of functioning.

When 2-year-old Jay is hospitalized for tonsilitis, he will drink only from a bottle, even though his Mom states he has been drinking from a cup for 6 months.

Repression:
The involuntary blocking of unpleasant feelings and experiences from one's awareness.

An accident victim can remember nothing about his accident.

Defense Mechanism / Definition	Example
intellectual processes of logic, reasoning, and analysis.	...ing to her parents the advantages associated with the move.
Introjection: Integrating the beliefs and values of another individual into one's own ego structure.	Children integrate their parents' value system into the process of conscience formation. Child says to friend, "Don't cheat. It's wrong."
Isolation: Separating a thought or memory from the feeling tone or emotion associated with it.	A young woman describes being attacked and raped without showing any emotion.
Sublimation: Rechanneling of drives or impulses that are personally or socially unacceptable into activities that are constructive.	A mother whose son was killed by a drunk driver channels her anger and energy into being the president of Mothers Against Drunk Drivers.
Suppression: The voluntary blocking of unpleasant feelings and experiences from one's awareness.	Scarlet O'Hara says, "I don't want to think about that now. I'll think about that tomorrow."
Undoing: Symbolically negating or cancelling out an experience that one finds intolerable.	Joe was nervous about his new job and yelled at his wife. On his way home he stops and buys her some flowers.

From Townsend, 1996, p. 23, with permission.

425

Appendix C

LEVELS OF ANXIETY

Level	Perceptual Field	Ability to Learn	Physical Characteristics	Emotional/Behavioral Characteristics
Mild	Heightened perception (e.g., noises may seem louder; details within the environment are clearer) Increased awareness Increased alertness	Learning is enhanced	Restlessness Irritability	May remain superficial with others Rarely experienced as distressful Motivation is increased

Moderate	Reduction in perceptual field Less alert to environmental events (e.g., someone talking may not be heard; part of the room may not be noticed)	Learning still occurs, but not at optimal ability Decreased attention span Decreased ability to concentrate	Increased restlessness Increased heart and respiration rate Increased perspiration rate Gastric discomfort Increased muscular tension Increase in speech rate volume, and pitch	A feeling of discontent May lead to a degree of impairment in interpersonal relationships as individual begins to focus on self and the need to relieve personal discomfort
Severe	Greatly diminished Only extraneous details are perceived, or fixation on a single detail may occur May not take notice of an event even when attention is directed by another	Extremely limited attention span Unable to concentrate or problem-solve Effective learning cannot occur	Headaches Dizziness Nausea Trembling Insomnia Palpitations Tachycardia Hyperventilation Urinary frequency Diarrhea	Feelings of dread, loathing, horror Total focus on self and intense desire to relieve the anxiety

(continued)

Panic	Unable to focus on even one detail within the environment Misperceptions of the environment are common (e.g., a perceived detail may be elaborated and out of proportion)	Learning cannot occur Unable to concentrate Unable to comprehend even simple directions	Dilated pupils Labored breathing Severe trembling Sleeplessness Palpitations Diaphoresis and pallor Muscular incoordination Immobility or purposeless hyperactivity Incoherence or inability to verbalize	Sense of impending doom Terror Bizarre behavior, including shouting, screaming, running about wildly, clinging to anyone or anything from which a sense of safety and security is derived Hallucinations; delusions Extreme withdrawal into the self

From Townsend, 1993, p. 20, with permission.

Appendix D

STAGES OF GRIEF

A Comparison of Models by Elisabeth Kubler-Ross, John Bowlby, and George Engel

Stages			Possible Time Dimension	Behaviors
Kubler-Ross	Bowlby	Engel		
I. Denial	I. Numbness/ protest	I. Shock/ disbelief	Occurs immediately on experiencing the loss. Usually lasts no more than 2 weeks.	Individual refuses to acknowledge that the loss has occurred.
II. Anger	II. Disequilibrium	II. Developing awareness	In most cases begins within hours of the loss. Peaks within 2 to 4 weeks.	Anger is directed toward self or others. Ambivalence and guilt may be felt toward the lost object.

(continued)

III. Bargaining				The individual fervently seeks alternatives to improve current situation.
		III. Restitution		Attends to various rituals associated with the culture in which the loss has occurred.
IV. Depression	III. Disorganization and despair	IV. Resolution of the loss	A year or more.	The actual work of grieving. Preoccupation with the lost object. Feelings of helplessness and loneliness occur in response to realization of the loss. Feelings associated with the loss are confronted.

V. Acceptance	IV. Reorganization	V. Recovery
		Resolution is complete. The bereaved person experiences a reinvestment in new relationships and new goals. In the case of the terminally ill person, he or she expresses a readiness to die.

From Townsend, 1993, p. 346, with permission.

Appendix E

RELATIONSHIP DEVELOPMENT AND THERAPEUTIC COMMUNICATION

PHASES OF A THERAPEUTIC NURSE-CLIENT RELATIONSHIP

Psychiatric nurses use interpersonal relationship development as the primary intervention with clients in various psychiatric and mental health settings. This is congruent with Peplau's (1962) identification of *counseling* as the major subrole of nursing in psychiatry. If what Sullivan (1953) believed is true, that is, that all emotional problems stem from difficulties with interpersonal relationships, then this role of the nurse in psychiatry becomes especially meaningful and purposeful. It becomes an integral part of the total therapeutic regimen.

The therapeutic interpersonal relationship is the means by which the nursing process is implemented. Through the relationship, problems are identified and resolution is sought. Tasks of the relationship have been categorized into four phases: the preinteraction phase, the orientation (introductory) phase, the working phase, and the termination phase. Although each phase is presented as specific and distinct from the others, there may be some overlapping of tasks, particularly when the interaction is limited.

THE PREINTERACTION PHASE

The preinteraction phase involves preparation for the first encounter with the client. Tasks include the following:

1. Obtaining available information about the client from the chart, significant others, or other health-team members. From this information, the initial assessment is begun. From this initial information, the nurse may also become aware of personal responses to knowledge about the client.
2. Examining one's feelings, fears, and anxieties about working with a particular client. For example, the nurse may have been reared in an alcoholic family and have ambivalent feelings about caring for a client who is alcohol dependent. All individuals bring attitudes and feelings from prior experiences to the clinical setting. The nurse needs to be aware of how these preconceptions may affect his or her ability to care for individual clients.

THE ORIENTATION (INTRODUCTORY) PHASE

During the orientation phase, the nurse and client become acquainted. Tasks include the following:

1. Creating an environment for the establishment of trust and rapport.
2. Establishing a contract for intervention that details the expectations and responsibilities of both the nurse and client.
3. Gathering assessment information to build a strong client data base.
4. Identifying the client's strengths and limitations.
5. Formulating nursing diagnoses.
6. Setting goals that are mutually agreeable to the nurse and client.
7. Developing a plan of action that is realistic for meeting the established goals.
8. Exploring feelings of both the client and the nurse in terms of the introductory phase. Introductions are often uncomfortable, and the participants may experience some anxiety until a degree of rapport has been established. Interactions may remain on a superficial level until anxiety subsides. Several interactions may be required to fulfill the tasks associated with this phase.

THE WORKING PHASE

The therapeutic work of the relationship is accomplished during this phase. Tasks include the following:

1. Maintaining the trust and rapport that was established during the orientation phase.
2. Promoting the client's insight and perception of reality.
3. Problem solving in an effort to bring about change in the client's life.
4. Overcoming resistance behaviors on the part of the client as the level of anxiety rises in response to discussion of painful issues.
5. Continuously evaluating progress toward goal attainment.

THE TERMINATION PHASE

Termination of the relationship may occur for a variety of reasons: the mutually agreed on goals may have been reached, the client may be discharged from the hospital, or in the case of a student nurse, it may be the end of a clinical rotation. Termination can be a difficult phase for both the client and nurse. Tasks include the following:

1. Bringing a therapeutic conclusion to the relationship. This occurs when
   a. Progress has been made toward attainment of mutually set goals.
   b. A plan for continuing care or for assistance during stressful life experiences is mutually established by the nurse and client.
   c. Feelings about termination of the relationship are recognized and explored. Both the nurse and client may experience feelings of sadness and loss. The nurse should share his or her feelings with the client. Through these interactions, the client learns that it is acceptable to undergo these feelings at a time of separation. Through this knowledge, the client experiences growth during the process of termination.
   Note: When the client feels sadness and loss, behaviors to delay termination may become evident. If the nurse experiences the same feelings, he or she may allow the client's behaviors to delay termination. For therapeutic closure, the nurse must establish the reality of the separation and resist being manipulated into repeated delays by the client.

Therapeutic Communication Techniques

Technique	Explanation/Rationale	Examples
Using silence	Gives the client the opportunity to collect and organize thoughts, to think through a point, or to consider introducing a topic of greater concern than the one being discussed.	
Accepting	Conveys an attitude of reception and regard.	"Yes, I understand what you said." Eye contact; nodding.
Giving recognition	Acknowledging; indicating awareness. Better than complimenting, which reflects the nurse's judgment.	"Hello, Mr. J. I noticed that you made a ceramic ash tray in OT." "I see you made your bed."
Offering self	Making oneself available on an unconditional basis increases client's feelings of self-worth.	"I'll stay with you a while." "We can eat our lunch together." "I'm interested in you."
Giving broad openings	Allows the client to take the initiative in introducing the topic. Emphasizes the importance of the client's role in the interaction.	"What would you like to talk about today?" "Tell me what you are thinking." *(continued)*

Offering general leads	Offers the client encouragement to continue.	"Yes, I see." "Go on." "And after that?"
Placing the event in time or sequence	Clarifies the relationship of events in time so that the nurse and client can view them in perspective.	"What seemed to lead up to . . . ?" "Was this before or after . . . ?" "When did this happen?"
Making observations	Verbalizing what is observed or perceived. This encourages the client to recognize specific behaviors and compare perceptions with the nurse.	"You seem tense." "I notice you are pacing a lot." "You seem uncomfortable when you . . ."
Encouraging description of perceptions	Asking the client to verbalize what is being perceived. Often used with clients experiencing hallucinations.	"Tell me what is happening now." "Are you hearing the voices again?" "What do the voices seem to be saying?"
Encouraging comparison	Asking the client to compare similarities and differences in ideas, experiences, or interpersonal relationships. Helps the client recognize life experiences that tend to recur as well as those aspects of life that are changeable.	"Was this something like . . . ?" "How does this compare to the time when . . . ?" "What was your response the last time this situation occurred?"

Restating	The main idea of what the client has said is repeated. Lets the client know whether or not an expressed statement has been understood and gives him or her the chance to continue, or to clarify if necessary.	Pt: "I can't study. My mind keeps wandering." Ns: "You have difficulty concentrating." Pt: "I can't take that new job. What if I can't do it?" Ns: "You're afraid you will fail in this new position."
Reflecting	Questions and feelings are referred back to the client so that they may be recognized and accepted, and so that the client may recognize that his or her point of view has value. A good technique to use when the client asks the nurse for advice.	Pt: "What do you think I should do about my wife's drinking problem?" Ns: "What do *you* think you should do?" Pt: "My sister won't help a bit toward my mother's care. I have to do it all!" Ns: "You feel angry when she doesn't help."

(continued)

437

Focusing	Taking notice of a single idea or even a single word. Works especially well with a client who is moving rapidly from one thought to another. This technique is *not* therapeutic, however, with the client who is very anxious. Focusing should not be pursued until the anxiety level has subsided.	"This point seems worth looking at more closely. Perhaps you and I can discuss it together."
Exploring	Delving further into a subject, idea, experience, or relationship. Especially helpful with clients who tend to remain on a superficial level of communication. However, if the client chooses not to disclose further information, the nurse should refrain from pushing or probing in an area that obviously creates discomfort.	"Please explain that situation in more detail." "Tell me more about that particular situation."
Seeking clarification and validation	Striving to explain that which is vague or incomprehensible and searching for mutual understanding. Clarifying the meaning of what has been said facilitates and increases understanding for both client and nurse.	"I'm not sure that I understand. Would you please explain." "Tell me if my understanding agrees with yours." "Do I understand correctly that you said . . . ?"

Presenting reality	When the client has a misperception of the environment, the nurse defines reality or indicates his or her perception of the situation for the client.	"I understand that the voices seem real to you, but I do not hear any voices." "There is no one else in the room but you and me."
Voicing doubt	Expressing uncertainty as to the reality of the client's perceptions. Often used with clients experiencing delusional thinking.	"I find that hard to believe." "That seems rather doubtful to me."
Verbalizing the implied	Putting into words what the client has only implied or said indirectly. Can also be used with the client who is mute or is otherwise experiencing impaired verbal communication. Clarifies that which is *implicit* rather than *explicit*.	Pt: "It's a waste of time to be here. I can't talk to you or anyone." Ns: "Are you feeling that no one understands?" Pt: (Mute) Ns: "It must have been very difficult for you when your husband died in the fire."
Attempting to translate words into feelings	When feelings are expressed indirectly, the nurse tries to "desymbolize" what has been said and find clues to the underlying true feelings.	Pt: "I'm way out in the ocean." Ns: "You must be feeling very lonely now."

(continued)

439

| Formulating a plan of action | When a client has a plan in mind for dealing with what is considered to be a stressful situation, it may serve to prevent anger or anxiety from escalating to an unmanageable level. | "What could you do to let your anger out harmlessly?" "Next time this comes up, what might you do to handle it more appropriately?" |

Nontherapeutic Communication Techniques

Technique	Explanation/Rationale	Examples
Giving reassurance	Indicates to the client that there is no cause for anxiety, thereby devaluing the client's feelings. May discourage the client from further expression of feelings if he or she believes they will only be downplayed or ridiculed.	"I wouldn't worry about that if I were you." "Everything will be all right." **Better to say:** "We will work on that together."
Rejecting	Refusing to consider or showing contempt for the client's ideas or behavior. This may cause the client to discontinue interaction with the nurse for fear of further rejection.	"Let's not discuss . . ." "I don't want to hear about . . ." **Better to say:** "Let's look at that a little closer."

Giving approval or disapproval	Sanctioning or denouncing the client's ideas or behavior. Implies that the nurse has the right to pass judgment on whether the client's ideas or behaviors are "good" or "bad," and that the client is expected to please the nurse. The nurse's acceptance of the client is then seen as conditional, depending upon the client's behavior.	"That's good. I'm glad that you . . ." "That's bad. I'd rather you wouldn't . . ." **Better to say:** "Let's talk about how your behavior invoked anger in the other clients at dinner."
Agreeing/disagreeing	Indicating accord with or opposition to the client's ideas or opinions. Implies that the nurse has the right to pass judgment on whether the client's ideas or opinions are "right" or "wrong." Agreement prevents the client from later modifying his or her point of view without admitting error. Disagreement implies inaccuracy, provoking the need for defensiveness on the part of the client.	"That's right. I agree." "That's wrong. I disagree." "I don't believe that." **Better to say:** "Let's discuss what you feel is unfair about the new community rules."

(continued)

Giving advice

Telling the client what to do or how to behave implies that the nurse knows what is best, and that the client is incapable of any self-direction. Nurtures the client in the dependent role by discouraging independent thinking.

"I think you should . . ."
"Why don't you . . ."
Better to say: "What do you think you should do?"

Probing

Persistent questioning of the client. Pushing for answers to issues the client does not wish to discuss. Causes the client to feel used and valued only for what is shared with the nurse. Places the client on the defensive.

"Tell me how your mother abused you when you were a child."
"Tell me how you feel toward your mother now that she is dead."
"Now tell me about . . ."

Better technique: The nurse should be aware of the client's response and discontinue the interaction at the first sign of discomfort.

Defending	Attempting to protect someone or something from verbal attack. To defend what the client has criticized is to imply that he or she has no right to express ideas, opinions, or feelings. Defending does not change the client's feelings and may cause the client to think the nurse is taking sides with those being criticized and against the client.	"No one here would lie to you." "You have a very capable physician. I'm sure he only has your best interests in mind." **Better to say:** "I will try to answer your questions and clarify some issues regarding your treatment."
Requesting an explanation	Asking the client to provide the reasons for thoughts, feelings, behavior, and events. Asking "Why?" a client did something or feels a certain way can be very intimidating, and implies that the client must defend his or her behavior or feelings.	"Why do you think that?" "Why do you feel this way?" "Why did you do that?" **Better to say:** "Describe what you were feeling just before that happened."
Indicating the existence of an external source of power	Attributing the source of thoughts, feelings, and behavior to others or to outside influences. This encourages the client to project blame for his or her thoughts or behaviors on others rather than accepting the responsibility personally.	"What makes you say that?" "What made you do that?" "What made you so angry last night?" **Better to say:** "You became angry when your brother insulted your wife."

(continued)

Belittling feelings expressed	When the nurse misjudges the degree of the client's discomfort, a lack of empathy and understanding may be conveyed. The nurse may tell the client to "perk up" or "snap out of it." This causes the client to feel insignificant or unimportant. When one is experiencing discomfort, it is no relief to hear that others are or have been in similar situations.	Pt: "I have nothing to live for. I wish I were dead." Ns: "Everybody gets down in the dumps at times. I feel that way myself sometimes." **Better to say:** "You must be very upset. Tell me what you are feeling right now."
Making stereotyped comments	Cliches and trite expressions are meaningless in a nurse-client relationship. For the nurse to make empty conversation is to encourage a like response from the client.	"I'm fine, and how are you?" "Hang in there. It's for your own good." "Keep your chin up." **Better to say:** "The therapy must be difficult for you at times. How do you feel about your progress at this point?"

Using denial

When the nurse denies that a problem exists, he or she blocks discussion with the client and avoids helping the client identify and explore areas of difficulty.

Pt: "I'm nothing."

Ns: "Of course you're something. Everybody is somebody."

Better to say: "You're feeling like no one cares about you right now."

Interpreting

With this technique the therapist seeks to make conscious that which is unconscious, to tell the client the meaning of his experience.

"What you really mean is . . ."

"Unconsciously you're saying . . ."

Better technique: The nurse must leave interpretation of the client's behavior to the psychiatrist. The nurse has not been prepared to perform this technique, and in attempting to do so, may endanger other nursing roles with the client.

(continued)

| Introducing an unrelated topic | Changing the subject causes the nurse to take over the direction of the discussion. This may occur in order to get to something that the nurse wants to discuss with the client or to get away from a topic that he or she would prefer not to discuss. | Pt: "I don't have anything to live for." Ns: "Did you have visitors this weekend?" **Better technique:** The nurse must remain open and free to hear the client, to take in all that is being conveyed, both verbally and nonverbally. |

Adapted from Hays and Larson, 1963.

Appendix F

PSYCHOSOCIAL THERAPIES

GROUP THERAPY

Group therapy is a type of psychosocial therapy with a number of clients at one time. The group is founded in a specific theoretical framework, with the goal being to encourage improvement in interpersonal functioning.

Nurses often lead "therapeutic groups," which are based to a lesser degree in theory. The focus of therapeutic groups is more on group relations, interactions among group members, and the consideration of a selected issue.

Types of groups include *task groups*, in which the function is to accomplish a specific outcome or task; *teaching groups*, in which knowledge or information is conveyed to a number of individuals; *supportive-therapeutic groups*, which help prevent future upsets by teaching participants effective ways of dealing with emotional stress arising from situational or developmental crises; and *self-help groups* of individuals with similar problems who meet to help each other with emotional distress associated with those problems.

Yalom (1985) identified 11 curative factors that individuals can achieve through interpersonal interactions within the group. They include the following:

1. The instillation of hope.
2. Universality (individuals come to understand that they are not alone in the problems they experience).
3. The imparting of information.
4. Altruism (mutual sharing and concern for each other)

5. The corrective recapitulation of the primary family group.
6. The development of socializing techniques
7. Imitative behavior.
8. Interpersonal learning
9. Group cohesiveness.
10. Catharsis (open expression of feelings).
11. Existential factors (the group is able to help individual members take direction of their own lives and to accept responsibility for the quality of their existence).

PSYCHODRAMA

Psychodrama is a specialized type of therapeutic group that employs a dramatic approach in which clients become "actors" in life-situation scenarios.

The group leader is called the *director*, group members are the *audience*, and the *set*, or *stage*, may be specially designed or may just be any room or part of a room selected for this purpose. Actors are members from the audience who agree to take part in the "drama" by role playing a situation about which they have been informed by the director. Usually the situation is an issue with which one individual client has been struggling. The client plays the role of himself or herself and is called the *protagonist*. In this role, the client is able to express true feelings toward individuals (represented by group members) with whom he or she has unresolved conflicts.

In some instances, the group leader may ask for a client to volunteer to be the protagonist for that session. The client may choose a situation he or she wishes to enact and select the audience members to portray the roles of others in the life situation.

The psychodrama setting provides the client with a safer and less threatening atmosphere than the real situation in which to express true feelings. Resolution of interpersonal conflicts is facilitated.

When the drama has been completed, group members from the audience discuss the situation they have observed, offer feedback, express their feelings, and relate their own similar experiences. In this way, all group members benefit from the session, either directly or indirectly.

Nurses often serve as actors, or role players, in psychodrama sessions. Leaders of psychodrama have graduate degrees in psychology, social work, nursing, or medicine with additional training in group therapy and specialty preparation to become a psychodramatist.

FAMILY THERAPY

In family therapy, the nurse-therapist works with the family as a group to improve communication and interaction patterns. Areas of assessment include communication, manner of self-concept reinforcement, family members' expectations, handling differences, family interaction patterns, and the "climate" of the family (a blend of feelings and experiences that are the result of sharing and interacting).

The Family as a System. General systems theory is a way of organizing thought according to the holistic perspective. A system is considered greater than the sum of its parts. A family can be viewed as a system composed of various subsystems. The systems approach to family therapy is composed of eight major concepts: (1) differentiation of self, (2) triangles, (3) nuclear family emotional process, (4) family projection process, (5) multigenerational transmission process, (6) sibling position profiles, (7) emotional cutoff, and (8) societal regression. The goal is to increase the level of differentiation of self, while remaining in touch with the family system.

The Structural Model. In this model, the family is viewed as a social system within which the individual lives and to which the individual must adapt. The individual both contributes to and responds to stresses within the family. Major concepts include systems, subsystems, transactional patterns, and boundaries. The goal of therapy is to facilitate change in the family structure. The therapist does this by joining the family, evaluating the family system, and restructuring the family.

The Strategic Model. This model uses the interactional or communications approach. Functional families are open systems where clear and precise messages, congruent with the situation, are sent and received. Healthy communication patterns promote nurturance and individual self-worth. In dysfunctional families, viewed as partially closed systems, communication is vague, and messages are often inconsistent and incongruent with the situation. Destructive patterns of communication tend to inhibit healthful nurturing and decrease individual feelings of self-worth. Concepts of this model include double-bind communication, pseudomutuality and pseudohostility, marital schism, and marital skew. The goal of therapy is to create change in destructive behavior and communication patterns among family members. This is accomplished by using paradoxical intervention (prescribing the symptom) and reframing (changing the setting or viewpoint in relation to which a situation is experienced and placing it in another more positive frame of reference).

MILIEU THERAPY

In psychiatry, milieu therapy, or a therapeutic community, constitutes a manipulation of the environment in an effort to create behavioral changes and to improve the psychological health and functioning of the individual. The goal of therapeutic community is for the client to learn adaptive coping, interaction, and relationship skills that can be generalized to other aspects of his or her life. The community environment itself serves as the primary tool of therapy.

According to Skinner (1979), a therapeutic community is based on seven basic assumptions:

1. The health in each individual is to be realized and encouraged to grow.
2. Every interaction is an opportunity for therapeutic intervention.
3. The client owns his own environment.
4. Each client owns his behavior.
5. Peer pressure is a useful and a powerful tool.
6. Inappropriate behaviors are dealt with as they occur.
7. Restrictions and punishment are to be avoided.

Since the goals of milieu therapy relate to helping the client learn to generalize that which is learned to other aspects of his or her life, the conditions that promote a therapeutic community in the hospital setting are similar to the types of conditions that exist in real-life situations. They include the following:

1. The fulfillment of basic physiologic needs.
2. Physical facilities that are conducive to the achievement of the goals of therapy.
3. The existence of a democratic form of self-government.

4. The assignment of unit responsibilities according to client capabilities.
5. A structured program of social and work-related activities.
6. The inclusion of community and family in the program of therapy in an effort to facilitate discharge from the hospital.

The program of therapy on the milieu unit is conducted by the interdisciplinary treatment (IDT) team. The team includes some, or all, of the following disciplines, and may include others that are not specified here: psychiatrist, clinical psychologist, psychiatric clinical nurse specialist, psychiatric nurse, mental health technician, psychiatric social worker, occupational therapist, recreational therapist, art therapist, music therapist, psychodramatist, dietitian, and chaplain.

Nurses play a crucial role in the management of a therapeutic milieu. They are involved in the assessment, diagnosis, outcome identification, planning, implementation, and evaluation of all treatment programs. They have significant input into the IDT plans that are developed for all clients. They are responsible for ensuring that clients' basic needs are fulfilled, for continual assessment of physical and psychosocial status, for medication administration, for the development of trusting relationships, for setting limits on unacceptable behaviors, for client education, and ultimately, for helping clients, within the limits of their capability, become productive members of society.

CRISIS INTERVENTION

A *crisis* is a situation that produces "psychological disequilibrium in a person who confronts a hazardous circumstance that for him constitutes an important problem, which he can for the time being neither escape nor solve with his customary problem-solving resources" (Caplan, 1964). All individuals experience crises at one time or another. This does not necessarily indicate psychopathology.

Crises are precipitated by specific, identifiable events and are determined by an individual's personal perception of the situation. They are acute, not chronic, and generally last no more than 4 to 6 weeks.

Crises occur when an individual is exposed to a stressor and previous problem-solving techniques are ineffective. This causes the level of anxiety to rise. Panic may ensue when new techniques are employed and resolution fails to occur.

Six types of crises have been identified. They include dispositional crises, crises of anticipated life transitions, crises resulting from traumatic stress, maturational or developmental crises, crises reflecting psychopathology, and psychiatric emergencies. The type of crisis determines the method of intervention selected.

Crisis intervention is designed to provide rapid assistance for individuals who have an urgent need. Aguilera and Messick (1982) have identified the minimum therapeutic goal of crisis intervention as "psychological resolution of the individual's immediate crisis and restoration to at least the level of functioning that existed before the crisis period. A maximum goal is improvement in functioning above the precrisis level."

Nurses regularly respond to individuals in crisis in all types of settings. Nursing process is the vehicle by which nurses assist individuals in crisis with a short-term problem-solving approach to change. A four-phase technique is used: assessment/analysis, planning of therapeutic intervention, intervention, and evaluation of crisis resolution and anticipatory planning. Through this structured method of assistance, nurses assist individuals in crisis to develop more adaptive coping strategies for dealing with stressful situations in the future.

RELAXATION THERAPY

Stress is a part of our everyday lives. It can be positive or negative, but it cannot be eliminated. Keeping stress at a manageable level is a lifelong process.

Individuals under stress respond with a physiologic arousal that can be dangerous over long periods. Indeed, the stress response has been shown to be a major contributor, either directly or indirectly, to coronary heart disease, cancer, lung ailments, accidental injuries, cirrhosis of the liver, and suicide—six of the leading causes of death in the United States.

Relaxation therapy is an effective means of reducing the stress response in some individuals. The degree of anxiety that an individual experiences in response to stress is related to certain predisposing factors, such as characteristics of temperament with which he or she was born, past experiences resulting in learned patterns of responding, and existing conditions, such as health status, coping strategies, and adequate support systems.

Deep relaxation can counteract the physiologic and behavioral manifestations of stress. Various methods of relaxation include the following:

Deep-Breathing Exercises. Tension is released when the lungs are allowed to breathe in as much oxygen as possible. Deep-breathing exercises involve inhaling slowly and deeply through the nose, holding the breath for a few seconds, then exhaling slowly through the mouth, pursing the lips as if trying to whistle.

Progressive Relaxation. This method of deep-muscle relaxation is based on the premise that the body responds to anxiety-provoking thoughts and events with muscle tension. Each muscle group is tensed for 5 to 7 seconds and then relaxed for 20 to 30 seconds, during which time the individual concentrates on the difference in sensations between the two conditions. Soft, slow background music may facilitate relaxation. A modified version of this technique (called passive progressive relaxation) involves relaxation of the muscles by concentrating on the feeling of relaxation within the muscle, rather than the actual tensing and relaxing of the muscle.

Meditation. The goal of meditation is to gain mastery over attention. It brings on a special state of consciousness as attention is concentrated solely on one thought or object. During meditation, as the individual becomes totally preoccupied with the selected focus, the respiration rate, heart rate, and blood pressure decrease. The overall metabolism declines, and the need for oxygen consumption is reduced.

Mental Imagery. Mental imagery uses the imagination in an effort to reduce the body's response to stress. The frame of reference is very personal, based on what each individual considers to be a relaxing environment. The relaxing scenario is most useful when taped and played back at a time when the individual wishes to achieve relaxation.

Biofeedback. Biofeedback is the use of instrumentation to become aware of processes in the body that usually go unnoticed and to help bring them under voluntary control. Biologic conditions, such as muscle tension, skin surface temperature, blood pressure, and heart rate, are monitored by the biofeedback equipment. With special training, the individual learns to use relaxation and voluntary control to modify the biologic condition, in turn indicating a modification of the autonomic function it represents. Bio-feedback is often used together with other relaxation techniques such as deep breathing, progressive relaxation, and mental imagery.

ASSERTIVENESS TRAINING

Assertive behavior helps individuals feel better about themselves by encouraging them to stand up for their own basic human rights. These rights have equal representation for all individuals. But along with rights comes an equal number of responsibilities. Part of being assertive includes living up to these responsibilities.

Assertive behavior increases self-esteem and the ability to develop satisfying interpersonal relationships. This is accomplished through honesty, directness, appropriateness, and respecting one's own rights, as well as the rights of others.

Individuals develop patterns of responding in various ways, such as role modeling, by receiving positive or negative reinforcement, or by conscious choice. These patterns can take the form of nonassertiveness, assertiveness, aggressiveness, or passive-aggressiveness.

Nonassertive individuals seek to please others at the expense of denying their own basic human rights. *Assertive* individuals stand up for their own rights while protecting the rights of others. Those who respond *aggressively* defend their own rights by violating the basic rights of others. Individuals who respond in a *passive-aggressive* manner defend their own rights by expressing resistance to social and occupational demands.

Some important behavioral considerations of assertive behavior include eye contact, body posture, personal distance, physical contact, gestures, facial expression, voice, fluency, timing, listening, thoughts, and content. Various techniques have been developed to assist individuals in the process of becoming more assertive.

1. **Standing up for one's basic human rights.**
   Example: "I have the right to express my opinion."
2. **Assuming responsibility for one's own statements.**
   Example: "I *don't want to* go out with you tonight," instead of "I *can't* go out with you tonight." The latter implies a lack of power or ability.

3. **Responding as a "broken record."** Persistently repeating in a calm voice what is wanted.
   Example:

Telephone salesperson:	"I want to help you save money by changing long-distance services."
Assertive response:	"I don't want to change my long-distance service."
Telephone salesperson:	"I can't believe you don't want to save money!"
Assertive response:	"I don't want to change my long-distance service."

4. **Agreeing assertively.** Assertively accepting negative aspects about oneself. Admitting when an error has been made.
   Example:

Ms. Jones:	"You sure let that meeting get out of hand. What a waste of time."
Ms. Smith:	"Yes, I didn't do a very good job of conducting the meeting today."

5. **Inquiring assertively.** Seeking additional information about critical statements.
   Example:

Male board member:	"You made a real fool of yourself at the board meeting last night."
Female board member:	"Oh, really? Just what about my behavior offended you?"
Male board member:	"You were so damned pushy!"
Female board member:	"Were you offended that I spoke up for my beliefs, or was it because my beliefs are in direct opposition to yours?"

6. **Shifting from content to process.** Changing the focus of the communication from discussing the topic at hand to analyzing what is actually going on in the interaction.
   Example:

Wife:	"Would you please call me if you will be late for dinner?"

Husband: "Why don't you just get off my back! I
           always have to account for every minute
           of my time with you!"

Wife: "Sounds to me like we need to discuss
           some other things here. What are you
           really angry about?"

7. **Clouding/fogging.** Concurring with the critic's argument without becoming defensive and without agreeing to change.
   Example:

   Nurse No. 1: "You make so many mistakes. I don't
                 know how you ever got this job!"

   Nurse No. 2: "You're right. I have made some
                 mistakes since I started this job."

8. **Defusing.** Putting off further discussion with an angry individual until he or she is calmer.
   Example:
   "You are very angry right now. I don't want to discuss this matter with you while you are so upset. I will discuss it with you in my office at 3 o'clock this afternoon."

9. **Delaying assertively.** Putting off further discussion with another individual until one is calmer.
   Example:
   "That's a very challenging position you have taken, Mr. Brown. I'll need time to give it some thought. I'll call you later this afternoon."

10. **Responding assertively with irony.**
    Example:

    Man: "I bet you're one of them so-called
              'women's libbers,' aren't you?"

    Woman: "Yes, thank you for noticing."

COGNITIVE THERAPY

Cognitive therapy, developed by Aaron Beck, is commonly used in the treatment of mood disorders. In cognitive therapy, the individual is taught to control thought distortions that are considered to be a factor in the development and maintenance of mood disorders. In the cognitive model, depression is characterized by a triad of negative distortions related to expectations of the environment, self, and future. The environment and activities within it are viewed as unsatisfying, the self is unrealistically devalued, and the future is perceived as hopeless. In the same model, mania is characterized by a positive cognitive triad—the self is seen as highly valued and powerful, experiences within the environment are viewed as overly positive, and the future is seen as one of unlimited opportunity (Leahy and Beck, 1988).

The general goals in cognitive therapy are to obtain symptom relief as quickly as possible, to assist the client in identifying dysfunctional patterns of thinking and behaving, and to guide the client to evidence and logic that effectively tests the validity of the dysfunctional thinking. Therapy focuses on changing "automatic thoughts" that occur spontaneously and contribute to the distorted affect. Examples of "automatic thoughts" in depression include the following:

1. **Personalizing:** "I'm the only one who failed."
2. **All or nothing:** "I'm a complete failure."
3. **Mind reading:** "He thinks I'm foolish."
4. **Discounting positives:** "The other questions were so easy. Any dummy could have gotten them right."

Examples of "automatic thoughts" in mania include the following:

1. **Personalizing:** "She's this happy only when she's with me."
2. **All or nothing:** "Everything I do is great."
3. **Mind reading:** "She thinks I'm wonderful."
4. **Discounting negatives:** "None of those mistakes are really important."

The client is asked to describe evidence that both supports and disputes the automatic thought. The logic underlying the inferences is then reviewed with the client. Another technique involves evaluating what would most likely happen if the client's automatic thoughts were true. Implications of the consequences are then discussed.

Clients should not become discouraged if one technique seems not to be working. There is no single technique that works with all clients. He or she should be reassured that there are a number of techniques that may be used, and both therapist and client may explore these possibilities. Cognitive therapy has been shown to be an effective treatment for mood disorders, particularly in conjunction with psychopharmacologic intervention.

Appendix G

ELECTRO-CONVULSIVE THERAPY

DEFINED

Electroconvulsive therapy (ECT) is a type of somatic treatment in which electric current is applied to the brain through electrodes placed on the temples. The current is sufficient to induce a grand mal seizure, from which the desired therapeutic effect is achieved.

INDICATIONS

ECT is primarily used in the treatment of severe depression. It is sometimes administered in conjunction with antidepressant medication, but most physicians prefer to perform this treatment only after an unsuccessful trial of drug therapy (Mulaik, 1979).

ECT may also be used as a fast-acting treatment for very hyperactive manic clients in danger of physical exhaustion, and with individuals who are extremely suicidal.

ECT was originally attempted in the treatment of schizophrenia, but with little success in most instances. There has been evidence, however, of its effectiveness in the treatment of acute psychoses and catatonia (Mulaik, 1979) and schizophrenia that is accompanied by affective symptomatology (Kaplan and Sadock, 1985).

CONTRAINDICATIONS

ECT should not be used if there is increased intracranial pressure (from brain tumor, recent cardiovascular accident, or other cerebrovascular lesion).

MECHANISM OF ACTION

The exact mechanism of action is unknown. However, it is thought that ECT produces biochemical changes in the brain—an increase in the levels of norepinephrine, serotonin, and dopamine—similar to the effects of antidepressant medications.

SIDE EFFECTS AND NURSING IMPLICATIONS

TEMPORARY MEMORY LOSS AND CONFUSION
- These are the most common side effects of ECT. It is important for the nurse to be present when the client awakens in order to alleviate the fears that accompany this loss of memory.
- Provide reassurance that memory loss is only temporary.
- Describe to client what has occurred.
- Reorient client to time and place.
- Allow client to verbalize fears and anxieties related to receiving ECT.
- To minimize confusion, provide a good deal of structure for client's routine activities.

RISKS INVOLVED

1. **Death.** The mortality rate from ECT falls in the range of 0.01% to 0.04% (Abrams, 1988). The major cause is cardiovascular complications, such as acute myocardial infarction or cardiac arrest.
2. **Brain Damage.** Brain damage is considered to be a risk, but evidence is largely unsubstantiated.
3. **Permanent Memory Loss.** Prolonged or permanent

memory loss has been reported by some individuals (Freeman et al, 1980).

Although the potential for these effects appears to be minimal, the client must be made aware of the risks involved before consenting to treatment.

POTENTIAL NURSING DIAGNOSES ASSOCIATED WITH ECT

1. Risk for injury related to certain risks associated with ECT.
2. Risk for aspiration related to altered level of consciousness immediately following treatment.
3. Decreased cardiac output related to vagal stimulation occurring during the ECT.
4. Altered thought processes related to side effects of temporary memory loss and confusion.
5. Knowledge deficit related to necessity for, and side effects and risks of, ECT.
6. Anxiety (moderate to severe) related to impending therapy.
7. Self-care deficit related to incapacitation during post-ictal stage.
8. Risk for activity intolerance related to post-ECT confusion and memory loss.

NURSING INTERVENTIONS FOR CLIENT RECEIVING ECT

1. Ensure that physician has obtained informed consent and that a signed permission form is on the chart.
2. Ensure that most recent laboratory reports (CBC, urinalysis) and results of ECG and x-ray examination are available.
3. Client should be NPO on the morning of the treatment.
4. Prior to the treatment, client should void, dress in night clothes (or other loose clothing), and remove dentures and eyeglasses or contact lenses. Bedrails should be raised.
5. Take baseline vital signs and blood pressure.
6. Administer cholinergic blocking agent (atropine sulfate, glycopyrrolate) approximately 30 minutes before

treatment, as ordered by the physician, to decrease secretions and increase heart rate (which is suppressed in response to vagal stimulation caused by the ECT).

7. Assist physician and/or anesthesiologist as necessary in the administration of intravenous medications. A short-acting anesthetic, such as methohexital sodium (Brevital sodium), is given along with the muscle relaxant succinylcholine chloride (Anectine).

8. Administer oxygen and provide suctioning as required.

9. After the procedure, take vital signs and blood pressure every 15 minutes for the first hour. Position client on side to prevent aspiration.

10. Stay with client until he or she is fully awake.

Appendix H

MEDICATION ASSESSMENT TOOL

Date _____ Client's Name _____ Age _____
Marital Status _____ Children _____ Occupation _____
Presenting Symptoms (subjective and objective) _____

Diagnosis (DSM-IV) _____
Current Vital Signs: Blood Pressure Sitting ___ / ___ Standing ___ / ___ Pulse ___ Respirations ___

CURRENT/PAST USE OF PRESCRIPTION DRUGS (Indicate with c or p beside name of drug whether current or past use):

Name	Dosage	How Long Used	Why Prescribed	By Whom	Side Effects/Results

CURRENT/PAST USE OF OVER-THE-COUNTER DRUGS (Indicate with c or p beside name of drug whether current or past use):

Name	Dosage	How Long Used	Why Prescribed	By Whom	Side Effects/Results

CURRENT/PAST USE OF STREET DRUGS, ALCOHOL, NICOTINE, AND/OR CAFFEINE:

Name	Amount Used	How Often Used	When Last Used	Effects Produced

Any allergies to food or drugs?

Any special diet considerations?

Do you have (or have you ever had) any of the following? If yes, provide explanation on the back of this sheet.

	Yes	No			Yes	No
1. Difficulty swallowing	—	—	8. Headaches		—	—
2. Delayed wound			9. Dizziness		—	—
healing	—	—	10. High blood pressure		—	—
3. Constipation			11. Palpitations		—	—
problems	—	—	12. Chest pain		—	—
4. Urination problems	—	—	13. Blood clots/pain in			
5. Recent change in			legs		—	—
elimination patterns	—	—	14. Fainting spells		—	—
6. Weakness or tremors	—	—	15. Swollen ankles/legs/		—	—
7. Seizures	—	—	hands			
			16. Asthma		—	—
			17. Varicose veins		—	—
			18. Numbness/tingling		—	—
			(state location)			
			19. Ulcers		—	—
			20. Nausea/vomiting		—	—
			21. Problems with			
			diarrhea		—	—
			22. Shortness of breath		—	—
			23. Sexual dysfunction		—	—

(continued)

24. Lumps in your breasts —— ——
25. Blurred or double vision —— ——

26. Ringing in the ears —— ——
27. Insomnia —— ——
28. Skin Rashes —— ——
29. Diabetes —— ——

30. Hepatitis (or other liver disease) —— ——
31. Kidney disease —— ——
32. Glaucoma —— ——

Are you pregnant or breast feeding? _____ Date of last menses _____ Type of contraception used _____
Describe any restrictions/limitations that might interfere with your use of medication for your current problem.

Prescription orders: _____ Patient teaching related to medications prescribed:

Laboratory work ordered:

_____   _____
Nurse's Signature   Client's Signature

Appendix I

CULTURAL ASSESSMENT TOOL

Client's Name _____ Ethnic Origin _____

Address _____ Birth Date _____

Name of Significant Other _____ Relationship _____

Primary Language Spoken _____ Second Language Spoken _____

How does client usually communicate with people who speak a different language? _____

Is an interpreter required? _____ Available? _____

Highest level of education achieved _____ Occupation _____

Presenting Problem _____

Has this problem ever occurred before? _____

If so, in what manner was it handled previously? _____

What is client's usual manner of coping with stress? _____

Who is(are) the client's main support system(s)? _____

Describe the family living arrangements _____

Who is the major decision maker in the family? _____

(continued)

Describe client's/family members' roles within the family _____

Describe religious beliefs and practices _____

Are there any religious requirements or restrictions that place limitations on the client's care? _____

If so, describe _____

Who in the family takes responsibility for health concerns? _____

Describe any special health beliefs and practices _____

From whom does family usually seek medical assistance in time of need? _____

Describe client's usual emotional/behavioral response to:

Anxiety _____

Anger _____

Loss/change/failure _____

Pain _____

Fear _____

Describe any topics that are particularly sensitive or that the client is unwilling to discuss (because of cultural taboos) _____

Describe any activities in which the client is unwilling to participate (because of cultural customs or taboos) _____

What are the client's personal feelings regarding touch? _____

What are the client's personal feelings regarding eye contact? _____

What is the client's personal orientation to time? (past, present, future) _____

466

Describe any particular illnesses to which the client may be bioculturally susceptible
(e.g., hypertension and sickle cell anemia in African Americans) _____

Describe any nutritional deficiencies to which the client may be bioculturally susceptible
(e.g., lactose intolerance in Native and Asian Americans) _____

Describe client's favorite foods _____

Are there any foods the client requests or refuses because of cultural beliefs related to this illness?
(e.g., "hot" and "cold" foods for Hispanic and Asian Americans). If so, please describe _____

Describe client's perception of the problem and expectations of health care _____
_____
_____

From Townsend, 1996, p. 822, with permission.

Appendix J*

DSM-IV CLASSIFICATION: AXES I AND II CATEGORIES AND CODES

DISORDERS USUALLY FIRST DIAGNOSED IN INFANCY, CHILDHOOD, OR ADOLESCENCE

Mental Retardation

317   Mild Mental Retardation
318.0   Moderate Retardation
318.1   Severe Retardation
318.2   Profound Mental Retardation
319   Mental Retardation, Severity Unspecified

Learning Disorders

315.00   Reading Disorder
315.1   Mathematics Disorder
315.2   Disorder of Written Expression
315.9   Learning Disorder Not Otherwise Specified (NOS)

*Reprinted with permission from the *Diagnostic and Statistical Manual of Mental Disorders, Fourth Edition.* Copyright 1994 American Psychiatric Association.

Motor Skills Disorder

315.4   Developmental Coordination Disorder

Communication Disorders

315.31 Expressive Language Disorder
315.31 Mixed Receptive/Expressive Language Disorder
315.39 Phonological Disorder
307.0   Stuttering
315.39 Communication Disorder NOS

Pervasive Developmental Disorders

299.00 Autistic Disorder
299.80 Rett's Disorder
299.10 Childhood Disintegrative Disorder
299.80 Asperger's Disorder
299.80 Pervasive Developmental Disorder NOS

Attention-Deficit and Disruptive Behavior Disorders

314.xx Attention-Deficit/Hyperactivity Disorder
314.01   Combined type
314.00   Predominantly inattentive type
314.01   Predominantly hyperactive-impulsive type
314.9   Attention-Deficit/Hyperactivity Disorder NOS
312.8   Conduct Disorder
           Specify Childhood- or Adolescent-Onset
           Type
313.81 Oppositional Defiant Disorder
312.9   Disruptive Behavior Disorder NOS

Feeding and Eating Disorders of Infancy or Early Childhood

307.52 Pica
307.53 Rumination Disorder
307.59 Feeding Disorder of Infancy or Early Childhood

Tic Disorders

307.23 Tourette's Disorder
307.22 Chronic Motor or Vocal Tic Disorder
307.21 Transient Tic Disorder
307.20 Tic Disorder NOS

Elimination Disorders

—   Encopresis
787.6   With constipation and overflow incontinence
307.7   Without constipation and overflow incontinence
307.6   Enuresis (Not Due to a General Medical Condition)

Other Disorders of Infancy, Childhood, or Adolescence

309.21 Separation Anxiety Disorder
313.23 Selective Mutism
313.89 Reactive Attachment Disorder of Infancy or Early Childhood
307.3 Stereotypic Movement Disorder
313.9 Disorder of Infancy, Childhood, or Adolescence NOS

DELIRIUM, DEMENTIA, AMNESTIC AND OTHER COGNITIVE DISORDERS

Delirium

293.0 Delirium Due to (indicate the general medical condition)
—   Substance Intoxication Delirium (refer to Substance-Related Disorders for substance-specific codes)
—   Substance Withdrawal Delirium (refer to Substance-Related Disorders for substance-specific codes)
—   Delirium Due to Multiple Etiologies (code each of the specific etiologies)
780.09 Delirium NOS

Dementia

290.xx Dementia of the Alzheimer's Type
        With Early Onset: if onset at age 65 or below
290.10   Uncomplicated
290.11   With delirium
290.12   With delusions
290.13   With depressed mood
290.xx Dementia of the Alzheimer's Type
        With Late Onset: if onset after age 65
290.00   Uncomplicated
290.3   With delirium
290.20   With delusions
290.21   With depressed mood
290.xx Vascular Dementia
290.40   Uncomplicated
290.41   With delirium
290.42   With delusions
290.43   With depressed mood
294.9   Dementia Due to Human Immunodeficiency
        Virus (HIV) Disease
294.1   Dementia Due to Head Trauma
294.1   Dementia Due to Parkinson's Disease
294.1   Dementia Due to Huntington's Disease
290.10 Dementia Due to Pick's Disease
290.10 Dementia Due to Creutzfeldt-Jakob Disease
294.1   Dementia Due to (indicate the general medical
        condition not listed above)
—   Substance-Induced Persisting Dementia (refer
        to Substance-Related Disorders for substance-
        specific codes)
—   Dementia Due to Multiple Etiologies
        (code each of the specific etiologies)
294.8   Dementia NOS

Amnestic Disorders

294.0   Amnestic Disorder Due to (indicate the general
        medical condition)
—   Substance-induced Persisting Amnestic
        Disorder (refer to specific substance for code)
294.8   Amnestic Disorder NOS

Other Cognitive Disorders

294.9   Cognitive Disorder NOS

MENTAL DISORDERS DUE TO A GENERAL MEDICAL CONDITION NOT ELSEWHERE CLASSIFIED

293.89 Catatonic Disorder Due to (indicate the general medical condition)
310.1 Personality Change Due to (indicate the general medical condition)
293.9 Mental Disorder NOS Due to (indicate the general medical condition)

SUBSTANCE-RELATED DISORDERS

ALCOHOL-RELATED DISORDERS

Alcohol Use Disorders

303.90 Alcohol Dependence
305.00 Alcohol Abuse

Alcohol-Induced Disorders

303.00 Alcohol Intoxication
291.8 Alcohol Withdrawal
291.0 Alcohol Intoxication Delirium
291.0 Alcohol Withdrawal Delirium
291.2 Alcohol-Induced Persisting Dementia
291.1 Alcohol-Induced Persisting Amnestic Disorder
291.x Alcohol-Induced Psychotic Disorder
291.5 　　With Delusions
291.3 　　With Hallucinations
291.8 Alcohol-Induced Mood Disorder
291.8 Alcohol-Induced Anxiety Disorder
292.8 Alcohol-Induced Sexual Dysfunction
292.89 Alcohol-Induced Sleep Disorder
291.9 Alcohol Related Disorder NOS

AMPHETAMINE (OR AMPHETAMINE-LIKE)-RELATED DISORDERS

Amphetamine Use Disorders

304.40 Amphetamine Dependence
305.70 Amphetamine Abuse

Amphetamine-Induced Disorders

292.89 Amphetamine Intoxication
292.0   Amphetamine Withdrawal
292.81 Amphetamine Intoxication Delirium
292.xx Amphetamine-Induced Psychotic Disorder
292.11   With Delusions
292.12   With Hallucinations
292.84 Amphetamine-Induced Mood Disorder
292.89 Amphetamine-Induced Anxiety Disorder
292.89 Amphetamine-Induced Sexual Dysfunction
292.89 Amphetamine-Induced Sleep Disorder
292.9   Amphetamine-Related Disorder NOS

CAFFEINE-RELATED DISORDERS

Caffeine-Induced Disorders

305.90 Caffeine Intoxication
292.89 Caffeine-Induced Anxiety Disorder
292.89 Caffeine-Induced Sleep Disorder
292.9   Caffeine-Related Disorder NOS

CANNABIS-RELATED DISORDERS

Cannabis Use Disorders

304.30 Cannabis Dependence
305.20 Cannabis Abuse

Cannabis-Induced Disorders

292.89 Cannabis Intoxication
292.81 Cannabis Intoxication Delirium
292.xx Cannabis-Induced Psychotic Disorder
292.11   With Delusions
292.12   With Hallucinations
292.89 Cannabis-Induced Anxiety Disorder
292.9   Cannabis-Related Disorder NOS

COCAINE-RELATED DISORDERS

Cocaine Use Disorders

304.20 Cocaine Dependence
305.60 Cocaine Abuse

Cocaine-Induced Disorders

292.89 Cocaine Intoxication
292.0 Cocaine Withdrawal
292.81 Cocaine Intoxication Delirium
292.xx Cocaine-Induced Psychotic Disorder
292.11 With Delusions
292.12 With Hallucinations
292.84 Cocaine-Induced Mood Disorder
292.89 Cocaine-Induced Anxiety Disorder
292.89 Cocaine-Induced Sexual Dysfunction
292.89 Cocaine-Induced Sleep Disorder
292.9 Cocaine-Related Disorder NOS

HALLUCINOGEN-RELATED DISORDERS

Hallucinogen Use Disorders

304.50 Hallucinogen Dependence
305.30 Hallucinogen Abuse

Hallucinogen-Induced Disorders

292.89 Hallucinogen Intoxication
292.89 Hallucinogen Persisting Perception Disorder
(Flashbacks)
292.81 Hallucinogen Intoxication Delirium
292.xx Hallucinogen-Induced Psychotic Disorder
292.11 With Delusions
292.12 With Hallucinations
292.84 Hallucinogen-Induced Mood Disorder
292.89 Hallucinogen-Induced Anxiety Disorder
292.9 Hallucinogen-Related Disorder NOS

INHALANT-RELATED DISORDERS

Inhalant Use Disorders

304.60 Inhalant Dependence
305.90 Inhalant Abuse

Inhalant-Induced Disorders

292.89 Inhalant Intoxication
292.81 Inhalant Intoxication Delirium

292.82 Inhalant-Induced Persisting Dementia
292.xx Inhalant-Induced Psychotic Disorder
292.11   With Delusions
292.12   With Hallucinations
292.84 Inhalant-Induced Mood Disorder
292.89 Inhalant-Induced Anxiety Disorder
292.9   Inhalant-Related Disorder NOS

NICOTINE-RELATED DISORDERS

Nicotine Use Disorders

305.10 Nicotine Dependence

Nicotine-Induced Disorders

292.0   Nicotine Withdrawal
292.9   Nicotine-Related Disorder NOS

OPIOID-RELATED DISORDERS

Opioid Use Disorders

304.00 Opioid Dependence
305.50 Opioid Abuse

Opioid-Induced Disorders

292.89 Opioid Intoxication
292.0   Opioid Withdrawal
292.81 Opioid Intoxication Delirium
292.xx Opioid-Induced Psychotic Disorder
292.11   With Delusions
292.12   With Hallucinations
292.84 Opioid-Induced Mood Disorder
292.89 Opioid-Induced Sexual Dysfunction
292.89 Opioid-Induced Sleep Disorder
292.9   Opioid-Related Disorder NOS

PHENCYCLIDINE (OR PHENCYCLIDINE-LIKE)-RELATED DISORDERS

Phencyclidine Use Disorders

304.90 Phencyclidine Dependence
305.90 Phencyclidine Abuse

Phencyclidine-Induced Disorders

292.89 Phencyclidine Intoxication
292.81 Phencyclidine Intoxication Delirium
292.xx Phencyclidine-Induced Psychotic Disorder
292.11   With Delusions
292.12   With Hallucinations
292.84 Phencyclidine-Induced Mood Disorder
292.89 Phencyclidine-Induced Anxiety Disorder
292.9   Phencyclidine-Related Disorder NOS

SEDATIVE-, HYPNOTIC-, OR ANXIOLYTIC-RELATED DISORDERS

Sedative, Hypnotic, or Anxiolytic Substance Use Disorders

304.10 Sedative, Hypnotic, or Anxiolytic Dependence
305.40 Sedative, Hypnotic, or Anxiolytic Abuse

Sedative-, Hypnotic-, or Anxiolytic-Induced Disorders

292.89 Sedative, Hypnotic, or Anxiolytic Intoxication
292.0   Sedative, Hypnotic, or Anxiolytic Withdrawal
292.81 Sedative, Hypnotic, or Anxiolytic Intoxication Delirium
292.81 Sedative, Hypnotic, or Anxiolytic Withdrawal Delirium
292.82 Sedative-, Hypnotic-, or Anxiolytic-Induced Persisting Dementia
292.83 Sedative-, Hypnotic-, or Anxiolytic-Induced Persisting Amnestic Disorder
292.xx Sedative-, Hypnotic-, or Anxiolytic-Induced Psychotic Disorder

292.11   With Delusions
292.12   With Hallucinations
292.84 Sedative-, Hypnotic-, or Anxiolytic-Induced Mood Disorder
292.89 Sedative-, Hypnotic-, or Anxiolytic-Induced Anxiety Disorder
292.89 Sedative-, Hypnotic-, or Anxiolytic-Induced Sexual Dysfunction
292.89 Sedative-, Hypnotic-, or Anxiolytic-Induced Sleep Disorder
292.9   Sedative-, Hypnotic-, or Anxiolytic-Related Disorder NOS

POLYSUBSTANCE-RELATED DISORDER

304.80 Polysubstance Dependence

OTHER (OR UNKNOWN) SUBSTANCE-RELATED DISORDERS

Other (or Unknown) Substance Use Disorders

304.90 Other (or Unknown) Substance Dependence
305.90 Other (or Unknown) Substance Abuse

Other (or Unknown) Substance-Induced Disorders

292.89 Other (or Unknown) Substance Intoxication
292.0   Other (or Unknown) Substance Withdrawal
292.81 Other (or Unknown) Substance-Induced Delirium
292.82 Other (or Unknown) Substance-Induced Persisting Dementia
292.83 Other (or Unknown) Substance-Induced Persisting Amnestic Disorder
292.xx Other (or Unknown) Substance-Induced Psychotic Disorder
292.11   With Delusions
292.12   With Hallucinations
292.84 Other (or Unknown) Substance-Induced Mood Disorder
292.89 Other (or Unknown) Substance-Induced Anxiety Disorder

292.89   Other (or Unknown) Substance-Induced Sexual Dysfunction

292.89   Other (or Unknown) Substance-Induced Sleep Disorder

292.9   Other (or Unknown) Substance-Related Disorder NOS

SCHIZOPHRENIA AND OTHER PSYCHOTIC DISORDERS

295.xx   Schizophrenia
295.30   Paranoid type
295.10   Disorganized type
295.20   Catatonic type
295.90   Undifferentiated type
295.60   Residual type
295.40   Schizophreniform Disorder
295.70   Schizoaffective Disorder
297.1   Delusional Disorder
298.8   Brief Psychotic Disorder
297.3   Shared Psychotic Disorder (Folie a Deux)
293.xx   Psychotic Disorder Due to a General Medical Condition
293.81   With Delusions
293.82   With Hallucinations
—   Substance-Induced Psychotic Disorder (refer to Substance-Related Disorders for substance-specific codes)
298.9   Psychotic Disorder NOS

MOOD DISORDERS

(Code current state of Major Depressive Disorder or Bipolar Disorder in fifth digit: 0 = unspecified; 1 = mild; 2 = moderate; 3 = severe, without psychotic features; 4 = severe, with psychotic features; 5 = in partial remission; 6 = in full remission.)

Depressive Disorders

296.xx   Major Depressive Disorder
296.2x   Single episode

296.3x   Recurrent
300.4   Dysthymic Disorder
311   Depressive Disorder NOS

Bipolar Disorders

296.xx Bipolar I Disorder
296.0x   Single manic episode
296.40   Most recent episode hypomanic
296.4x   Most recent episode manic
296.6x   Most recent episode mixed
296.5x   Most recent episode depressed
296.7   Most recent episode unspecified
296.89 Bipolar II Disorder
     (Specify current or most recent episode:
     Hypomanic or Depressed)
301.13 Cyclothymic Disorder
296.80 Bipolar Disorder NOS
293.83 Mood Disorder Due to (indicate the general
     medical condition)
—   Substance-Induced Mood Disorder (refer to
     Substance-Related Disorders for substance-
     specific codes)
296.90 Mood Disorder NOS

ANXIETY DISORDERS

300.01 Panic Disorder without Agoraphobia
300.21 Panic Disorder with Agoraphobia
300.22 Agoraphobia Without History of Panic Disorder
300.29 Specific Phobia
300.23 Social Phobia
300.3   Obsessive-Compulsive Disorder
309.81 Posttraumatic Stress Disorder
308.3   Acute Stress Disorder
300.02 Generalized Anxiety Disorder
293.89 Anxiety Disorder Due to (indicate the general
     medical condition)
—   Substance-Induced Anxiety Disorder (refer to
     Substance-Related Disorders for substance-
     specific codes)
300.00 Anxiety Disorder NOS

SOMATOFORM DISORDERS

300.81   Somatization Disorder
300.11   Conversion Disorder
300.7   Hypochondriasis
300.7   Body Dysmorphic Disorder
307.xx   Pain Disorder
307.80   Associated with Psychological Factors
307.89   Associated with Both Psychological Factors
         and a General Medical Condition
300.81   Undifferentiated Somatoform Disorder
300.81   Somatoform Disorder NOS

FACTITIOUS DISORDERS

300.xx   Factitious Disorder
300.16   With predominantly psychological signs and
             symptoms
300.19   With predominantly physical signs and
             symptoms
300.19   With combined psychological and physical
             signs and symptoms
300.19   Factitious Disorder NOS

DISSOCIATIVE DISORDERS

300.12   Dissociative Amnesia
300.13   Dissociative Fugue
300.14   Dissociative Identity Disorder
300.6   Depersonalization Disorder
300.15   Dissociative Disorder NOS

SEXUAL AND GENDER IDENTITY DISORDERS

SEXUAL DYSFUNCTIONS

Sexual Desire Disorders

302.71   Hypoactive Sexual Desire Disorder
302.79   Sexual Aversion Disorder

Sexual Arousal Disorders

302.72 Female Sexual Arousal Disorder
302.72 Male Erectile Disorder

Orgasmic Disorders

302.73 Female Orgasmic Disorder
302.74 Male Orgasmic Disorder
302.75 Premature Ejaculation

Sexual Pain Disorders

302.76 Dyspareunia (Not Due to a General Medical Condition)
306.51 Vaginismus (Not Due to a General Medical Condition)

Sexual Dysfunctions Due to a General Medical Condition

625.8 Female Hypoactive Sexual Desire Disorder Due to (indicate the general medical condition)
608.89 Male Hypoactive Sexual Desire Disorder Due to (indicate the general medical condition)
607.84 Male Erectile Disorder Due to (indicate the general medical condition)
625.0 Female Dyspareunia Due to (indicate the general medical condition)
608.89 Male Dyspareunia Due to (indicate the general medical condition)
625.8 Other Female Sexual Dysfunction Due to (indicate the general medical condition)
608.89 Other Male Sexual Dysfunction Due to (indicate the general medical condition)
— Substance-Induced Sexual Dysfunction (refer to Substance-Related Disorders for substance-specific codes)
302.70 Sexual Dysfunction NOS

PARAPHILIAS

302.4   Exhibitionism
302.81   Fetishism
302.89   Frotteurism
302.2   Pedophilia
302.83   Sexual Masochism
302.84   Sexual Sadism
302.3   Transvestic Fetishism
302.82   Voyeurism
302.9   Paraphilia NOS

GENDER IDENTITY DISORDERS

302.xx   Gender Identity Disorder
302.6   In Children
302.85   In Adolescents or Adults
302.6   Gender Identity Disorder NOS

302.9   Sexual Disorder NOS

EATING DISORDERS

307.1   Anorexia Nervosa
307.51   Bulimia Nervosa
307.50   Eating Disorder NOS

SLEEP DISORDERS

PRIMARY SLEEP DISORDERS

Dyssomnias

307.42   Primary Insomnia
307.44   Primary Hypersomnia
347   Narcolepsy
780.59   Breathing-Related Sleep Disorder
307.45   Circadian Rhythm Sleep Disorder
307.47   Dyssomnia NOS

Parasomnias

307.47   Nightmare Disorder
307.46   Sleep Terror Disorder

307.46 Sleepwalking Disorder
307.47 Parasomnia NOS

SLEEP DISORDERS RELATED TO ANOTHER MENTAL DISORDER

307.42 Insomnia Related to (indicate the Axis I or Axis II disorder)
307.44 Hypersomnia Related to (indicate the Axis I or Axis II disorder)

OTHER SLEEP DISORDERS

780.xx Sleep Disorder Due to (indicate the general medical condition)
780.52   Insomnia type
780.54   Hypersomnia type
780.59   Parasomnia type
780.59   Mixed type
—   Substance-Induced Sleep Disorder (refer to Substance-Related Disorders for substance-specific codes)

IMPULSE CONTROL DISORDERS NOT ELSEWHERE CLASSIFIED

312.34 Intermittent Explosive Disorder
312.32 Kleptomania
312.33 Pyromania
312.31 Pathological Gambling
312.39 Trichotillomania
312.30 Impulse Control Disorder NOS

ADJUSTMENT DISORDERS

309.xx Adjustment Disorder
309.0   With Depressed Mood
309.24   With Anxiety
309.28   With Mixed Anxiety and Depressed Mood
309.3   With Disturbance of Conduct
309.4   With Mixed Disturbance of Emotions and Conduct
309.9   Unspecified

PERSONALITY DISORDERS

Note: These are coded on Axis II.

301.0   Paranoid Personality Disorder
301.20 Schizoid Personality Disorder
301.22 Schizotypal Personality Disorder
301.7   Antisocial Personality Disorder
301.83 Borderline Personality Disorder
301.50 Histrionic Personality Disorder
301.81 Narcissistic Personality Disorder
301.82 Avoidant Personality Disorder
301.6   Dependent Personality Disorder
301.4   Obsessive-Compulsive Personality Disorder
301.9   Personality Disorder NOS

OTHER CONDITIONS THAT MAY BE A FOCUS OF CLINICAL ATTENTION

(Psychological Factors) Affecting Medical Condition

316   *Choose name based on nature of factors:*
Mental Disorder Affecting Medical Condition
Psychological Symptoms Affecting Medical Condition
Personality Traits or Coping Style Affecting Medical Condition
Maladaptive Health Behaviors Affecting Medical Condition
Stress-Related Physiological Response Affecting Medical Condition
Other or Unspecified Psychological Factors Affecting Medical Condition

Medication-Induced Movement Disorders

332.1   Neuroleptic-Induced Parkinsonism
333.92 Neuroleptic Malignant Syndrome
333.7   Neuroleptic-Induced Acute Dystonia
333.99 Neuroleptic-Induced Acute Akathisia
333.82 Neuroleptic-Induced Tardive Dyskinesia
333.1   Medication-Induced Postural Tremor
333.90 Medication-Induced Movement Disorder NOS

Other Medication-Induced Disorder

995.2   Adverse Effects of Medication NOS

Relational Problems

V61.9   Relational Problem Related to a Mental
         Disorder or General Medical Condition
V61.20   Parent-Child Relational Problem
V61.1   Partner Relational Problem
V61.8   Sibling Relational Problem
V62.81   Relational Problem NOS

Problems Related to Abuse or Neglect

V61.21   Physical Abuse of Child
V61.21   Sexual Abuse of Child
V61.21   Neglect of Child
V61.1   Physical Abuse of Adult
V61.1   Sexual Abuse of Adult

Additional Conditions That May Be a Focus of Clinical Attention

V15.81   Noncompliance with Treatment
V65.2   Malingering
V71.01   Adult Antisocial Behavior
V71.02   Childhood or Adolescent Antisocial Behavior
V62.89   Borderline Intellectual Functioning (coded on
         Axis II)
780.9   Age-Related Cognitive Decline
V62.82   Bereavement
V62.3   Academic Problem
V62.2   Occupational Problem
313.82   Identity Problem
V62.61   Religious or Spiritual Problem
V62.4   Acculturation Problem
V62.89   Phase of Life Problem

ADDITIONAL CODES

300.9   Unspecified Mental Disorder (nonpsychotic)
V71.09   No Diagnosis or Condition on Axis I

799.9   Diagnosis or Condition Deferred on Axis I
V71.09 No Diagnosis on Axis II
799.9   Diagnosis Deferred on Axis II

DSM-IV CRITERIA SETS AND AXES PROVIDED FOR FURTHER STUDY

Text and criteria for these disorders will be provided to facilitate systematic clinical research:

Postconcussional disorder
Mild neurocognitive disorder
Caffeine withdrawal
Alternative dimensional descriptors for schizophrenia
Postpsychotic depression of schizophrenia
Simple schizophrenia
Minor depressive disorder
Alternative criteria B for dysthymic disorder
Recurrent brief depressive disorder
Premenstrual dysphoric disorder
Mixed anxiety-depressive disorder
Factitious disorder by proxy
Dissociative trance disorder
Binge eating disorder
Depressive personality disorder
Passive aggressive personality disorder (negativistic personality disorder)
Medication-induced movement disorders
Defensive Functioning Scale
Global Assessment of Relational Functioning (GARF) Scale
Social and Occupational Functioning Assessment Scale (SOFAS)

Appendix K*

MENTAL STATUS ASSESSMENT

Gathering the correct information about the client's mental status is essential to the development of an appropriate plan of care. The mental status examination is a description of all the areas of the client's mental functioning (Scheiber, 1994). The following are the components that are considered critical in the assessment of a client's mental status.

IDENTIFYING DATA

1. Name
2. Sex
3. Age
4. Race/culture
5. Occupational/financial status
6. Educational level
7. Significant other
8. Living arrangements
9. Religious preference
10. Allergies
11. Special diet considerations
12. Chief complaint
13. Medical diagnosis

---

*From Townsend, 1996, pp. 859–861, with permission.

GENERAL DESCRIPTION

APPEARANCE

1. Grooming and dress
2. Hygiene
3. Posture
4. Height and weight
5. Level of eye contact
6. Hair color and texture
7. Evidence of scars, tattoos, or other distinguishing skin marks
8. Evaluation of client's appearance compared with chronological age

MOTOR ACTIVITY

1. Tremors
2. Tics or other stereotypical movements
3. Mannerisms and gestures
4. Hyperactivity
5. Restlessness or agitation
6. Aggressiveness
7. Rigidity
8. Gait patterns
9. Echopraxia
10. Psychomotor retardation
11. Freedom of movement (range of motion)

SPEECH PATTERNS

1. Slowness or rapidity of speech
2. Pressure of speech
3. Intonation
4. Volume
5. Stuttering or other speech impairments
6. Aphasia

GENERAL ATTITUDE

1. Cooperative/uncooperative
2. Friendly/hostile/defensive
3. Uninterested/apathetic

4. Attentive/interested
5. Guarded/suspicious

EMOTIONS

MOOD

1. Sad
2. Depressed
3. Despairing
4. Irritable
5. Anxious
6. Elated
7. Euphoric
8. Fearful
9. Guilty
10. Labile

AFFECT

1. Congruence with mood
2. Constricted or blunted (diminished amount/range and intensity of emotional expression)
3. Flat (absence of emotional expression)
4. Appropriate or inappropriate (defines congruence of affect with the situation or with the client's behavior)

THOUGHT PROCESSES

FORM OF THOUGHT

1. Flight of ideas
2. Associative looseness
3. Circumstantiality
4. Tangentiality
5. Neologisms
6. Concrete thinking
7. Clang associations
8. Word salad
9. Perseveration
10. Echolalia
11. Mutism

12. Poverty of speech (restriction in the amount of speech)
13. Ability to concentrate
14. Attention span

CONTENT OF THOUGHT

1. Delusions
   a. Persecutory
   b. Grandiose
   c. Reference
   d. Control or influence
   e. Somatic
   f. Nihilistic
2. Suicidal or homicidal ideas
3. Obsessions
4. Paranoia/suspiciousness
5. Magical thinking
6. Religiosity
7. Phobias
8. Poverty of content (vague, meaningless responses)

PERCEPTUAL DISTURBANCES

1. Hallucinations
   a. Auditory
   b. Visual
   c. Tactile
   d. Olfactory
   e. Gustatory
2. Illusions
3. Depersonalization (altered perception of the self)
4. Derealization (altered perception of the environment)

SENSORIUM AND COGNITIVE ABILITY

1. Level of alertness/consciousness
2. Orientation
   a. Time
   b. Place
   c. Person
   d. Circumstances

3. Memory
   a. Recent
   b. Remote
   c. Confabulation
4. Capacity for abstract thought

IMPULSE CONTROL

1. Ability to control impulses related to the following:
   a. Aggression
   b. Hostility
   c. Fear
   d. Guilt
   e. Affection
   f. Sexual feelings

JUDGMENT AND INSIGHT

1. Ability to solve problems
2. Ability to make decisions
3. Knowledge about self
   a. Awareness of limitations
   b. Awareness of consequences of actions
   c. Awareness of illness
4. Adaptive/maladaptive use of coping strategies and ego defense mechanisms

REFERENCES

Schieber, SC: The psychiatric interview, psychiatric history, and mental status examination. In Hales, RE, Yudofsky, SC, and Talbott, JA (eds): *Textbook of Psychiatry,* ed 2. American Psychiatric Press, Washington, DC, 1994.

BIBLIOGRAPHY

Hamilton, DB: Psychiatric nursing: Content review and tests. In Beare, PG (ed): Davis's NCLEX-RN Review. FA Davis, Philadelphia, 1991.
Kaplan, HI, Sadock, BJ, and Grebb, JA: Kaplan and Sadock's Synopsis of Psychiatry, ed 7. Williams & Wilkins, Baltimore, 1994.
Reynolds, JI, and Logsdon, JB: Assessing your patient's mental status. Nursing 79, 9(8):26–33, 1979.

INDEX OF NURSING DIAGNOSES